MW01670687

I acknowledge receipt of the Hazardous Materials Compliance Pocketbook (120-ORS) which details driver responsibilities and duties in the transportation of hazardous materials, as prescribed by the U.S. Department of Transportation in Title 49 CFR Parts 107, 171-180 and 390-397.

REMOVABLE PAGE - PULL SLOWLY FROM TOP RIGHT CORNER

______________________ ______________

Driver's Signature   Date

____

Company

____

Company Supervisor's Signature

10/05

NOTE: This receipt shall be read and signed by the driver. A responsible company supervisor shall countersign the receipt and place in the driver's file.

HAZARDOUS MATERIALS COMPLIANCE POCKETBOOK

©2005

J. J. Keller & Associates, Inc.
3003 W. Breezewood Lane, P.O. Box 368
Neenah, Wisconsin 54957-0368
USA
Phone: (800) 327-6868
Fax: (800) 727-7516
www.jjkeller.com

ISBN 1-59042-634-7

Canadian Goods and Services Tax (GST) Number: R123-317687

Printed in the U.S.A.

All rights reserved. Neither the Hazardous Materials Compliance Pocketbook nor any part thereof may be reproduced in any manner without written permission of the Publisher.

Due to the constantly changing nature of government regulations, it is impossible to guarantee absolute accuracy of the material contained herein. The Publisher and Editors, therefore, cannot assume any responsibility for omissions, errors, misprinting, or ambiguity contained within this publication and shall not be held liable in any degree for any loss or injury caused by such omission, error, misprinting or ambiguity presented in this publication.

This publication is designed to provide reasonably accurate and authoritative information in regard to the subject matter covered. It is sold with the understanding that the Publisher is not engaged in rendering legal, accounting, or other professional service. If legal advice or other expert assistance is required, the services of a competent professional person should be sought.

The Editorial Staff is available to provide information generally associated with this publication to a normal and reasonable extent, and at the option of, and as a courtesy of, the Publisher.

---

120 ORS **10/05**

TABLE OF CONTENTS

The Law Affects You Directly

The current Hazardous Materials Regulations can be traced to the Transportation Safety Act of 1974, the hazardous materials regulations "consolidation" of 1976, the Hazardous Materials Transportation Uniform Safety Act of 1990, and the numerous amendments issued to date. Carriers are subject to both the Hazardous Materials Regulations and Motor Carrier Safety Regulations (49 CFR Parts 105-107, 171-180 & 390-397).

In turn, carriers (employers) are responsible for training, testing and certifying drivers and other employees in proper hazardous materials handling, and for providing necessary documents and information to drivers hauling hazardous materials loads.

Drivers are responsible for following the procedures prescribed in the regulations. Drivers can be fined for not complying with parts of the regulations that relate to them. A person who violates a requirement in the regulations is liable for a penalty of not more than $32,500 and not less than $275 for each violation.

The regulations for transporting hazardous materials are based on good common sense, and are designed to protect the safety of all concerned. It makes good sense for you to follow them carefully!

Besides obeying requirements specifically aimed at them, responsible drivers can do a lot to ensure that hazardous materials shipments are handled properly by all concerned. The following checklist for drivers rounds up the ways you can help.

Checklist

1. **Be able to recognize discrepancies in documents, packaging, labeling and compatibility.**

2. **Inspect all hazardous material shipments before loading and contact carrier management for instructions if there are any suspicious shipments offered.**

3. **Refuse to accept hazardous material freight from shippers or interline carriers, if the shipping papers**

are improperly prepared or don't check out with the freight. Also refuse leaking containers, those that might be damaged or any that appear improper.

4. Be sure that packages bearing POISON (TOXIC) or POISON INHALATION HAZARD labels are not loaded with foodstuffs, animal feeds or any other edible cargo intended for consumption by humans or animals unless they are packaged and loaded according to the regulations.

5. Be sure that all hazardous material is properly blocked and secured for transportation. Be sure containers won't be damaged by any other freight or by nails, rough floors, etc.

6. Be sure any required placards are in place before starting.

7. Have all necessary shipping papers (bills of lading, hazardous waste manifest, etc.) in good order, in your possession and available for immediate use in case of accident or inspection.

8. Know your responsibilities for attending your vehicle while carrying hazardous materials.

9. Know the procedures (and have them in writing if possible) for disposing of (or decontaminating) the hazardous cargo if there is an accident or some incident involving your hazardous cargo.

10. Be prepared to provide the required information to police, firemen, or other authorities in case of emergency.

11. Report the full details on any hazardous materials incident to your superior as quickly as possible. Include detailed information on cause, container damage, identification of specific containers and any corrective action which was taken.

How to Comply with the Law

How can you be sure that you can successfully comply with the provisions of the Hazardous Materials Regulations? It does take some study and responsibility on your part and you should have received training and testing from your employer. Requirements vary somewhat, depending on the type of operation you are working for. The following brief descriptions cover various types of operations which might be involved at some time with hauling hazardous goods.

Road Drivers

You should have a broad knowledge of the hazardous materials regulations.

You must have proper shipping papers for any hazardous shipment (except for ORM-D, Consumer Commodity). The papers must be properly stored and be available for immediate reference in case of accident.

You should be able to recognize improper shipping papers, and take appropriate action to get the situation corrected.

You should be able to match the freight being hauled with the correct documents, and be able to question the shipment if it does not appear to comply with the rules for hazardous shipments.

You must understand and comply with the attendance requirements for vehicles hauling hazardous materials.

You must report leaking containers, defective valves, etc. or any accident that occurs during a trip. If you receive written instructions from the carrier on emergency procedures, etc., you are required to follow them carefully.

Pick-Up and Delivery Drivers

If you fall into this category, you also need to be acquainted with the regulations concerning transportation of hazardous materials. Knowing the basics will help you identify any discrepancies you might find in shipments.

You should be advised in advance that you will be picking up hazardous materials.

Before the vehicle is loaded, you must inspect the hazardous materials to be hauled. If you suspect that the shipment may not be in compliance with regulations, you should contact the terminal for instructions before proceeding.

You must comply with any special blocking and securing requirements for the type of cargo you will be hauling.

You should also know proper procedures to follow in accidents or emergencies during transit. Finally, you must comply with attendance requirements for vehicles hauling hazardous materials.

Passenger-Carrying Vehicles

In general, no hazardous materials **at all** should be hauled on any for-hire passenger vehicle, if any other practicable means of transportation is available. Extremely dangerous Division 6.1 (poisonous) or Division 2.3 (poisonous gas) liquids, or any paranitraniline may **not** be hauled in passenger vehicles. However, in instances where there is no other means of transportation available, certain quantities of some types of hazardous materials may be hauled in passenger vehicles. In general, any hazardous material (with the exception of small arms ammunition) hauled on a passenger-carrying vehicle must be hauled outside the passenger compartment. The following may be hauled:

- **Up to 45 kg (99 pounds) gross weight of Class 1 (explosives) that are permitted to be transported by passenger-carrying aircraft or rail car.**
- **Not more than 100 detonators, Division 1.4 (explosives) per vehicle.**
- **Not more than 2 lab samples of Class 1 (explosives) materials per vehicle.**
- **Not more than 225 kg (496 pounds) of other types of hazardous materials, with no more than 45 kg (99 pounds) of any class.**

- A cylinder not exceeding 113 kg (250 pounds) that is secured against movement.
- Not more than 45 kg (99 pounds) of non-liquid, Division 6.1 (poisonous) materials.
- Class 7 (radioactive) materials requiring labels, when no other practicable means of transportation is available, and then only in full compliance with specific loading requirements.
- Emergency shipments of drugs, chemicals, and hospital supplies.
- Department of Defense materials under special circumstances.

How to Identify a Hazardous Materials Shipment

If you, as a driver, are to handle hazardous materials safely, you must be able to recognize them easily. HM shipments are recognizable by entries on the shipping papers, labels, markings on the packages, and placards.

Terms

Hazardous Material

A hazardous material is a substance or material which has been determined by the Secretary of Transportation to be capable of posing an unreasonable risk to health, safety, and property when transported in commerce, and which has been so designated. This includes hazardous substances, hazardous wastes, marine pollutants, and elevated temperature materials.

Hazardous materials fall into the following categories:

Class 1 (explosives) — is divided into six divisions as follows:

Division 1.1 — explosives that have a mass explosion hazard.

Division 1.2 — explosives that have a projection hazard.

Division 1.3 — explosives that have a fire hazard and either a minor blast hazard or a minor projection hazard or both.

Division 1.4 — explosive devices that present a minor blast hazard.

Division 1.5 — very insensitive explosives.

Division 1.6 — extremely insensitive detonating substances.

Class 2 (gases) — is divided into three divisions as follows:

Division 2.1 — gases that are flammable.

Division 2.2 — gases that are non-flammable and non-poisonous.

Division 2.3 — gases that are poisonous by inhalation.

Class 3 (flammable and combustible liquids) — A flammable liquid has a flash point of not more than 60.5°C (141°F). A combustible liquid has a flash point above 60.5°C (141°F) and below 93°C (200°F).

Class 4 (flammable solids) — is divided into three divisions as follows:

Division 4.1 — solids that are flammable.

Division 4.2 — material that is spontaneously combustible.

Division 4.3 — material that is dangerous when wet.

Class 5 (oxidizers and organic peroxides) — is divided into two divisions as follows:

Division 5.1 — oxidizer.

Division 5.2 — organic peroxide.

Class 6 (poisons) — is divided into two divisions as follows:

Division 6.1 — material that is poisonous.

Division 6.2 — material that is an infectious substance (eiologic agent).

Class 7 (radioactive materials) — material having a specific radioactive activity greater than 0.002 microcuries per gram.

Class 8 (corrosives) — material that causes visible destruction or irreversible alteration to human skin or a liquid that has a severe corrosion rate on steel or aluminum.

Class 9 (miscellaneous) — material which presents a hazard during transport, but which is not included in any other hazard class (such as a hazardous substance or a hazardous waste).

ORM–D (other regulated material) — material which although otherwise subject to the regulations, presents a limited hazard during transportation due to its form, quantity and packaging (consumer commodities).

Elevated Temperature Materials

An elevated temperature material is a material offered for transportation in a **BULK** packaging and meets one of the following criteria:

1. Is a liquid at a temperature at or above 100°C (212°F);
2. Is a liquid with a flash point at or above 37.8°C (100°F) that is intentionally heated and transported at or above its flash point; or
3. Is in a solid phase and at a temperature at or above 240°C (464°F).

Hazardous Substances

A hazardous substance is a material, including its mixtures or solutions, that is listed in Appendix A to §172.101 and is in a quantity, in one package, that equals or exceeds the reportable quantity (RQ) listed in Appendix A.

Hazardous Wastes

A hazardous waste is any material that is subject to the hazardous waste manifest requirements of the U.S. Environmental Protection Agency specified in 40 CFR 262.

Marine Pollutants

A marine pollutant is a material that is listed in Appendix B to §172.101 and when in a solution or mixture of one or more marine pollutants, is packaged in a concentration which equals or exceeds:

1. Ten percent by weight of the solution or mixture; or
2. One percent by weight of the solution or mixture for materials that are identified as severe marine pollutants (PP) in Appendix B.

Marine pollutants transported by water, in any size packaging, are subject to all the applicable requirements. Marine pollutants transported by highway, rail or air are subject to the requirements when transported in **BULK** packaging.

Bulk Packaging

A bulk packaging has no intermediate form of containment and has:

1. A maximum capacity greater than 450 L (119 gallons) as a receptacle for a liquid;
2. A maximum net mass greater than 400 kg (882 pounds) and a maximum capacity greater than 450 L (119 gallons) as a receptacle for a solid; or
3. A water capacity greater than 454 kg (1,000 pounds) as a receptacle for a gas.

Shipping Papers

A look at the shipping papers will help you identify a hazardous materials shipment and the hazard(s) you will be dealing with in a particular shipment. Hazardous materials are required to be indicated on shipping papers in one of three ways.

1. The hazardous materials may be listed **first**, before any non-hazardous materials, or

Number of packages	DESCRIPTION OF ARTICLES	Weight
10 drums	Gasoline, 3, UN1203, II	3,400 lbs.
3 skids	100# Sorex paper 36″ x 40″	3,000 lbs.

2. they may be listed in a **color** that clearly contrasts with entries for materials that are not subject to the hazardous materials regulations (hazardous material entries may be highlighted **only** on reproductions of the shipping paper), or

	Number of packages	DESCRIPTION OF ARTICLES	Weight
Black →	3 skids	100# Sorex paper 36″ x 40″	3,000 lbs.
Red →	10 drums	Gasoline, 3, UN1203, II	3,400 lbs.
Black →	100	36″ x 40″ wooden skids	3,000 lbs.

3. by placing an "**X**" in a column captioned "HM".

No. of packages	Type of package	HM	Description of articles (proper shipping name)	Hazard Class	I.D. Number	PG	Weight
10	drums	X	Gasoline	3	UN1203	II	3,400 lbs.
3	skids		100# Sorex paper 36″ x 40″				3,000 lbs.

Each hazardous material that is offered for transport must be clearly described on the shipping paper using the applicable information from the Hazardous Materials Table. This shipping description must include the material's:

- Proper shipping name;
- Hazard class or division number;
- Subsidiary Hazard Class(es) or Division number(s) entered in parentheses (mandatory October 1, 2005);
- UN or NA identification number;
- Packing group, if any;
- Total quantity, by net or gross mass, capacity, or as otherwise appropriate; and
- Number and type of packages (mandatory October 1, 2007).

Example: 2 drums, Acetyl chloride, 3, (8), UN1717, II, 180 lbs.

The total quantity is **not** required for hazardous material packaging containing only residue (i.e., one that has not been cleaned/purged or refilled with a non-hazardous material), cylinders, and bulk packagings. However, some indication of total quantity must be shown for cylinders and bulk packagings (10 cylinders or 1 cargo tank).

The first five (5) items — often referred to as the material's basic description — must be shown in sequence, with no additional information interspersed unless authorized by the regulations. The identification number must include the letters "UN" or "NA", as appropriate. The packing group must be shown in Roman numerals and may be preceded by the letters "PG".

Examples: Gasoline, 3, UN1203, PG II
Diallylamine, 3, (6.1, 8), UN2359, II

The basic description may be shown in an alternate sequence with the identification number listed first.

Examples: UN1203, Gasoline, 3, PG II
UN2359, Diallylamine, 3, (6.1, 8), II

Proper shipping names with a "G" in Column 1 of the Hazardous Materials Table must have the technical name of the hazardous material entered in parentheses in association with the basic description. If a hazardous material is a mixture or solution the technical names of at least two components most predominately contributing to the hazards of the mixture or solution must be entered.

Examples: Corrosive liquids, n.o.s. (Caprylyl chloride), 8, UN1760, II

Flammable liquid, corrosive, n.o.s., 3, (8), UN2924, II (methanol, potassium hydroxide)

Although there are a number of additional descriptions which may be required on shipping papers, there are several of special significance.

1. If the material is a hazardous substance, the letters "**RQ**" must appear either before or after the basic description. The letters "RQ" may be entered in the HM Column in place of the "X".

No. of packages	Type of package	HM	Description of articles (proper shipping name)	Hazard Class	I.D. Number	PG	Weight
10	drums	RQ	Aldrin, liquid	6.1	NA2762	II	2,000 lbs.

2. For materials being shipped under a limited quantity exception, the words "Limited Quantity" or the abbreviation "Ltd. Qty" must be entered following the basic description.

3. For all materials meeting the poisonous by inhalation criteria, the words "Poison-Inhalation Hazard" or "Toxic-Inhalation Hazard" and the words "Zone A", "Zone B", "Zone C", or "Zone D", for gases or "Zone A" or "Zone B" for liquids,

as appropriate, must be added on the shipping paper immediately following the shipping description. For anhydrous ammonia transported within the U.S., only the words "Inhalation Hazard" must be added in association with the shipping description.

4. The fact that a material is an elevated temperature material must be indicated in the shipping name or the word "HOT" must immediately precede the proper shipping name.

5. If a material is a marine pollutant the words "Marine Pollutant" must be entered in association with the basic shipping description, unless the proper shipping name indicates that it is a marine pollutant.

In most cases, an emergency response phone number must be entered on the shipping paper. It can be immediately following the description of each hazardous material or if the number applies to every hazardous material entered on the shipping paper, entered once on the shipping paper in a clearly visible location.

Each shipping paper should include the date of acceptance by the carrier. This date is a required part of the shipping paper retention requirements.

Finally, check for the Shipper's Certification which states the shipment has been properly classified, described, packaged, marked and labeled/placarded.

Labels

Labels can help you identify a hazardous materials shipment and the hazard(s) present.

When hazard warning labels are required on packages, the shipper is required to affix the labels before offering the shipment. The driver should not accept the shipment unless the required labels are affixed to the packages.

The Hazardous Materials Table in this book provides a ready reference to the labels required for each proper shipping name.

If more than one label is indicated by the label codes listed in Column 6 of the Hazardous Materials Table, the first one listed is the primary label and any others are subsidiary labels. When primary and subsidiary labels are required they must be displayed next to each other (within 6 inches).

The hazard warning labels are diamond-shaped and should measure at least 100 mm (3.9 inches) on each side. Labels must be printed on or affixed to a surface (other than the bottom) of the package containing the hazardous material. If possible, the label should be located on the same surface and near the proper shipping name marking. Labels must be clearly visible and not obscured by markings or attachments. The package pictured, has labels properly affixed.

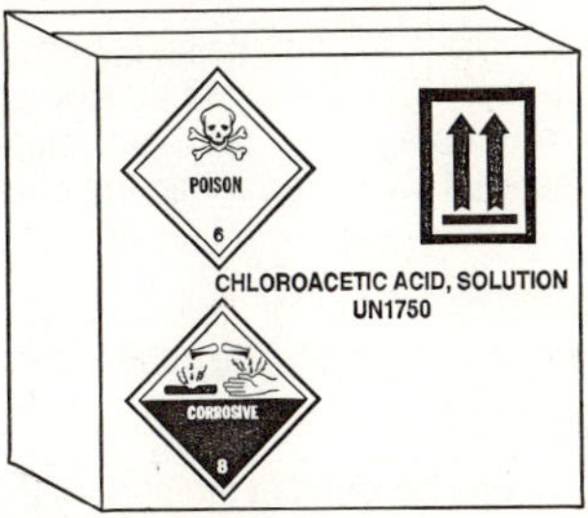

A label may be printed on or placed on a securely affixed tag, or may be affixed by other suitable means to:

- A package that contains no radioactive material and which has dimensions less than those of the required label; or
- A cylinder; or
- A package which has such an irregular surface that a label cannot be satisfactorily affixed.

Generally, only one of each different required label must be displayed on a package. However, duplicate labels must be displayed on at least two sides or two ends (other than the bottom) of the following:

- Each package or overpack having a volume of 1.8 m^3 (64 ft^3) or more;
- Each non-bulk package containing a radioactive material;
- Each DOT 106 or 110 multi-unit tank car tank. Labels must be displayed on each end;
- Each portable tank of less than 3,785 L (1,000 gallons) capacity; and
- Each freight container or aircraft unit load device having a volume of 1.8 m^3 (64 ft^3) or more, but less than 18 m^3 (640 ft^3). One of each required label must be displayed on or near the closure.

When two or more packages containing compatible hazardous materials are placed within the same outside container or overpack, the outside container or overpack must be labeled for each class of material contained within the outside container or overpack.

Text is not required on a label for Classes 1, 2, 3, 4, 5, 6, and 8. However, the label must meet the other specifications in the regulations.

Label illustrations can be found at the back of this pocketbook.

Markings

Markings are also helpful in identifying a hazardous materials shipment. The type of marking(s) displayed is often different for non-bulk and bulk packagings.

Non-Bulk Packagings

Almost all non-bulk packagings (119 gallons or less) **must be marked with the proper shipping name and** the four digit UN/NA **identification number** as shown in the Hazardous Materials Table and illustrated on page 21. Most n.o.s. and other generic proper shipping names must also have the technical name(s) entered in parentheses in association with the proper shipping name. In addition, other markings may be required, such as package orientation arrows illustrated on page 21.

Several other important markings may also be required. If the non-bulk package contains a hazardous substance (meets or exceeds the reportable quantity) the letters "RQ" must be marked in association with the proper shipping name.

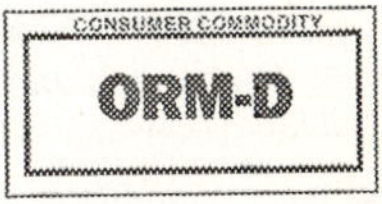

Packagings that contain a material classed as "ORM-D" must be marked on at least one side or end with the ORM-D designation — immediately following or below the proper shipping name. If the shipment is to be by air, the marking must be ORM-D-AIR.

A package containing a limited quantity of hazardous materials must be marked in one of the following two ways.

1. Marked with the proper shipping name and no identification number.

   OR

2. Marked with the identification number in a square-on-point border and no proper shipping name. The identification number must be preceded by the letters "UN" or "NA", as appropriate.

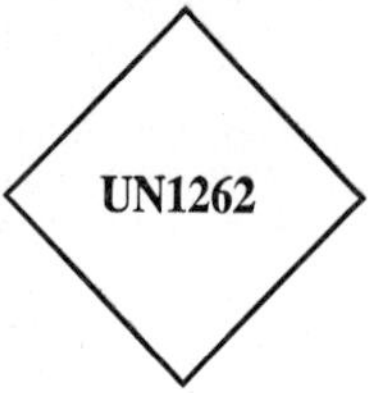

When two or more hazardous materials with different identification numbers are contained in the package, the package must be marked with either individual square-on-points bearing a single identification number, or a single square-on-point large enough to include each applicable identification number.

For transportation by aircraft, packages containing self-reactive substances of Division 4.1 or organic peroxides of Division 5.2 must be marked with the KEEP AWAY FROM HEAT handling mark.

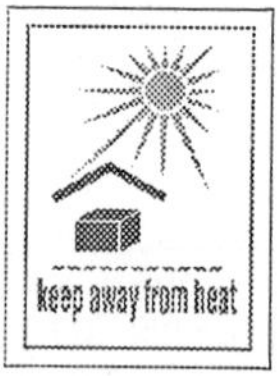

For those materials meeting the poisonous by inhalation criteria, the words "Inhalation Hazard" must appear in association with the hazard warning labels or shipping name, when required. The INHALATION HAZARD marking is not required on packages that display a label with the words "INHALATION HAZARD" on the label.

Finally, packagings (except for cylinders, Class 7 packagings and bulk packagings) for most hazardous materials must meet the United Nations Performance-Oriented Packaging Standards and be marked by the manufacturer in a manner such as illustrated below for a fiberboard box with an inner packaging.

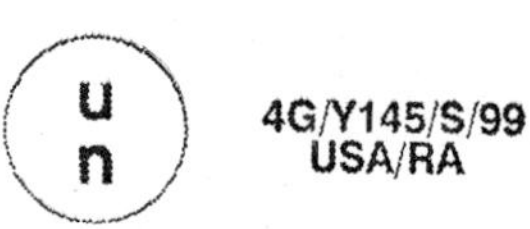

Large Quantities of Non-Bulk Packagings

A transport vehicle or freight container containing only a single hazardous material in non-bulk packages must be marked, on each side and each end with the material's identification number, subject to the following:

- Each package must be marked with the same proper shipping name and identification number;
- The aggregate gross weight of the hazardous material is 4,000 kg (8,820 pounds) or more;
- All of the hazardous material is loaded at one loading facility; and
- The transport vehicle or freight container contains no other material, hazardous or non-hazardous.

This does not apply to Class 1 materials, Class 7 materials, or non-bulk packagings for which identification numbers are not required (such as limited quantities or ORM–D).

A transport vehicle or freight container loaded at one loading facility with 1,000 kg (2,205 pounds) or more of non-bulk packages containing material that is poisonous by inhalation (in Hazard Zone A or B), having the same proper shipping name and identification number, must be marked on each side and each end with the identification number for the material. If the transport vehicle or freight container contains more than one inhalation hazard material that meets this requirement, it must be marked with the identification number for only one material. That one identification number is determined by the following:

- For different materials in the same hazard zone, the identification number of the material having the greatest aggregate gross weight.
- For different materials in both Hazard Zone A or B, the identification number for the Hazard Zone A material.

Bulk Packagings

Unless excepted, all bulk packagings (more than 119 gallons) of hazardous materials must be marked with the UN or NA identification number(s) of the contents. The identification number marking may be displayed on an orange panel, primary hazard placard, or a white square-on-point configuration.

A bulk package containing Poison Inhalation Hazard material must be marked "Inhalation Hazard" in association with any required labels, placards, or shipping name, when required. The INHALATION HAZARD marking is not required on packages that display a label or placard with the words "INHALATION HAZARD" on the label or placard.

This marking must be at least 25 mm (1.0 inch) in height for portable tanks with capacities of less than 3,785 L (1,000 gallons) and at least 50 mm (2.0 inches) in height for cargo tanks and other bulk packages. Bulk packaging must be marked on two opposing sides with this marking.

Bulk packagings of anhydrous ammonia transported in the U.S. must be marked with "INHALATION HAZARD" on two opposing sides.

Most bulk packages containing elevated temperature materials must be marked on two opposing sides with the word "HOT". However, if the package contains molten aluminum or molten sulfur the package must be marked "MOLTEN ALUMINUM" or "MOLTEN SULFUR" instead of the word "HOT".

The "HOT" marking must be on the package itself or in black lettering on a white square-on-point configuration that is the same size as a placard. The lettering must be at least 50 mm (2 inches) high.

The word "HOT" may be displayed in the upper corner of a white-square-on-point configuration that also displays the required identification number.

A package containing solid elevated temperature material is **not subject** to any of the Hazardous Materials Regulations, **except** that the word "HOT" **must** be on the package.

Bulk packages containing marine pollutants must be marked, on all four sides, with the MARINE POLLUTANT marking, unless they are labeled or placarded.

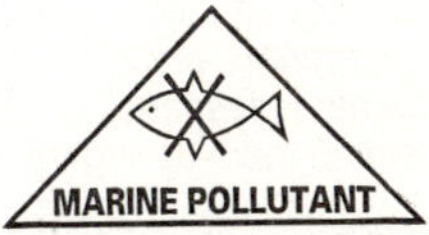

A bulk packaging containing a regulated medical waste must be marked with the BIOHAZARD marking, visible from the direction it faces:

- on two opposing sides or ends if the packaging has a capacity of less than 1,000 gallons (3,785 L), or
- on each end and each side if the packaging has a capacity of 1,000 gallons (3,785 L) or more.

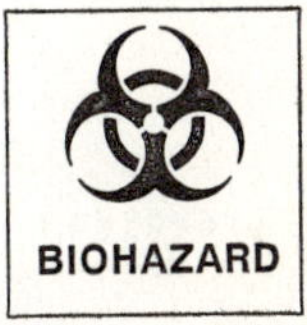

If the BIOHAZARD markings on a bulk packaging are not visible, the vehicle or freight container containing the bulk packaging must be marked on each side and each end with the BIOHAZARD marking. The BIOHAZARD marking may be displayed on a white square-on-point configuration.

Each truck body or trailer, rail car or freight container containing lading that has been fumigated or treated with any material must have a FUMIGANT marking displayed so that it can be seen by any person attempting to enter the vehicle or container.

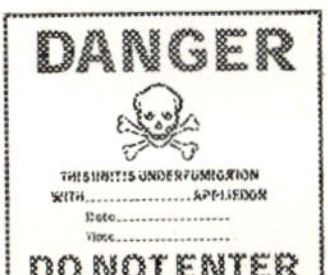

Placards

Placards can help you identify a hazardous materials shipment and the hazard(s) present.

Most vehicles, freight containers, and bulk packagings hauling hazardous materials are required to be placarded. In most cases placards must be displayed on all four sides. Placards must not be displayed when hazardous materials are not present.

In most situations the shipper is responsible for providing the appropriate placards to the motor carrier for a shipment. The carrier is responsible for applying them to the vehicle and maintaining them during transport.

Placards are diamond-shaped and should measure at least 273 mm (10.8 inches) on each side. Placards must be displayed on-point with the words or identification number displayed horizontally, reading from left to right.

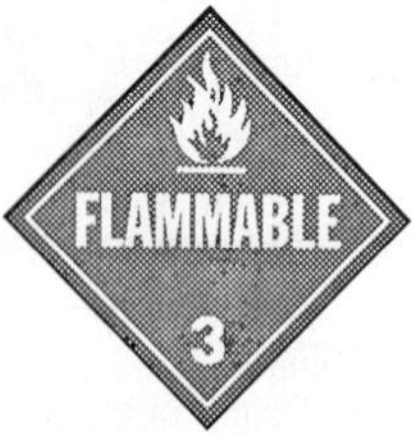

More information on placards can be found starting on page 33.

Placard illustrations can be found at the back of this pocketbook.

Materials of Trade

A Material of trade is a hazardous material that is carried on a motor vehicle:

- For the purpose of protecting the health and safety of the motor vehicle operator or passengers (such as insect repellant or self-contained breathing apparatus);
- For the purpose of supporting the operation or maintenance of a motor vehicle, including its auxiliary equipment (such as a spare battery or engine starting fluid); or
- By a private motor carrier (including vehicles operated by a rail carrier) in direct support of a principal business that is other than transportation by motor vehicle (such as lawn care, plumbing, welding, or farm operations).

A material of trade (not including self-reactive material, poisonous by inhalation material, or hazardous waste) is limited to:

- A Class 3, 8, 9, Division 4.1, 5.1, 5.2, 6.1, or ORM–D material contained in a packaging having a gross mass or capacity not over—
  - 0.5 kg (1 pound) or 0.5 L (1 pint) for Packing Group I material,
  - 30 kg (66 pounds) or 30 L (8 gallons) for a Packing Group II, III, or ORM–D material,
  - 1500 L (400 gallons) for a diluted mixture, not to exceed 2 percent concentration, of a Class 9 material;
- A Division 2.1 or 2.2 material in a cylinder with a gross weight not over 100 kg (220 pounds);
- A non-liquefied Division 2.2 material with no subsidiary hazard in a permanently mounted tank manufactured to the ASME Code at not more than 70 gallons water capacity; or

- A Division 4.3 material in Packing Group II or III contained in a packaging having a gross capacity not exceeding 30 mL (1 ounce).
- A Division 6.2 material, other than a Risk Group 4 material, that is a diagnostic specimen, biological product, or regulated medical waste in combination packaging conforming to the following:
  - For a diagnostic specimen or biological product:
    1. in a single inner packaging with a gross mass or capacity not exceeding 16 kg (35.2 lb) or 16 L (4.2 gal) in a single outer packaging; or
    2. in one or more inner packagings where the gross mass or capacity of each inner packaging does not exceed 0.5 kg (1.1 lb), or 0.5 L (17 ounces), and an outer packaging having a gross mass or capacity not exceeding 4 kg (8.8 lb) or 4 L (1 gal).
  - For a regulated medical waste, in one or more inner packagings having a gross mass or capacity not exceeding 4 kg (8.8 lb) or 4 L (1 gal), and an outer packaging having a gross mass or capacity not exceeding 16 kg (35.2 lb) or 16 L (4.2 gal).

For liquids, the inner packagings must be leak tight, and the outer packaging must contain sufficient absorbent material to absorb the entire contents of the inner packaging. For sharps, the inner packaging must be constructed of a rigid material resistant to punctures and leaks.

The gross weight of all materials of trade on a motor vehicle may not exceed 200 kg (440 pounds), not including 1,500 L (400 gallons) or less of a diluted mixture of Class 9 material, as mentioned above.

A non-bulk packaging, other than a cylinder, must be marked with a common name or proper shipping name to identify the material it contains. The letters "RQ" must be included if the packaging contains a reportable quantity of a hazardous substance.

Packaging for materials of trade must be leak tight for liquids and gases, sift proof for solids, and be securely closed, secured against shifting, and protected against damage. Each material must be packaged in the manufacturer's original packaging or a packaging of equal or greater strength and integrity. Packaging for gasoline must be made of metal or plastic and conform to the Hazardous Materials Regulations or OSHA regulations.

Outer packagings are not required for receptacles (e.g. cans and bottles) that are secured against shifting in cages, carts, bins, boxes or compartments.

A cylinder or other pressure vessel containing a Division 2.1 or 2.2 material must conform to the packaging, qualification, maintenance, and use requirements of the Hazardous Materials Regulations, except that outer packagings are not required.

The operator of a motor vehicle that contains a material of trade must be informed of the presence of the material and must be informed of the materials of trade requirements in the regulations.

General Requirements When Hauling Hazardous Materials

This chapter briefly details the requirements for vehicles transporting hazardous materials. Areas covered include **hazmat endorsement, shipping papers, emergency response information, placards, identification numbers, cargo heaters, and special documents.**

Hazardous Materials Endorsement

The driver of a commercial motor vehicle that is required to be placarded for hazardous materials or that transports any quantity of a material listed as a select agent or toxin in 42 CFR part 73, must have a hazardous materials endorsement on their Commercial Driver's License.

Shipping Papers

Most hazardous materials shipments must be accompanied by proper shipping papers, such as bills of lading, hazardous waste manifests, etc. During the course of the trip, the driver is responsible for maintaining the shipping papers according to requirements, so that they are easily accessible to authorities in case of accidents or inspection.

The hazardous materials shipping paper requirements do not apply to materials (other than hazardous wastes or hazardous substances) identified by the letter "A" or "W" in column 1 of the 172.101 Table unless they are intended for transportation by air or water. Materials classed as ORM–D are not subject to the HM shipping paper requirements unless they are intended for transportation by air.

Hazardous materials shipping papers must be retained by the shipper and the carrier for 375 days (one year and 10 days) after the material is accepted by the carrier. The date of acceptance must be included. This may be a paper copy or an electronic image of the shipping paper. Hazardous waste manifests must be retained for three years.

Emergency Response Information

Most hazardous material shipments (except those that do not require shipping papers) must have emergency response information on or in association with the shipping paper. If the information is in association with the shipping paper it may be in the form of the Emergency Response Guidebook, a Material Safety Data Sheet, or any other form that provides all the information required in §172.602.

In most cases, an emergency response phone number must be entered on the shipping paper. It can be immediately following the description of each hazardous material or if the number applies to every hazardous material entered on the shipping paper, entered once on the shipping paper in a clearly visible location and identified as an emergency response information number.

Placards

The Hazardous Materials Regulations require most vehicles hauling hazardous goods to be placarded. **The shipper is responsible for providing the appropriate placards** to the motor carrier for a shipment. **The carrier is responsible for applying them correctly to the vehicle** and maintaining them during transport. In addition, carriers are responsible for any placarding necessitated by aggregate shipment which collect at their terminals. Large freight containers (640 cubic feet or more) must be placarded by the shipper.

Placards must be affixed on all four sides of the vehicle, trailer or cargo carrier. The front placard may be on the front of the tractor or the cargo body. Placards must be removed from any vehicle not carrying hazardous materials.

In general, some basic rules apply to placards:

- **Placards must be securely attached to the vehicle or placed in a proper placard holder.**
- **Placards must be located at least 76.0 mm (3 inches) from any other type of marking on the vehicle.**
- **Words and numbers on placards must read horizontally.**

- **Placards must be clearly visible and maintained in a legible condition throughout the trip.**

As a rule, a driver may not move a vehicle that is not properly placarded, if placards are demanded by the cargo carried in the vehicle. However, in certain emergency situations, a vehicle not properly placarded may be moved if at least one of these three conditions is met:

- **Vehicle is escorted by a state or local government representative.**
- **Carrier has received permission from the Department of Transportation.**
- **Movement is necessary to protect life and property.**

Placards are chosen according to tables found in §172.504. Table 1 lists categories of hazardous materials which require placarding no matter what amount of material is being hauled. **Any quantity of hazardous material covered by Table 1 must be placarded** as specified in Table 1.

Table 2 also lists categories of hazardous materials and the placards required, but, there are some exceptions.

When the gross weight of hazardous materials in non-bulk packages covered by Table 2 is **less than 454 kg (1,001 pounds), no placard is required** on a transport vehicle or freight container. This does not apply to bulk packagings (such as portable tanks or cargo tanks) or hazardous materials subject to §172.505–Placarding for subsidiary hazards.

Non-bulk packaging that contains only the residue of Table 2 materials does not have to be included in determining placarding, except for materials subject to §172.505, subsidiary placarding.

A transport vehicle or freight container which contains non-bulk packagings with two or more categories of materials, requiring different placards specified in Table 2, may be placarded DANGEROUS in place of the separate placarding specified for each of the categories in Table 2. However, when 1,000 kg (2,205 pounds) or more of **one category** of materials is loaded at **one**

loading facility on **one transport vehicle** or container, the placard specified for that category in Table 2 must be applied.

Placard illustrations can be found at the back of this pocketbook.

In the following tables the **bold face entry** describes the category of the hazardous material, the light face entry indicates the placard required for that type of shipment.

TABLE 1

CATEGORY OF MATERIAL	*PLACARD*
1.1	EXPLOSIVES 1.1
1.2	EXPLOSIVES 1.2
1.3	EXPLOSIVES 1.3
2.3	POISON GAS
4.3	DANGEROUS WHEN WET
5.2 (Organic peroxide, Type B, liquid *or* solid, temperature controlled)	ORGANIC PEROXIDE
6.1 (material poisonous by inhalation (see §171.8 of this subchapter))	POISON INHALATION HAZARD
7 (Radioactive Yellow III label only)	RADIOACTIVE[1]

[1]RADIOACTIVE placard also required for exclusive use shipments of low specific activity material and surface contaminated objects transported in accordance with §173.427(b)(4) and (5) or (c) of this subchapter.

TABLE 2

CATEGORY OF MATERIAL	*PLACARD*
1.4	EXPLOSIVES 1.4
1.5	EXPLOSIVES 1.5
1.6	EXPLOSIVES 1.6
2.1	FLAMMABLE GAS
2.2	NON-FLAMMABLE GAS
3	FLAMMABLE
Combustible liquid	COMBUSTIBLE
4.1	FLAMMABLE SOLID
4.2	SPONTANEOUSLY COMBUSTIBLE
5.1	OXIDIZER

TABLE 2, Continued

CATEGORY OF MATERIAL	*PLACARD*
5.2 (Other than organic peroxide, Type B, liquid or solid, temperature controlled)	ORGANIC PEROXIDE
6.1 (other than material poisonous by inhalation)	POISON
6.2	(None)
8	CORROSIVE
9	CLASS 9
ORM–D	(None)

Placarding exceptions.

1. When more than one division placard is required for Class 1 materials on a transport vehicle, rail car, freight container or unit load device, only the placard representing the lowest division number must be displayed.

2. A FLAMMABLE placard may be used in place of a COMBUSTIBLE placard on—

   (i) A cargo tank or portable tank.

   (ii) A compartmented tank car which contains both flammable and combustible liquids.

3. A NON-FLAMMABLE GAS placard is not required on a transport vehicle which contains non-flammable gas if the transport vehicle also contains flammable gas or oxygen and it is placarded with FLAMMABLE GAS or OXYGEN placards, as required.

4. OXIDIZER placards are not required for Division 5.1 materials on freight containers, unit load devices, transport vehicles or rail cars which also contain Division 1.1 or 1.2 materials and which are placarded with EXPLOSIVES 1.1 or 1.2 placards, as required.

5. For transportation by transport vehicle or rail car only, an OXIDIZER placard is not required for Division 5.1 materials on a transport vehicle, rail car or freight container which also contains Division 1.5 explosives and is placarded with EXPLOSIVES 1.5 placards, as required.

6. The EXPLOSIVE 1.4 placard is not required for those Division 1.4 Compatibility Group S (1.4S) materials that are not required to be labeled 1.4S.

7. For domestic transportation of oxygen, compressed or oxygen, refrigerated liquid, the OXYGEN placard in §172.530 of this subpart may be used in place of a NON-FLAMMABLE GAS placard.

8. For domestic transportation, a POISON INHALATION HAZARD placard is not required on a transport vehicle or freight container that is already placarded with the POISON GAS placard.

9. For Class 9, a CLASS 9 placard is not required for domestic transportation, including that portion of international transportation, defined in §171.8 of this subchapter, which occurs within the United States. However, a bulk packaging must be marked with the appropriate identification number on a CLASS 9 placard, an orange panel, or a white square-on-point display configuration as required by subpart D of this part.

10. For Division 6.1, PG III materials, a POISON placard may be modified to display the text "PG III" below the mid line of the placard.

11. For domestic transportation, a POISON placard is not required on a transport vehicle or freight container required to display a POISON INHALATION HAZARD or POISON GAS placard.

The compatibility group letter must be displayed on placards for shipments of Class 1 materials when transported by aircraft or vessel. When more than one compatibility group placard is required for Class 1 materials, only one placard is required to be displayed as follows:

1. Explosive articles of compatibility groups C, D or E may be placarded displaying compatibility group E.

2. Explosive articles of compatibility groups C, D, or E, when transported with those in compatibility group N, may be

placarded displaying compatibility group D.

3. Explosive substances of compatibility groups C and D may be placarded displaying compatibility group D.

4. Explosive articles of compatibility groups C, D, E or G, except for fireworks, may be placarded displaying compatibility group E.

Each transport vehicle, portable tank, freight container, or unit load device that contains a material subject to the Poison-Inhalation Hazard shipping paper description must be placarded POISON INHALATION HAZARD or POISON GAS, as appropriate, on each side and each end if not so placarded under §172.504.

Placards for subsidiary hazards are required when certain hazardous materials are transported. The subsidiary placards that you will most likely encounter are DANGEROUS WHEN WET, POISON INHALATION HAZARD, POISON GAS and CORROSIVE.

On placards, text indicating the hazard (such as CORROSIVE) is only required on RADIOACTIVE, OXYGEN, and DANGEROUS placards. Identification numbers may be displayed on most placards. However, identification numbers must not be displayed on DANGEROUS, subsidiary, RADIOACTIVE, EXPLOSIVES 1.1, 1.2, 1.3, 1.4, 1.5, or 1.6 placards.

Identification Numbers

Hazardous materials UN/NA identification numbers are required on non-bulk packagings of hazardous materials, unless excepted by the regulations. The identification number must be marked on the package near the proper shipping name. The number must be preceded by "UN" or "NA", as appropriate. Identification numbers are not required on packages which contain ORM–D or limited quantity materials.

A transport vehicle or freight container that is loaded at one loading facility with 4,000 kg (8,820 pounds) or more of non-bulk packages of hazardous material having the same proper shipping name and identification number, and no other material (hazardous or non-hazardous), must be marked on each side and each end with the identification number. This does not apply to Class 1 materials, Class 7 materials, or non-bulk packagings for which identification numbers are not required.

A transport vehicle or freight container loaded at one loading facility with 1,000 kg (2,205 pounds) or more of non-bulk packages containing material that is poisonous by inhalation (in Hazard Zone A or B), having the same proper shipping name and identification number, must be marked on each side and each end with the identification number for the material. If more than one inhalation material is present, the identification number for the material in the most severe hazard zone or if in the same zone, the material having the largest gross weight, must be displayed.

When the four digit identification number is required to be displayed on vehicles, containers, or bulk packagings it may be displayed on an "Orange Panel" [160 mm (6.3 inches) by 400 mm (15.7 inches)], or on a white square-on-point display configuration having the same outside dimensions as a placard, or across the center of the proper placard in place of the hazard wording. Identification numbers must not be displayed on DANGEROUS, subsidiary, RADIOACTIVE, EXPLOSIVES 1.1, 1.2, 1.3, 1.4, 1.5, or 1.6 placards.

UN/NA identification numbers must be displayed on bulk packagings such as portable tanks, cargo tanks, and tank cars. Identification numbers are required to be displayed on each side and each end of a bulk packaging which has a capacity of 3,785 L (1,000 gallons) or more. Bulk packagings that have a capacity of less than 3,785 L (1,000 gallons) only need the identification numbers displayed on two opposing sides.

Identification numbers are not required on the ends of portable tanks and cargo tanks having more than one compartment if hazardous materials having different identification numbers are transported in the compartments. The identification numbers on the sides of the tank must be displayed in the same sequence as the compartments containing the materials they identify.

Cargo Heaters

If a cargo heater is located in a vehicle that will be used to transport hazardous materials, various restrictions apply.

When transporting Class 1 (explosives), any cargo heater must be made inoperable by draining or removing the heater's fuel tank and disconnecting its power source.

When transporting Class 3 (flammable liquid) or Division 2.1 (flammable gas), any cargo heater in the vehicle must meet the following specifications:

- **It is a catalytic heater.**
- **Surface temperature on the heater cannot exceed 54°C (129°F) on a thermostatically controlled heater or on a heater without thermostat control when the outside temperature is 16°C (60°F) or less.**
- **The heater is not ignited in a loaded vehicle.**
- **There is no flame on the catalyst or anywhere else in the heater.**
- **Heater is permanently marked by the manufacturer with "MEETS DOT REQUIREMENTS FOR CATALYTIC HEATERS USED WITH FLAMMABLE LIQUID AND GAS" and also "DO NOT LOAD INTO OR USE IN CARGO COMPARTMENTS CONTAINING FLAMMABLE LIQUID OR GAS IF FLAME IS VISIBLE ON CATALYST OR IN HEATER."**

There are also special restrictions on the use of **automatic cargo space heating temperature control devices.** Such devices may be used in transporting Class 3 (flammable liquid) or Division 2.1 (flammable gas) materials only if all the following conditions are met:

- **Electrical apparatus in the cargo compartment is explosion-proof or non-sparking.**

- **No combustion apparatus is located in the cargo compartment.**
- **No air-return connection exists between the cargo compartment and the combustion apparatus.**
- **The system is not capable of heating any part of the cargo to more than 54°C (129°F).**

If the temperature control device in question does not meet the previous four specifications, the following steps must be taken before the vehicle can be used to transport flammable liquid or flammable gas:

- **Any cargo heater fuel tank (other than LPG) must be emptied or removed.**
- **LPG tanks must have all discharge valves closed and fuel feed lines disconnected.**

Special Documents

Certificate of Registration

Any person who offers for transport, or transports in foreign, interstate or intrastate commerce, any of the following, is subject to the DOT hazardous materials registration and fee requirements.

- **Any highway route-controlled quantity of a Class 7 (radioactive) material;**
- **More than 25 kg (55 pounds) of a Division 1.1, 1.2, 1.3 (explosive) material;**
- **More than one L (1.06 quarts) per package of a material extremely toxic by inhalation (i.e., "material poisonous by inhalation," as defined in §171.8, that meets the criteria for "hazard zone A," as specified in §§173.116(a) or 173.133(a));**
- **A hazardous material in a bulk packaging having a capacity equal to or greater than 13,248 L (3,500**

gallons) for liquids or gases, or more than 13.24 cubic meters (468 cubic feet) for solids;

- **A shipment in other than a bulk packaging (being offered or loaded at one loading facility using one transport vehicle) of 2,268 kg (5,000 pounds) gross weight or more of one class of hazardous materials for which placarding is required; or**
- **A quantity of hazardous material that requires placarding.** Except farmers in direct support of farming operations.

Motor carriers subject to the registration requirements must carry, on board **each** vehicle that is transporting a hazardous material requiring registration:

- **A copy of the carriers' current Certificate of Registration; or**
- **Another document bearing the registration number identified as the "U.S. DOT Hazmat Reg. No.".**

Class 1 (Explosive) Shipments

Some special documents are required to be carried by drivers of vehicles transporting Division 1.1, 1.2, or 1.3 (explosive) materials:

- **A copy of Part 397, Transportation of Hazardous Materials; Driving and Parking Rules (Federal Motor Carrier Safety Regulations).** Part 397 can be found at the back of this pocketbook.
- **Instructions on procedures to be followed in case of an accident or delay. This must include the nature of the explosives being hauled, the names and phone numbers of persons to be contacted and precautions to be taken.**

Drivers are required to sign a receipt for these documents. The carrier must maintain the receipt for one year.

In addition to the above documents drivers must also have the following documents:

- **Proper shipping papers.**
- **A written route plan for the shipment. (In some cases, this plan may be prepared by the driver, if the trip begins at some other point than the carrier's terminal.)**

Hazardous Waste Shipment

A driver **must not** accept a shipment of hazardous waste unless it is accompanied by a properly prepared Uniform Hazardous Waste Manifest!

Delivery of hazardous wastes **must be** made ONLY to the facility or alternate facility designated on the hazardous waste manifest. If delivery can not be made, the driver should contact his dispatcher or other designated official, immediately.

Loading and Unloading Rules for All Hazardous Materials Shipments

There are some regulations for the safe and secure loading and unloading of hazardous materials shipments which apply to all hazardous commodities shipments. They are included in this chapter, and should be interpreted as general common sense rules to follow in the operation of your vehicle. Specifics on loading and unloading certain particular hazardous materials are contained in a later chapter.

Securing Packages

Any package containing any hazardous material that is not permanently attached to a vehicle must be secured against any movement, including motion between packages, within the vehicle during normal transportation conditions. Packages having valves or other fittings must be loaded in a manner to minimize the likelihood of damage during transportation

Each package bearing orientation arrow markings must be loaded on a vehicle or within a freight container in accordance with the arrow markings. The package must remain in this position during transportation.

No Smoking

Smoking on or near any vehicle while loading or unloading any Class 1 (explosive), Class 3 (flammable liquid), Class 4 (flammable solid), Class 5 (oxidizer), or Division 2.1 (flammable gas) materials is forbidden. Further, care should be taken to keep all fire sources — matches and smoking materials in particular — away from vehicles hauling any of the above materials.

Set Handbrake

During the loading and unloading of any hazardous materials shipment the handbrake on the vehicle must be set, and all precautions taken to prevent movement of the vehicle.

Tools

Any tools used in loading or unloading hazardous material must be used with care not to damage the closures on any packages or containers, or to harm packages of Class 1 (explosive) material and other hazardous materials in anyway.

Attending Vehicles

There are attendance requirements for **cargo tanks** that are being loaded and unloaded with hazardous materials. Such a tank must be attended at all times during loading and unloading by a qualified person. The person who is responsible for loading the cargo is also responsible for seeing that the vehicle is attended. However, the carrier's obligation to oversee unloading ceases when all these conditions are met:

- **The carrier's transportation obligation is completed.**
- **The cargo tank is placed on the consignee's premises.**
- **Motive power is removed from the cargo tank and the premises.**

A person qualified to attend the cargo tank during loading and/or unloading must be:

- **Alert.**
- **Within 7.62 m (25 feet) of the cargo tank.**
- **Have an unobstructed view of the cargo tank and delivery hose to the maximum extent practicable.**
- **Aware of the nature of the hazardous material.**
- **Instructed in emergency procedures.**
- **Authorized to and capable of moving the cargo tank if necessary.**

Forbidden Articles

No motor carrier may accept for transportation or transport any goods classed as "Forbidden" in the §172.101 Hazardous Materials Table or goods not prepared in accordance with the regulations.

Carrier personnel are also responsible for rejecting packages of hazardous materials which show signs of leakage or other damage.

Commodity Compatibility

The Hazardous Materials Regulations contain segregation requirements which indicate which hazardous materials may not be loaded, transported or stored together.

Materials which are in packages that require labels, in a compartment within a multi-compartmented cargo tank, or in a portable tank loaded in a transport vehicle or freight container are subject to the segregation requirements. In addition to the following Tables and §173.12(e), cyanides or cyanide mixtures or solutions may not be stored, loaded and transported with acids, and Division 4.2 materials may not be stored, loaded and transported with Class 8 liquids.

Except as mentioned in the previous paragraph hazardous materials may not be stored, loaded, or transported together, except as provided in the following Tables:

SEGREGATION TABLE FOR HAZARDOUS MATERIALS

Class or Division		Notes	1.1, 1.2	1.3	1.4	1.5	1.6	2.1	2.2	2.3 gas Zone A	2.3 gas Zone B	3	4.1	4.2	4.3	5.1	5.2	6.1 liquids PG I Zone A	7	8 liquids only
Explosives	1.1 and 1.2	A	*	*	*	*	*	x	x	x	x	x	x	x	x	x	x	x	x	x
Explosives	1.3		*	*	*	*	*	x		x	x	x		x	x	x	x	x		x
Explosives	1.4		*	*	*	*	*	o		o	o	o		o				o		o
Very insensitive explosives.	1.5	A	*	*	*	*	*	x	x	x	x	x	x	x	x	x	x	x	x	x
Extremely insensitive explosives.	1.6		*	*	*	*	*													
Flammable gases	2.1		x	x	o	x				x	o							o	o	
Non-toxic, non-flammable gases.	2.2		x			x														
Poisonous gas Zone A	2.3		x	x	o	x		x				x	x	x	x	x	x			x
Poisonous gas Zone B	2.3		x	x	o	x		o				o	o	o	o	o	o			o
Flammable liquids	3		x	x	o	x				x	o					o		x		
Flammable solids	4.1		x			x				x	o							x		o
Spontaneously combustible materials.	4.2		x	x	o	x				x	o							x		x
Dangerous when wet materials.	4.3		x	x		x				x	o							x		o
Oxidizers	5.1	A	x	x		x				x	o	o						x		o
Organic peroxides	5.2		x	x		x				x	o							x		o
Poisonous liquids PG I Zone A.	6.1		x	x	o	x		o				x	x	x	x	x	x			x
Radioactive materials .	7		x			x		o												
Corrosive liquids	8		x	x	o	x				x	o		o	x	o	o	o	x		

Instructions for using the segregation table for hazardous materials are as follows:

1. The absence of any hazard class or division or a blank space in the Table indicates that no restrictions apply.

2. The letter "X" in the Table indicates that these materials may not be loaded, transported, or stored together in the same transport vehicle or storage facility during the course of transportation.

3. The letter "O" in the Table indicates that these materials may not be loaded, transported, or stored together in the same transport vehicle or storage facility during the course of transportation unless separated in a manner that, in the event of leakage from packages under conditions normally incident to transportation, commingling of hazardous materials would not occur. Notwithstanding the methods of separation employed, Class 8 (corrosive) liquids may not be loaded above or adjacent to Class 4 (flammable) or Class 5 (oxidizing) materials; except that shippers may load truckload shipments of such materials together when it is known that the mixture of contents would not cause a fire or a dangerous evolution of heat or gas.

4. The "*" in the Table indicates that segregation among different Class 1 (explosive) materials is governed by the compatibility table for Class 1 (explosive) materials.

5. The note "A" in the second column of the Table means that, notwithstanding the requirements of the letter "X", ammonium nitrate (UN1942) and ammonium nitrate fertilizer may be loaded or stored with Division 1.1 (explosive) or Division 1.5 materials.

6. When the §172.101 Table or §172.402 of this subchapter requires a package to bear a subsidiary hazard label, segregation appropriate to the subsidiary hazard must be applied when that segregation is more restrictive than that required by the primary hazard. However, hazardous materials of the same class may be stowed together without regard to segregation required for any secondary haz-

ard if the materials are not capable of reacting dangerously with each other and causing combustion or dangerous evolution of heat, evolution of flammable, poisonous, or asphyxiant gases, or formation of corrosive or unstable materials.

Class 1 (explosive) materials shall not be loaded, transported, or stored together, except as provided in this section, and in accordance with the following Table:

COMPATIBILITY TABLE FOR CLASS 1 (EXPLOSIVE) MATERIALS.

Compatibility group	A	B	C	D	E	F	G	H	J	K	L	N	S
A		x	x	x	x	x	x	x	x	x	x	x	x
B	x		x	$x_{(4)}$	x	x	x	x	x	x	x	x	4/5
C	x	x		2	2	x	6	x	x	x	x	3	4/5
D	x	$x_{(4)}$	2		2	x	6	x	x	x	x	3	4/5
E	x	x	2	2		x	6	x	x	x	x	3	4/5
F	x	x	x	x	x		x	x	x	x	x	x	4/5
G	x	x	6	6	6	x		x	x	x	x	x	4/5
H	x	x	x	x	x	x	x		x	x	x	x	4/5
J	x	x	x	x	x	x	x	x		x	x	x	4/5
K	x	x	x	x	x	x	x	x	x		x	x	4/5
L	x	x	x	x	x	x	x	x	x	x	1	x	x
N	x	x	3	3	3	x	x	x	x	x	x		4/5
S	x	4/5	4/5	4/5	4/5	4/5	4/5	4/5	4/5	4/5	x	4/5	

Instructions for using the compatibility table for Class 1 (explosive) materials are as follows:

1. A blank space in the Table indicates that no restrictions apply.
2. The letter "X" in the Table indicates that explosives of different compatibility groups may not be carried on the same transport vehicle.
3. The numbers in the Table mean the following:
   - 1 means an explosive from compatibility group L shall only be carried on the same transport vehicle with an identical explosive.
   - 2 means any combination of explosives from compatibility groups C, D, or E is assigned to compatibility group E.
   - 3 means any combination of explosives from compatibility groups C, D, or E with those in compatibility group N is assigned to compatibility group D.
   - 4 means 'see §177.835(g)' when transporting detonators.
   - 5 means Division 1.4S fireworks may not be loaded on the same transport vehicle with Division 1.1 or 1.2 (explosive) materials.
   - 6 means explosive articles in compatibility group G, other than fireworks and those requiring special handling, may be loaded, transported and stored with other explosive articles of compatibility groups C, D and E, provided that explosive substances (such as those not contained in articles) are not carried in the same vehicle.

Except as provided in the next paragraph, explosives of the same compatibility group but of different divisions may be transported together provided that the whole shipment is transported as though its entire contents were of the lower numerical division (i.e., Division 1.1 being lower than Division 1.2). For example, a mixed shipment of Division 1.2 (explosive) materials and Division 1.4 (explosive) materials, both of compatibility group D, must be transported as Division 1.2 (explosive) materials.

When Division 1.5 materials, compatibility group D, are transported in the same freight container as Division 1.2 (explosive) materials, compatibility group D, the shipment must be transported as Division 1.1 (explosive) materials, compatibility group D.

TERMINAL INFORMATION

Omaha, NE
800-228-2240

Indianapolis, IN
888-259-7542

Allentown, PA
800-404-0995

Lakeland, FL
877-675-4790

Atlanta, GA
800-828-7556

Laredo, TX
877-675-4789

Dallas, TX
800-433-5655

Phoenix, AZ
800-522-2668

Denver, CO
800-338-6177

Portland, OR
877-210-0278

Fontana, CA
800-255-2194

Springfield, OH
800-221-5969

DRIVE SAFELY.

WERNER ENTERPRISES
SPECIALIZED CARRIER ®

IMPORTANT NUMBERS

BENEFITS

Allstate
877-282-0808

BCBS
Health/Dental: 800-356-3485

COBRA
866-895-2607

Hartford Insurance
877-282-0808

Pharmacy
Medco: 800-711-0917

401(k)/Stock Purchase Plan
800-228-2240, ext. 2257

Superior Vision
800-507-3800

Werner Benefits Department
877-856-7711

After Hours EMERGENCY
800-331-0361

Cargo Claims
800-362-3058

Driver Payroll & Bonds
800-227-6849

Driver Recruiting/Placement
800-346-2818

Driver Relations
800-567-8855

Fuel Dept/Surcharge
800-628-8143

Logs
800-646-0536

Owner/Operator Payroll
Advances: 800-937-6376
Settlements: 800-937-6375

Permits
800-362-3076

Road Breakdown
800-228-0013

Safety Hotline
800-331-0361

Work Comp
800-228-2240, ext. 2226

www.werner.com

www.superiorvision.com

www.bcbsne.com

www.hartfordlife.com

www.medco.com

Revised 11/05

On the Road with Hazardous Materials

Some general rules apply to drivers hauling hazardous materials during the actual time on the road. The following covers these driving rules for all hazardous materials shipments.

Shipping Papers

Hazardous materials shipments must be accompanied by proper shipping papers, such as bills of lading, hazardous waste manifests, etc. During the course of the trip, the driver is responsible for maintaining the shipping papers according to requirements, so that they are easily accessible to authorities in case of accidents or inspection.

1. **If the hazardous material shipping paper is carried with any other papers, it must be clearly distinguished, either by tabbing it or having it appear first.**
2. **When the driver is at the controls, the shipping papers must be within his immediate reach when he is restrained by the seat belt.**
3. **The shipping papers must be readily visible to someone entering the driver's compartment, or in a holder mounted on the inside of the door on the driver's side.**
4. **If the driver is not in the vehicle, the shipping papers must be either in the holder on the door or on the driver's seat.**

Emergency Response Information

Most hazardous material shipments (except those that do not require shipping papers) must have emergency response information on or in association with the shipping paper. If the information is in association with the shipping paper it may be in the form of the Emergency Response Guidebook, a Material Safety Data Sheet, or any other form that provides all the information required in §172.602.

In most cases, an emergency response phone number must be entered on the shipping paper. It can be immediately following the description of each hazardous material or if the number applies to every hazardous material entered on the shipping paper, entered once on the shipping paper in a clearly visible location.

Registration

Motor carriers that are subject to the federal DOT hazmat registration requirements (§107.601) must carry, on board **each** vehicle that is transporting a hazardous material requiring registration:

- A copy of the carriers' current Certificate of Registration;

  OR

- Another document bearing the registration number identified as the "U.S. DOT Hazmat Reg. No.".

Railroad Crossings

Any marked or placarded vehicle (except Divisions 1.5, 1.6, 4.2, 6.2, and Class 9), any cargo tank motor vehicle, loaded or empty, used to transport any hazardous material, or a vehicle carrying any amount of chlorine, must stop at railroad crossings.

Stops must be made within 50 feet of the crossing, but no closer than 15 feet. When you determine it is safe to cross the tracks, you may do so, but do not shift gears while crossing the tracks.

Stops need not be made at:

1. **Streetcar crossings or industrial switching tracks within a business district.**
2. **Crossings where a police officer or flagman is directing traffic.**

3. **Crossings which are controlled by a stop-and-go traffic light which is green.**

4. **Abandoned rail lines and industrial or spur line crossings clearly marked "exempt".**

Tunnels

Unless there is no other practicable route, marked or placarded shipments of hazardous materials should not be driven through tunnels. Operating convenience cannot be used as a determining factor in such decisions.

In addition, the provisions of the Hazardous Materials Regulations do not supersede state or local laws and ordinances which may be more restrictive concerning hazardous materials and urban vehicular tunnels used for mass transportation.

Routing

A motor carrier transporting hazardous materials required to be marked or placarded shall operate the vehicle over routes which do not go through or near heavily populated areas, places where crowds are assembled, tunnels, narrow streets, or alleys, except when:

- There is no practicable alternative;
- It is necessary to reach a terminal, points of loading or unloading, facilities for food, fuel, rest, repairs, or a safe haven; or
- A deviation is required by emergency conditions;

Operating convenience is not a basis for determining if a route can be used. A motor carrier shall also comply with the routing designations of States or Indian tribes as authorized by federal regulations.

Attending Vehicles

Any marked or placarded vehicle containing hazardous materials which is on a public street or highway or the shoulder of any such road must be attended by the driver. Except when transporting Division 1.1, 1.2, or 1.3 material, the vehicle does not have to be attended when the driver is performing duties necessary to the operation of the vehicle.

What exactly does "attended" mean? In terms of the regulations a motor vehicle is attended when the person in charge is on the vehicle and awake (cannot be in the sleeper berth) or is within 100 feet of the vehicle and has an unobstructed view of it.

Fueling

When a marked or placarded vehicle is being fueled, the engine must be shut off and a person must be in control of the fueling process at the point where the fuel tank is filled.

Parking

Marked or placarded vehicles containing hazardous materials should not be parked on or within five feet of the traveled portion of any roadway. If the vehicle does not contain Division 1.1, 1.2, or 1.3 material, it may be stopped for brief periods when operational necessity requires parking the vehicle, and it would be impractical to stop elsewhere. Further restrictions apply to vehicles hauling Division 1.1, 1.2, or 1.3 (explosive) materials. Standard warning devices are to be set out as required by law when a vehicle is stopped along a roadway.

Warning devices

Vehicles must be equipped with emergency warning devices such as reflective triangles, red lanterns, fusees or liquid-burning flares. Liquid-burning flares, fusees, oil lanterns, or any signal produced by a flame must not be carried on or used for any vehicle transporting Division 1.1, 1.2, 1.3 (explosives) materials, any cargo tank motor vehicle transporting Division 2.1 (flammable gas) or Class 3 (flammable liquid) materials, loaded or empty.

Emergency Carrier Information Contact

If you are transporting hazardous materials that require shipping papers your carrier must instruct you to contact them (e.g., by telephone or radio) in the event of an incident involving the hazardous material.

If a transport vehicle (semi-trailer or freight container-on-chassis) contains hazardous materials that require shipping papers and the vehicle is separated from its motive power and parked at a location [other than a facility operated by the consignor or consignee or a facility subject to the emergency response information requirements in §172.602(c)(2)] the carrier must:

- Mark the vehicle with the telephone number of the motor carrier on the front exterior near the brake hose and electrical connections, or on a label, tag, or sign attached to the vehicle at the brake hose or electrical connection; or
- Have the shipping paper and emergency response information readily available on the transport vehicle.

The above requirements do not apply if the vehicle is marked on an orange panel, a placard, or a plain white square-on-point configuration with the identification number of each hazardous material contained within. The identification number(s) must be visible on the outside of the vehicle.

Tire Checks

The driver of any vehicle which must be marked or placarded because it contains hazardous materials, must examine each tire on their vehicle at the beginning of each trip and each time the vehicle is parked.

If any defect is found in a tire, it should be repaired or replaced immediately. The vehicle may, however, be driven a short distance to the nearest safe place for repair.

If a hot tire is found, it must be removed from the vehicle immediately and taken to a safe distance. Such a vehicle may not be operated until the cause of the overheating is corrected.

No Smoking

No person may smoke or carry any lighted smoking materials on or within 25 feet of marked or placarded vehicles containing any Class 1 (explosive) materials, Class 5 (oxidizer) materials or flammable materials classified as Division 2.1, Class 3, Divisions 4.1 and 4.2, or any empty tank vehicle that has been used to transport Class 3 (flammable liquid) or Division 2.1 (flammable gas) materials.

Fires

A marked or placarded vehicle containing hazardous materials should not be driven near an open fire, unless careful precautions have been taken to be sure the vehicle can completely pass the fire without stopping. In addition, a marked or placarded vehicle containing hazardous materials should not be parked within 300 feet of any open fire.

Fire Extinguisher

If a power unit or a vehicle pulled by a power unit requires the display of markings or placards, the power unit must be equipped with a fire extinguisher having an Underwriters' Laboratories (UL) rating of 10 B:C or more. The fire extinguisher must be properly filled, securely mounted, and located so that it is readily accessible for use. It must be designed, constructed, and maintained to permit visual determination of whether it is fully charged.

Vehicle Maintenance

No person may use heat, flame or spark producing devices to repair or maintain the cargo or fuel containment system of a motor vehicle required to be placarded, other than COMBUSTIBLE. The containment system includes all vehicle components intended physically to contain cargo or fuel during loading or filling, transport, or unloading.

Damaged Packages

Packages of hazardous materials that are damaged or found leaking during transportation, and hazardous materials that have spilled or leaked during transportation, may be forwarded to their destination or returned to the shipper in a salvage drum in accordance with the regulations.

Packages may be repaired in accordance with the best and safest practice known and available.

Any package repaired in accordance with the requirements in the regulations may be transported to the nearest place where it may safely be disposed. This may be done only if the following requirements are met:

1. The package must be safe for transportation.
2. The repair of the package must be adequate to prevent contamination of other lading or producing a hazardous mixture with other lading transported on the same motor vehicle.
3. If the carrier is not the shipper, the consignee's name and address must be plainly marked on the repaired package.

In the event any leaking package or container cannot be safely and adequately repaired for transportation or transported, it shall be stored pending proper disposition in the safest and most expeditious manner possible.

Incident Reporting

As soon as possible, report any incident involving hazardous materials during transportation (including loading, unloading, and temporary storage) to your carrier. Any incident subject to the immediate telephone notification requirements or any unintentional release of hazardous materials must be reported in writing to the DOT on Form F 5800.1 (Hazardous Materials Incident Report) within 30 days of the date of discovery.

In some cases, immediate telephone notification to the DOT is required. In these cases, contact your carrier by phone as soon as possible, so the telephone report can be made to the Department of Transportation. Incidents which require this immediate notification include those in which:

- **As a direct result of hazardous materials**
  1. **A person is killed;**
  2. **A person receives an injury requiring hospitalization;**
  3. **An evacuation of the general public occurs lasting one or more hours;**
  4. **A major transportation artery or facility is closed or shut down for one hour or more; or**
  5. **The operational flight pattern or routine of an aircraft is altered.**
- **Fire, breakage, spillage or suspected radioactive contamination occurs involving radioactive material.**
- **Fire, breakage, spillage or suspected contamination occurs involving infectious substances other than a diagnostic specimen or regulated medical waste.**
- **There has been a release of a marine pollutant in a quantity exceeding 450 L (119 gallons) for liquids or 400 kg (882 pounds) for solids.**
- **Some other situation occurs which the person in possession of the hazardous material considers important enough to warrant immediate reporting.**

Loading, Unloading & on the Road with Specific Hazardous Materials

Following are sections on specific classes of hazardous materials, with special emphasis on the role **YOU, the driver,** play in their safe and lawful transportation.

- **Class 1 (Explosives)**
- **Class 2 (Gases)**
- **Class 3 (Flammable Liquids)**
- **Class 4 (Flammable Solids) and Class 5 (Oxidizers)**
- **Division 6.1 (Poisonous Materials) and Division 2.3 (Poisonous Gases)**
- **Class 7 (Radioactive Materials)**
- **Class 8 (Corrosive Liquids)**

Another helpful feature is the reminder checklist which closes each section.

Shipments of CLASS 1 (Explosives)

General loading, transportation and unloading requirements that apply to all hazardous materials shipments can be found in the two preceding chapters. The following information is specific to Class 1 materials.

Combination Vehicles

Division 1.1 or 1.2 (explosives) materials may not be loaded on any vehicle of a combination of vehicles if:

1. More than two cargo carrying vehicles are in the combination;
2. Any full trailer in the combination has a wheel base of less than 184 inches;
3. Any vehicle in the combination is a cargo tank which is required to be marked or placarded; or
4. The other vehicle in the combination contains any:
   - Substances, explosive, n.o.s., Division 1.1A (explosive) material (Initiating explosive),
   - Packages of Class 7 (radioactive) materials bearing "Yellow III" labels,
   - Division 2.3 (poison gas) Hazard Zone A or B or Division 6.1 (poison) PG I, Hazard Zone A materials, or
   - Hazardous materials in a portable tank or a DOT Spec. 106A or 110A tank.

Vehicle Condition

Vehicles transporting any Class 1 materials must be free of sharp projections into the body which could damage packages of explosives.

Vehicles carrying Division 1.1, 1.2, or 1.3 materials must have tight floors. They must be lined with non-metallic material or non-ferrous material in any portion that comes in contact with the load.

Motor vehicles carrying Class 1 materials should have either a closed body or have the body covered with a tarpaulin, so that the load is protected from moisture and sparks. However, explosives other than black powder may be hauled on flat-bed vehicles if the explosive portions of the load are packed in fire and water-resistant containers or are covered by a fire and water-resistant tarpaulin.

If the vehicle assigned to haul Class 1 materials is equipped with any kind of cargo heater, **it must be inoperable for the duration of that shipment.** Check to be sure the heater's fuel tank has been completely drained and the power source disconnected.

Loading & Unloading

Rules for loading Class 1 (explosive) materials are based on good common sense. They include:

1. **Be sure the engine of your vehicle is stopped before loading or unloading any Class 1 materials.**
2. **Don't use bale hooks or any other metal tool to handle Class 1 materials.**
3. **Don't roll any Class 1 materials packages, except barrels or kegs.**
4. **Be careful not to throw or drop packages of Class 1 materials.**
5. **Keep Class 1 materials well clear of any vehicle exhaust pipes at all times.**
6. **Be sure any tarpaulins are well-secured with ropes or wire tie-downs.**

7. **Loads of Class 1 materials must be contained entirely within the body of the vehicle, with no projection or overhang.**

8. **If there is a tailgate or tailboard, it should be securely in place throughout the trip.**

9. **Don't load Class 1 materials with any other materials that might damage packages during transit. In an allowable mixed load, bulkheads or other effective means must be used to separate cargo.**

Emergency Transfers

Division 1.1, 1.2, or 1.3 materials may not be transferred (from container to container, motor vehicle to motor vehicle, another vehicle to a motor vehicle) on any street, road or highway, except in emergencies.

In such cases all possible precautions must be taken to alert other drivers of the hazards involved in the transfer. Specifically, red electric lanterns, emergency reflectors or flags must be set out as prescribed for stopped or disabled vehicles.

Liquid-burning flares, fusees, oil lanterns, or any signal produced by a flame must not be used for protecting any stopped or disabled vehicle transporting Division 1.1, 1.2 or 1.3 materials.

Parking

Marked or placarded vehicles carrying Division 1.1, 1.2, or 1.3 materials must not be parked in the following locations:

- **On a public street or highway, or within five feet of the traveled portion of such a roadway.**
- **On private property (including truck stops and restaurants) without the knowledge and consent of the person in charge of the property and who is aware of the nature of the materials.**
- **Within 300 feet of any bridge, tunnel, dwelling, building or place where people work or assemble,**

except for brief periods necessary to the operation of the vehicle when parking elsewhere is not practical.

Marked or placarded vehicles containing Division 1.4, 1.5, or 1.6 materials should not be parked on or within five feet of the traveled portion of any public street or highway, except for brief periods necessary to vehicle operation.

Attending Vehicles

Marked or placarded vehicles containing Division 1.1, 1.2, or 1.3 materials must be attended at all times by their drivers or some qualified representative of the motor carrier, except in those situations where all the following conditions are met:

1. **Vehicle is located on the property of a carrier, shipper or consignee; in a safe haven; or on a construction or survey site (if the vehicle contains 50 pounds or less of Division 1.1, 1.2, or 1.3 materials).**
2. **A lawful bailee knows the nature of the vehicle's cargo and has been instructed in emergency procedures.**
3. **Vehicle is within the unobstructed field of vision of the bailee, or is in a safe haven.**

Marked or placarded vehicles containing Division 1.4, 1.5, or 1.6 materials, located on a public street or highway or the shoulder of the roadway, must be attended by the driver, except when the driver is performing necessary duties as operator of the vehicle.

No Smoking

An extra reminder! Don't smoke or carry a lighted cigarette, cigar or pipe on or within 25 feet of any vehicle containing Class 1 materials.

Required Documents

Motor carriers transporting Division 1.1, 1.2, or 1.3 materials must furnish drivers with the following required documents:

- **A copy of Part 397 — Transportation of Hazardous Materials; Driving and Parking Rules (Federal Motor Carrier Safety Regulations).** Part 397 can be found at the back of this pocketbook.
- **Instructions on procedures to be followed in case of an accident or delay. This must include the nature of the explosives being hauled, the names and phone numbers of persons to be contacted and precautions to be taken.**

Drivers are required to sign a receipt for these documents.

The carrier must maintain the receipt for one year.

In addition to the above documents drivers must also have the following documents:

- **Proper shipping papers.**
- **A written route plan for the shipment. (In some cases, this plan may be prepared by the driver, if the trip begins at some other point than the carrier's terminal.)**

The driver must be in possession of, be familiar with, and be in compliance with all four of the documents described above.

Class 1 Do's

1. Check vehicle thoroughly to be sure it meets specifications.
2. Stop engine while loading or unloading.
3. Handle cargo as specified.
4. Deliver only to authorized persons.

5. Know the vehicle attendance requirements.
6. Have all required documents in order before starting.

Class 1 Don'ts

1. Don't transfer Class 1 materials, except in emergencies.
2. Don't park a Class 1 materials vehicle in prohibited areas.
3. Don't smoke on or within 25 feet of a Class 1 materials vehicle.

Shipments of CLASS 2 (Gases)

General loading, transportation and unloading requirements that apply to all hazardous materials shipments can be found in the two preceding chapters. The following information is specific to Class 2 materials. For information on shipments of Division 2.3 (Poisonous Gases), see shipments of Division 6.1 & Division 2.3.

Vehicle Condition

Before any cylinders of Class 2 materials are loaded onto a motor vehicle, that vehicle should be inspected to determine that the floor or loading platform is essentially flat. If a solid floor or platform is not provided in the vehicle, there must be securely-fastened racks which will secure the cargo.

Loading & Unloading

Cylinders — To prevent shifting, overturning, or ejection from the vehicle under normal transport conditions, cylinders of Class 2 materials must be securely attached to the motor vehicle by one of the following ways:

1. **Securely restrained in an upright or horizontal position.**
2. **Loaded into racks.**
3. **Packed in boxes or crates.**

A pressure relief device, when installed, must be in communication with the vapor space of a cylinder containing a Division 2.1 (flammable) material.

Bulk packagings — Portable tank containers may be loaded on the flat floor or platform of a vehicle or onto a suitable frame. In either case, the containers must be blocked or held down in some way to prevent movement during transportation, including sudden starts or stops and changes in direction of the vehicle

Containers may even be stacked, if they are secured to prevent any motion.

If a Division 2.1 (flammable gas) material is being loaded or unloaded from a tank motor vehicle, the engine must be stopped. The only exception occurs if the engine is used to operate the transfer pump. The engine must also be off while filling or discharge connections are disconnected, unless the delivery hose is equipped with a shut-off valve.

Liquid discharge valves on cargo tanks must be closed securely after loading or unloading, before any movement of the vehicle.

Special handling provisions are specified for certain kinds of Class 2 materials. Information on these follows.

Liquefied Hydrogen

Specification DOT-4L cylinders filled with liquefied hydrogen, cryogenic liquid must be carried on vehicles with open bodies equipped with racks or supports having clamps or bands to hold the cylinders securely upright. These arrangements must be capable of withstanding acceleration of 2 "g" in any horizontal direction.

Cylinders of liquefied hydrogen are marked with venting rates. The combined total venting rates on all cylinders on a single motor vehicle must not exceed 60 standard cubic feet per hour.

Only private and contract carriers may haul liquefied hydrogen on the highway and the transportation must be a direct movement from origin to destination.

Vehicles hauling liquefied hydrogen may not be driven through tunnels.

Chlorine

Any shipment of chlorine in a cargo tank must be accompanied by a gas mask (approved for chlorine service by the National Institute of Occupational Safety and Health (NIOSH)) and an emergency kit to control leaks in the fittings on the dome cover plate.

Do not move, couple or uncouple any chlorine tank vehicle while loading or unloading connections are attached.

Do not leave any trailer or semitrailer without a power unit, unless it has been chocked or some adequate means provided to prevent it from moving.

No Smoking

Smoking on or near the vehicle while you are loading or unloading Division 2.1 material is forbidden.

Attending Vehicles

Marked or placarded vehicles located on a public street or highway or the shoulder of the roadway, must be attended by the driver, except when the driver is performing necessary duties as operator of the vehicle.

In addition, cargo tanks must be attended by a qualified person at all times during loading and unloading.

Parking

Marked or placarded vehicles containing Class 2 materials should not be parked on or within five feet of the traveled portion of any public roadway, except for brief periods necessary to vehicle operation.

Warning Devices

Liquid-burning flares, fusees, oil lanterns, or any signal produced by a flame must not be carried on or used for protecting any stopped cargo tank motor vehicle transporting Division 2.1 materials, loaded or empty.

Class 2 Do's

1. Be sure vehicle is adequately equipped to haul Class 2 materials safely.

2. Stop engine while loading or unloading Division 2.1 materials.
3. Be sure liquid discharge valves are closed before moving vehicle.
4. Know special provisions for handling liquefied hydrogen and chlorine.

Class 2 Don'ts

1. Don't drive a vehicle hauling liquefied hydrogen through a tunnel.
2. Don't move chlorine tanks with loading or unloading connections attached.
3. Don't smoke on or near vehicles containing Division 2.1 materials.

Shipments of CLASS 3 (Flammable Liquids)

General loading, transportation and unloading requirements that apply to all hazardous materials shipments can be found in the two preceding chapters. The following information is specific to Class 3 materials.

Loading & Unloading

There are some common sense rules to follow when loading and unloading Class 3 materials:

- **Engine should be stopped. Two possible exceptions are:**
  - **If the engine is used to operate a pump used in the loading or unloading process, or**
  - **A diesel engine may be left running during loading or unloading if the temperature is at or below 10°F (-12°C).**
- **Tanks, barrels, drums, cylinders or other types of packaging containing Class 3 materials (and not permanently attached to the vehicle) must be secured to prevent movement during transportation.**
- **Keep fires (of all kinds and sizes) away!**

Bonding & Grounding

Containers other than cargo tanks not in metallic contact with each other must have metallic bonds or ground conductors attached to avoid the possibility of static charge. Attach bonding first to the vehicle to be filled, then to the container from which the flammable liquid will be loaded. **Attachment must be done in this order!** To prevent ignition of vapors, connection should be made at some distance from the opening where Class 3 material is discharged.

For cargo tanks, similar provisions apply, but they vary depending on loading procedure.

When loading through an open filling hole, attach one end of a bond wire to the stationary system piping or integral steel framing, the other end to the cargo tank shell. Make the connection before any filling hole is opened, and leave it in place until the last hole has been closed.

If nonmetallic flexible connections exist in the stationary system piping, additional bond wires are required.

When unloading from open filling holes using a suction piping system, electrical connection must be maintained from cargo tank to receiving tank.

When loading through a vaportight top or bottom connection, and where there is no release of vapor at any point where a spark could occur, no bonding or grounding is required. However, contact of the closed connection must be made before flow starts and must not be broken until flow is complete.

When unloading through a non-vaportight connection, into a stationary tank, no bonding or grounding is required if the metallic filling connection is in contact with the filling hole at all times.

No Smoking

Smoking on or within 25 feet of any vehicle containing Class 3 materials is forbidden during the loading and unloading process, as well as the rest of the trip. Keep anyone with any kind of smoking materials away from the vehicle! The rule also applies to empty tank vehicles used to transport Class 3 materials.

Cargo Tank Attendance

A cargo tank must be attended by a qualified person at all times while it is being loaded or unloaded. The person responsible for loading the tank is also responsible for seeing that the tank is attended. The person attending must be awake, have an unobstructed view and be within 7.62 meters (25 feet) of the tank.

The person must also know the nature of the hazard, be instructed in emergency procedures and be able to move the vehicle, if necessary.

Cargo Heaters

Vehicles equipped with combustion cargo heaters may transport Class 3 materials only if:

- **It is a catalytic heater.**
- **Heater surface cannot exceed 54°C (129°F) when the outside temperature is 16°C (61°F) or less.**
- **Heater is not ignited in a loaded vehicle.**
- **No flame is present anywhere in or on the heater.**
- **Heater must bear manufacturer's certification that it meets DOT specifications.**

There are also restrictions on the use of automatic cargo-space-heating temperature control devices. Such devices may be used in vehicles transporting Class 3 materials if the following conditions are met:

- **Any electrical apparatus in the cargo area must be non-sparking or explosive-proof.**
- **No combustion apparatus is located in the cargo area, and there is no connection for air return between the cargo area and the combustion apparatus.**
- **The heating system will not heat any part of the cargo to more than 54°C (129°F).**

If the above conditions are not met, the vehicle may still be used to transport Class 3 materials, if the device is rendered inoperable.

Parking & Attending Vehicles

Marked or placarded vehicles containing Class 3 materials should not be parked on or within five feet of the traveled portion of any public highway, except for brief periods necessary to vehicle operation. While such a vehicle is on the highway, it must be attended by the driver, except when the driver is performing necessary duties as operator of the vehicle.

Warning Devices

Liquid-burning flares, fusees, oil lanterns, or any signal produced by a flame must not be carried on or used for protecting any stopped cargo tank motor vehicle transporting Class 3 materials, loaded or empty.

Class 3 Do's

1. Stop engine while loading and unloading.
2. Know the bonding and grounding procedures.
3. Check smaller cargo packages to be sure they are secure.

Class 3 Don'ts

1. Don't smoke or allow others to smoke while handling flammable liquids.
2. Don't leave vehicle unattended while unloading.
3. Don't use any cargo heater without knowing the restrictions.

Shipments of CLASS 4 (Flammable Solids) & CLASS 5 (Oxidizers)

General loading, transportation and unloading requirements that apply to all hazardous materials shipments can be found in the two preceding chapters. The following information is specific to Class 4 and Class 5 materials.

Loading & Unloading

Logic dictates the rules that apply to the loading and unloading of Class 4 and Class 5 materials:

- **The entire load must be contained within the body of the vehicle.**
- **The load must be covered either by the vehicle body or tarpaulins or other similar means.**
- **If there is a tailgate or board, it must be closed securely.**
- **Care must be taken to load cargo while dry and to keep it dry.**
- **Provide adequate ventilation for cargos which are known to be subject to heating and/or spontaneous combustion, in order to prevent fires.**
- **Shipments of water-tight bulk containers do not have to be covered by a tarpaulin or other means.**

Pick-up & Delivery

Provisions concerning Class 4 and Class 5 loads being completely contained inside the body of the vehicle with the tailgate closed do not apply to pick-up and delivery vehicles used entirely for that purpose in and around cities.

Special provisions are necessary for some particular commodities. The following sections detail those requirements.

Charcoal

Charcoal screenings and ground, crushed, pulverized or lump charcoal become more hazardous when wet. Extra care should be taken to keep packages completely dry during loading and carriage.

In addition, these commodities must be loaded so that bags lay horizontally in the vehicle and piled so that there are spaces at least 10 cm (3.9 inches) wide for effective air circulation. These spaces must be maintained between rows of bags. No bags may be piled closer than 15 cm (5.9 inches) from the top of a vehicle with a closed body.

Smokeless Powder

Smokeless powder for small arms, Division 4.1, in quantities not exceeding 45.4 kg (100 pounds) net mass of material may be transported in a motor vehicle.

Nitrates

All nitrates (except ammonium nitrate with organic coating) must be loaded in vehicles that have been swept clean and are free of projections which could damage the bags. The vehicles may be closed or open-type. If open, the cargo must be covered securely.

Ammonium nitrate with organic coating should not be loaded in all-metal closed vehicles, except those made of aluminum or aluminum alloys.

No Smoking

Don't smoke or carry a lighted cigarette, cigar or pipe on or within 25 feet of a vehicle containing Class 4 or Class 5.

Parking & Attending Vehicles

A marked or placarded vehicle containing Class 4 and/or Class 5 materials should not be parked on or within five feet of the traveled portion of any public roadway, except for brief periods necessary to vehicle operation. While such a vehicle is on the highway, it must be attended by the driver, except when the driver is performing necessary duties as operator of the vehicle.

Class 4 & Class 5 Do's

1. Know loading and covering requirements for cargo.
2. Be sure ventilation is adequate for the cargo you're hauling.
3. Know the special handling requirements for your commodity, if any.

Class 4 & Class 5 Don'ts

1. Don't leave vehicle unattended for long periods.
2. Don't reload damaged cargo without following correct safety procedures to determine if all hazards have been eliminated.
3. Don't smoke on or near vehicle.

Shipments of DIVISION 6.1 (Poisonous Materials) & DIVISION 2.3 (Poisonous Gases)

General loading, transportation and unloading requirements that apply to all hazardous materials shipments can be found in the two preceding chapters. The following information is specific to Division 6.1 or Division 2.3 materials.

Loading & Unloading

No Division 6.1 or 2.3 materials may be hauled if there is any interconnection between packagings.

Except as provided in the following paragraph, a motor carrier may not transport a package bearing or required to bear a POISON (TOXIC) or POISON INHALATION HAZARD label or placard in the same motor vehicle with material that is marked as or known to be a foodstuffs, feed or edible material intended for consumption by humans or animals unless the poisonous material is:

- **(i)** Overpacked in a metal drum as specified in §173.25(c) of the regulations, or
- **(ii)** Loaded into a closed unit load device and the foodstuffs, feed, or other edible material are loaded into another closed unit load device.

A motor carrier may not transport a package bearing a POISON label displaying the text "PG III" or bearing a "PG III" mark adjacent to a POISON label, with materials marked as, or known to be, foodstuffs, feed or any other edible material intended for consumption by humans or animals, unless the package containing the Division 6.1, PG III material is separated in a manner that, in the event of leakage from packages under conditions normally incident to transportation, commingling of hazardous materials with foodstuffs, feed or any other edible material will not occur.

A motor carrier may not transport a package bearing or required to bear a POISON (TOXIC), POISON GAS or POISON INHALATION HAZARD label in the driver's compartment (including a sleeper berth) of a motor vehicle.

Arsenical Materials

Bulk arsenical compounds loaded and unloaded under certain conditions demand extra caution. These materials include:

- **arsenical dust**
- **arsenic trioxide**
- **sodium arsenate**

These materials may be loaded in siftproof steel hopper or dump vehicle bodies, if they are equipped with waterproof and dustproof covers secured on all openings. They must be loaded carefully, using every means to minimize the spread of the compounds into the atmosphere. Loading and unloading may not be done in any area where there might be persons not connected with the transportation. This includes all highways and other public places.

After a vehicle is used for transporting arsenicals, and before it may be used again for any other materials, the vehicle must be flushed with water or use other appropriate means to remove all traces of arsenical material.

Parking & Attending Vehicles

A marked or placarded vehicle containing Division 6.1 or 2.3 materials should not be parked on or within five feet of the traveled portion of any public roadway, except for brief periods necessary to vehicle operation. While such a vehicle is on the highway, it must be attended by the driver, except when the driver is performing necessary duties as an operator of the vehicle.

Division 6.1 & Division 2.3 Do's

1. Know provisions for hauling Division 6.1 materials with foodstuffs.
2. Know special provisions for hauling arsenicals.
3. Be aware of vehicle parking and attendance rules.

Division 6.1 & Division 2.3 Don'ts

1. Don't transport any package labeled poison, poison gas or poison inhalation hazard in the driver's compartment.
2. Don't haul any arsenical material unless vehicle is properly loaded and marked.

Shipments of CLASS 7 (Radioactive Materials)

General loading, transportation and unloading requirements that apply to all hazardous materials shipments can be found in the two preceding chapters. The following information is specific to Class 7 materials.

Loading & Unloading

The number of packages of Class 7 material which may be carried in a transport vehicle is limited by the total transport index number. This number is determined by adding together the transport index numbers given on the labels of individual packages. The total may not exceed 50, except in certain special "exclusive use" shipments that the regulations describe.

Class 7 material in a package labeled "RADIOACTIVE YELLOW-II" or "RADIOACTIVE YELLOW-III" may not be positioned closer to any area which may be continuously occupied by passengers, employees, animals, or packages of undeveloped film than indicated in the following table. If several packages are involved, distances are determined by the total transport index number.

Total transport index	Minimum separation distance in meters (feet) to nearest undeveloped film for various times of transit					Minimum distance in meters (feet) to area of persons, or minimum distance in meters (feet) from dividing partition of cargo compartments
	Up to 2 hours	2-4 hours	4-8 hours	8-12 hours	Over 12 hours	
None	0.0 (0)	0.0 (0)	0.0 (0)	0.0 (0)	0.0 (0)	0.0 (0)
0.1 to 1.0	0.3 (1)	0.6 (2)	0.9 (3)	1.2 (4)	1.5 (5)	0.3 (1)
1.1 to 5.0	0.9 (3)	1.2 (4)	1.8 (6)	2.4 (8)	3.4 (11)	0.6 (2)
5.1 to 10.0	1.2 (4)	1.8 (6)	2.7 (9)	3.4 (11)	4.6 (15)	0.9 (3)
10.1 to 20.0	1.5 (5)	2.4 (8)	3.7 (12)	4.9 (16)	6.7 (22)	1.2 (4)
20.1 to 30.0	2.1 (7)	3.0 (10)	4.6 (15)	6.1 (20)	8.8 (29)	1.5 (5)
30.1 to 40.0	2.4 (8)	3.4 (11)	5.2 (17)	6.7 (22)	10.1 (33)	1.8 (6)
40.1 to 50.0	2.7 (9)	3.7 (12)	5.8 (19)	7.3 (24)	11.0 (36)	2.1 (7)

Note: The distance in this table must be measured from the nearest point on the nearest packages of Class 7 (radioactive) material.

Shipments of low specific activity materials and surface contaminated objects must be loaded to avoid spilling and scattering loose materials.

Be sure packages are blocked and braced so they cannot change position during normal transportation conditions.

Fissile material, controlled shipments must be shipped as described in Section 173.457 of the hazardous materials regulations. No fissile material, controlled shipments may be loaded in the same vehicle with any other fissile Class 7 material. Fissile material, controlled shipments must be separated by at least 6 m (20 feet) from any other package or shipment labeled "Radioactive."

Keep the time spent in a vehicle carrying radioactive materials at an absolute minimum.

Vehicle Contamination

Vehicles used to transport Class 7 materials under exclusive use conditions must be checked after each use with radiation detection instruments. These vehicles may not be returned to use until the radiation dose at every accessible surface is 0.005 mSv per hour (0.5 mrem per hour) or less, and the removable radioactive surface contamination is not greater than prescribed in §173.443.

These contamination limitations do not apply to vehicles used only for transporting Class 7 materials, provided certain conditions are met:

- **Interior surface shows a radiation dose of no more than 0.1 mSv per hour (10 mrem per hour).**
- **Dose is no more than 0.02 mSv per hour (2 mrem per hour) at a distance of 1 m (3.3 feet) from any interior surface.**
- **The vehicle must be stenciled with "For Radioactive Materials Use Only" in letters at least 7.6 cm (3 inches) high in a conspicuous place, on both sides of the exterior of the vehicle.**
- **Vehicles must be kept closed at all times except during loading and unloading.**

Parking & Attending Vehicles

A marked or placarded vehicle containing Class 7 materials should not be parked on or within five feet of the traveled portion of any public roadway except for brief periods necessary to vehicle operation. While such a vehicle is on the highway, it must be attended by the driver, except when the driver is performing necessary duties as operator of the vehicle.

Class 7 Do's

1. Know how the transport index system works in limiting Class 7 shipments.
2. Be sure packages are blocked and braced correctly for shipment.
3. If your vehicle transports Class 7 materials only, know the special provisions for marking and acceptable radiation dose.

Class 7 Don'ts

1. Don't spend more time than absolutely necessary in a vehicle used for transporting Class 7 materials.
2. Don't leave vehicle unattended for long periods of time.
3. Don't handle damaged cargo unless you have been instructed in disposal procedures by authorized personnel.

Shipments of CLASS 8 (Corrosive Liquids)

General loading, transportation and unloading requirements that apply to all hazardous materials shipments can be found in the two preceding chapters. The following information is specific to Class 8 materials.

Nitric Acid

No package of nitric acid of 50 percent or greater concentration may be loaded above any packaging containing any other kind of material.

Storage Batteries

Storage batteries containing any electrolyte and hauled in a mixed load must be loaded so that they are protected from the possibility of other cargo falling on or against them. Battery terminals must be insulated and protected from the possibility of short circuits.

Parking & Attending Vehicles

A marked or placarded vehicle containing Class 8 materials should not be parked on or within five feet of the traveled portion of any public roadway, except for brief periods necessary for vehicle operation. While such a vehicle is on the highway, it must be attended by the driver, except when the driver is performing necessary duties as operator of the vehicle.

Class 8 Do's

1. Be sure vehicle condition meets requirements.
2. Know container handling requirements for loading by hand.
3. Be sure cargo is loaded in accordance with specifications.

4. If you are hauling batteries, be sure they are adequately protected during transit.

Class 8 Don'ts

1. Don't load nitric acid above other commodities.

2. Don't park on or near the roadway, or leave your vehicle unattended for more than very brief periods necessary to your duties.

ID Cross Reference

The identification number cross reference index to proper shipping names is useful in determining a shipping name when only an identification number is known. It is also useful in checking if an identification number is correct for a specific shipping description. This listing is for information purposes only, the §172.101 Hazardous Materials Table should be consulted for authorized shipping names and identification numbers

IDENTIFICATION NUMBER CROSS REFERENCE TO PROPER SHIPPING NAMES IN §172.101 HM TABLE

ID Number	Description
UN0004	Ammonium picrate
UN0005	Cartridges for weapons
UN0006	Cartridges for weapons
UN0007	Cartridges for weapons
UN0009	Ammunition, incendiary
UN0010	Ammunition, incendiary
UN0012	Cartridges for weapons, inert projectile or Cartridges, small arms
UN0014	Cartridges for weapons, blank or Cartridges, small arms, blank
UN0015	Ammunition, smoke
UN0016	Ammunition, smoke
UN0018	Ammunition, tear-producing
UN0019	Ammunition, tear-producing
UN0020	Ammunition, toxic
UN0021	Ammunition, toxic
NA0027	Black powder for small arms
UN0027	Black powder or Gunpowder
UN0028	Black powder, compressed or Gunpowder, compressed or Black powder, in pellets or Gunpowder, in pellets
UN0029	Detonators, non-electric
UN0030	Detonators, electric
UN0033	Bombs
UN0034	Bombs
UN0035	Bombs
UN0037	Bombs, photo-flash
UN0038	Bombs, photo-flash
UN0039	Bombs, photo-flash
UN0042	Boosters
UN0043	Bursters
UN0044	Primers, cap type
UN0048	Charges, demolition
UN0049	Cartridges, flash

ID Number	Description
UN0050	Cartridges, flash
UN0054	Cartridges, signal
UN0055	Cases, cartridge, empty with primer
UN0056	Charges, depth
UN0059	Charges, shaped
UN0060	Charges, supplementary explosive
UN0065	Cord, detonating
UN0066	Cord, igniter
UN0070	Cutters, cable, explosive
UN0072	Cyclotrimethylenetrinitramine, wetted or Cyclonite, wetted or Hexogen, wetted or RDX, wetted
UN0073	Detonators for ammunition
UN0074	Diazodinitrophenol, wetted
UN0075	Diethyleneglycol dinitrate, desensitized
UN0076	Dinitrophenol
UN0077	Dinitrophenolates
UN0078	Dinitroresorcinol
UN0079	Hexanitrodiphenylamine or Dipicrylamine or Hexyl
UN0081	Explosive, blasting, type A
UN0082	Explosive, blasting, type B
UN0083	Explosive, blasting, type C
UN0084	Explosive, blasting, type D
UN0092	Flares, surface
UN0093	Flares, aerial
UN0094	Flash powder
UN0099	Fracturing devices, explosive
UN0101	Fuse, non-detonating
UN0102	Cord detonating or Fuse detonating
UN0103	Fuse, igniter
UN0104	Cord, detonating, mild effect or Fuse, detonating, mild effect
UN0105	Fuse, safety
UN0106	Fuzes, detonating
UN0107	Fuzes, detonating
UN0110	Grenades, practice
UN0113	Guanyl nitrosaminoguanylidene hydrazine, wetted
UN0114	Guanyl nitrosaminoguanyltetrazene, wetted or Tetrazene, wetted
UN0118	Hexolite or Hexotol
UN0121	Igniters
NA0124	Jet perforating guns, charged oil well, with detonator
UN0124	Jet perforating guns, charged
UN0129	Lead azide, wetted
UN0130	Lead styphnate, wetted or Lead trinitroresorcinate, wetted
UN0131	Lighters, fuse
UN0132	Deflagrating metal salts of aromatic nitroderivatives, n.o.s

ID Number	Description
UN0133	Mannitol hexanitrate, wetted or Nitromannite, wetted
UN0135	Mercury fulminate, wetted
UN0136	Mines
UN0137	Mines
UN0138	Mines
UN0143	Nitroglycerin, desensitized
UN0144	Nitroglycerin, solution in alcohol
UN0146	Nitrostarch
UN0147	Nitro urea
UN0150	Pentaerythrite tetranitrate wetted or Pentaerythritol tetranitrate wetted or PETN, wetted, or Pentaerythrite tetranitrate, or Pentaerythritol tetranitrate, or PETN, desensitized
UN0151	Pentolite
UN0153	Trinitroaniline or Picramide
UN0154	Trinitrophenol or Picric acid
UN0155	Trinitrochlorobenzene or Picryl chloride
UN0159	Powder cake, wetted or Powder paste, wetted
UN0160	Powder, smokeless
UN0161	Powder, smokeless
UN0167	Projectiles
UN0168	Projectiles
UN0169	Projectiles
UN0171	Ammunition, illuminating
UN0173	Release devices, explosive
UN0174	Rivets, explosive
UN0180	Rockets
UN0181	Rockets
UN0182	Rockets
UN0183	Rockets
UN0186	Rocket motors
UN0190	Samples, explosive
UN0191	Signal devices, hand
UN0192	Signals, railway track, explosive
UN0193	Signals, railway track, explosive
UN0194	Signals, distress
UN0195	Signals, distress
UN0196	Signals, smoke
UN0197	Signals, smoke
UN0204	Sounding devices, explosive
UN0207	Tetranitroaniline
UN0208	Trinitrophenylmethylnitramine or Tetryl
UN0209	Trinitrotoluene or TNT
UN0212	Tracers for ammunition
UN0213	Trinitroanisole
UN0214	Trinitrobenzene

ID Number	Description
UN0215	Trinitrobenzoic acid
UN0216	Trinitro-meta-cresol
UN0217	Trinitronaphthalene
UN0218	Trinitrophenetole
UN0219	Trinitroresorcinol or Styphnic acid
UN0220	Urea nitrate
UN0221	Warheads, torpedo
UN0222	Ammonium nitrate
UN0224	Barium azide
UN0225	Boosters with detonator
UN0226	Cyclotetramethylenetetranitramine, wetted or HMX, wetted or Octogen, wetted
UN0234	Sodium dinitro-o-cresolate
UN0235	Sodium picramate
UN0236	Zirconium picramate
UN0237	Charges, shaped, flexible, linear
UN0238	Rockets, line-throwing
UN0240	Rockets, line-throwing
UN0241	Explosive, blasting, type E
UN0242	Charges, propelling, for cannon
UN0243	Ammunition, incendiary, white phosphorus
UN0244	Ammunition, incendiary, white phosphorus
UN0245	Ammunition, smoke, white phosphorus
UN0246	Ammunition, smoke, white phosphorus
UN0247	Ammunition, incendiary
UN0248	Contrivances, water-activated
UN0249	Contrivances, water-activated
UN0250	Rocket motors with hypergolic liquids
UN0254	Ammunition, illuminating
UN0255	Detonators, electric
UN0257	Fuzes, detonating
UN0266	Octolite or Octol
UN0267	Detonators, non-electric
UN0268	Boosters with detonator
UN0271	Charges, propelling
UN0272	Charges, propelling
UN0275	Cartridges, power device
NA0276	Model rocket motor
UN0276	Cartridges, power device
UN0277	Cartridges, oil well
UN0278	Cartridges, oil well
UN0279	Charges, propelling, for cannon
UN0280	Rocket motors
UN0281	Rocket motors

ID Number	Description
UN0282	Nitroguanidine or Picrite
UN0283	Boosters
UN0284	Grenades
UN0285	Grenades
UN0286	Warheads, rocket
UN0287	Warheads, rocket
UN0288	Charges, shaped, flexible, linear
UN0289	Cord, detonating
UN0290	Cord, detonating or Fuse, detonating
UN0291	Bombs
UN0292	Grenades
UN0293	Grenades
UN0294	Mines
UN0295	Rockets
UN0296	Sounding devices, explosive
UN0297	Ammunition, illuminating
UN0299	Bombs, photo-flash
UN0300	Ammunition, incendiary
UN0301	Ammunition, tear-producing
UN0303	Ammunition, smoke
UN0305	Flash powder
UN0306	Tracers for ammunition
UN0312	Cartridges, signal
UN0313	Signals, smoke
UN0314	Igniters
UN0315	Igniters
UN0316	Fuzes, igniting
UN0317	Fuzes, igniting
UN0318	Grenades, practice
UN0319	Primers, tubular
UN0320	Primers, tubular
UN0321	Cartridges for weapons
UN0322	Rocket motors with hypergolic liquids
NA0323	Model rocket motor
UN0323	Cartridges, power device
UN0324	Projectiles
UN0325	Igniters
UN0326	Cartridges for weapons, blank
UN0327	Cartridges for weapons, blank or Cartridges, small arms, blank
UN0328	Cartridges for weapons, inert projectile
UN0329	Torpedoes
UN0330	Torpedoes
NA0331	Ammonium nitrate-fuel oil mixture
UN0331	Explosive, blasting, type B or Agent blasting, Type B

ID Number	Description
UN0332	Explosive, blasting, type E or Agent blasting, Type E
UN0333	Fireworks
UN0334	Fireworks
UN0335	Fireworks
UN0336	Fireworks
NA0337	Toy caps
UN0337	Fireworks
UN0338	Cartridges for weapons, blank or Cartridges, small arms, blank
UN0339	Cartridges for weapons, inert projectile or Cartridges, small arms
UN0340	Nitrocellulose
UN0341	Nitrocellulose
UN0342	Nitrocellulose, wetted
UN0343	Nitrocellulose, plasticized
UN0344	Projectiles
UN0345	Projectiles
UN0346	Projectiles
UN0347	Projectiles
UN0348	Cartridges for weapons
UN0349	Articles, explosive, n.o.s.
UN0350	Articles, explosive, n.o.s.
UN0351	Articles, explosive, n.o.s.
UN0352	Articles, explosive, n.o.s.
UN0353	Articles, explosive, n.o.s.
UN0354	Articles, explosive, n.o.s.
UN0355	Articles, explosive, n.o.s.
UN0356	Articles, explosive, n.o.s.
UN0357	Substances, explosive, n.o.s.
UN0358	Substances, explosive, n.o.s.
UN0359	Substances, explosive, n.o.s.
UN0360	Detonator assemblies, non-electric
UN0361	Detonator assemblies, non-electric
UN0362	Ammunition, practice
UN0363	Ammunition, proof
UN0364	Detonators for ammunition
UN0365	Detonators for ammunition
UN0366	Detonators for ammunition
UN0367	Fuzes, detonating
UN0368	Fuzes, igniting
UN0369	Warheads, rocket
UN0370	Warheads, rocket
UN0371	Warheads, rocket
UN0372	Grenades, practice
UN0373	Signal devices, hand
UN0374	Sounding devices, explosive

ID Number	Description
UN0375	Sounding devices, explosive
UN0376	Primers, tubular
UN0377	Primers, cap type
UN0378	Primers, cap type
UN0379	Cases, cartridges, empty with primer
UN0380	Articles, pyrophoric
UN0381	Cartridges, power device
UN0382	Components, explosive train, n.o.s.
UN0383	Components, explosive train, n.o.s.
UN0384	Components, explosive train, n.o.s.
UN0385	5-Nitrobenzotriazol
UN0386	Trinitrobenzenesulfonic acid
UN0387	Trinitrofluorenone
UN0388	Trinitrotoluene and Trinitrobenzene mixtures or TNT and trinitrobenzene mixtures or TNT and hexanitrostilbene mixtures or Trinitrotoluene and hexanitrostilnene mixtures
UN0389	Trinitrotoluene mixtures containing Trinitrobenzene and Hexanitrostilbene or TNT mixtures containing trinitrobenzene and hexanitrostilbene
UN0390	Tritonal
UN0391	RDX and HMX mixtures, wetted, or RDX and HMX mixtures, desensitized
UN0392	Hexanitrostilbene
UN0393	Hexotonal
UN0394	Trinitroresorcinol, wetted or Styphnic acid, wetted
UN0395	Rocket motors, liquid fueled
UN0396	Rocket motors, liquid fueled
UN0397	Rockets, liquid fueled
UN0398	Rockets, liquid fueled
UN0399	Bombs with flammable liquid
UN0400	Bombs with flammable liquid
UN0401	Dipicryl sulfide
UN0402	Ammonium perchlorate
UN0403	Flares, aerial
UN0404	Flares, aerial
UN0405	Cartridges, signal
UN0406	Dinitrosobenzene
UN0407	Tetrazol-1-acetic acid
UN0408	Fuzes, detonating
UN0409	Fuzes, detonating
UN0410	Fuzes, detonating
UN0411	Pentaerythrite tetranitrate or Pentaerythritol tetranitrate or PETN
UN0412	Cartridges for weapons
UN0413	Cartridges for weapons, blank
UN0414	Charges, propelling, for cannon

ID Number	Description
UN0415	Charges, propelling
UN0417	Cartridges for weapons, inert projectile or Cartridges, small arms
UN0418	Flares, surface
UN0419	Flares, surface
UN0420	Flares, aerial
UN0421	Flares, aerial
UN0424	Projectiles
UN0425	Projectiles
UN0426	Projectiles
UN0427	Projectiles
UN0428	Articles, pyrotechnic
UN0429	Articles, pyrotechnic
UN0430	Articles, pyrotechnic
UN0431	Articles, pyrotechnic
UN0432	Articles, pyrotechnic
UN0433	Powder cake, wetted or Powder paste, wetted
UN0434	Projectiles
UN0435	Projectiles
UN0436	Rockets
UN0437	Rockets
UN0438	Rockets
UN0439	Charges, shaped
UN0440	Charges, shaped
UN0441	Charges, shaped
UN0442	Charges, explosive, commercial
UN0443	Charges, explosive, commercial
UN0444	Charges, explosive, commercial
UN0445	Charges, explosive, commercial
UN0446	Cases, combustible, empty, without primer
UN0447	Cases, combustible, empty, without primer
UN0448	5-Mercaptotetrazol-1-acetic acid
UN0449	Torpedoes, liquid fueled
UN0450	Torpedoes, liquid fueled
UN0451	Torpedoes
UN0452	Grenades practice
UN0453	Rockets, line-throwing
UN0454	Igniters
UN0455	Detonators, non-electric
UN0456	Detonators, electric
UN0457	Charges, bursting, plastics bonded
UN0458	Charges, bursting, plastics bonded
UN0459	Charges, bursting, plastics bonded
UN0460	Charges, bursting, plastics bonded
UN0461	Components, explosive train, n.o.s.

ID Number	Description
UN0462	Articles, explosive, n.o.s.
UN0463	Articles, explosive, n.o.s.
UN0464	Articles, explosive, n.o.s.
UN0465	Articles, explosive, n.o.s.
UN0466	Articles, explosive, n.o.s.
UN0467	Articles, explosive, n.o.s.
UN0468	Articles, explosive, n.o.s.
UN0469	Articles, explosive, n.o.s.
UN0470	Articles, explosive, n.o.s.
UN0471	Articles, explosive, n.o.s.
UN0472	Articles, explosive, n.o.s.
UN0473	Substances, explosive, n.o.s.
UN0474	Substances, explosive, n.o.s.
UN0475	Substances, explosive, n.o.s.
UN0476	Substances, explosive, n.o.s.
UN0477	Substances, explosive, n.o.s.
UN0478	Substances, explosive, n.o.s.
UN0479	Substances, explosives, n.o.s.
UN0480	Substances, explosives, n.o.s.
UN0481	Substances, explosive, n.o.s.
UN0482	Substances, explosive, very insensitive, n.o.s., or Substances, EVI, n.o.s.
UN0483	Cyclotrimethylenetrinitramine, desensitize or Cyclonite, desensitized or Hexogen, desensitized or RDX, desensitized
UN0484	Cyclotetramethylenetetrani-tramine, desensitized or Octogen, desensitized or HMX, desensitized
UN0485	Substances, explosive, n.o.s.
UN0486	Articles, explosive, extremely insensitive or Articles, EEI
UN0487	Signals, smoke
UN0488	Ammunition, practice
UN0489	Dinitroglycoluril or Dingu
UN0490	Nitrotriazolone or NTO
UN0491	Charges, propelling
UN0492	Signals, railway track, explosive
UN0493	Signals, railway track, explosive
NA0494	Jet perforating guns, charged oil well, with detonator
UN0494	Jet perforating guns, charged
UN0495	Propellant, liquid
UN0496	Octonal
UN0497	Propellant, liquid
UN0498	Propellant, solid
UN0499	Propellant, solid
UN0500	Detonator assemblies, non-electric
UN0501	Propellant, solid
UN0502	Rockets

ID Number	Description
UN0503	Air bag inflators, or Air bag modules, or Seat-belt pretensioners
UN0504	1H-Tetrazole
UN1001	Acetylene, dissolved
UN1002	Air, compressed
UN1003	Air, refrigerated liquid
UN1005	Ammonia, anhydrous
UN1006	Argon, compressed
UN1008	Boron trifluoride
UN1009	Bromotrifluoromethane or Refrigerant gas R 13B1
UN1010	Butadienes, stabilized or Butadienes and Hydrocarbon mixture, stabilized
UN1011	Butane
UN1012	Butylene
UN1013	Carbon dioxide
UN1014	Carbon dioxide and oxygen mixtures, compressed
UN1015	Carbon dioxide and nitrous oxide mixture
UN1016	Carbon monoxide, compressed
UN1017	Chlorine
UN1018	Chlorodifluoromethane or Refrigerant gas R22
UN1020	Chloropentafluoroethane or Refrigerant gas R115
UN1021	1-Chloro-1,2,2,2-tetrafluoroethane or Refrigerant gas R 124
UN1022	Chlorotrifluoromethane or Refrigerant gas R 13
UN1023	Coal gas, compressed
UN1026	Cyanogen
UN1027	Cyclopropane
UN1028	Dichlorodifluoromethane or Refrigerant gas R 12
UN1029	Dichlorofluoromethane or Refrigerant gas R 21
UN1030	1, 1-Difluoroethane or Refrigerant gas R 152a
UN1032	Dimethylamine, anhydrous
UN1033	Dimethyl ether
UN1035	Ethane
UN1036	Ethylamine
UN1037	Ethyl chloride
UN1038	Ethylene, refrigerated liquid
UN1039	Ethyl methyl ether
UN1040	Ethylene oxide or Ethylene oxide with nitrogen
UN1041	Ethylene oxide and Carbon dioxide mixtures
UN1043	Fertilizer ammoniating solution
UN1044	Fire extinguishers
UN1045	Fluorine, compressed
UN1046	Helium, compressed
UN1048	Hydrogen bromide, anhydrous
UN1049	Hydrogen, compressed
UN1050	Hydrogen chloride, anhydrous

ID Number	Description
UN1051	Hydrogen cyanide, stabilized
UN1052	Hydrogen fluoride, anhydrous
UN1053	Hydrogen sulfide
UN1055	Isobutylene
UN1056	Krypton, compressed
UN1057	Lighters or Lighter refills
UN1058	Liquefied gases
UN1060	Methyl acetylene and propadiene mixtures, stabilized
UN1061	Methylamine, anhydrous
UN1062	Methyl bromide
UN1063	Methyl chloride or Refrigerant gas R 40
UN1064	Methyl mercaptan
UN1065	Neon, compressed
UN1066	Nitrogen, compressed
UN1067	Dinitrogen tetroxide
UN1069	Nitrosyl chloride
UN1070	Nitrous oxide
UN1071	Oil gas, compressed
UN1072	Oxygen, compressed
UN1073	Oxygen, refrigerated liquid
UN1075	Petroleum gases, liquefied or Liquefied petroleum gas
UN1076	Phosgene
UN1077	Propylene
UN1078	Refrigerant gases, n.o.s.
UN1079	Sulfur dioxide
UN1080	Sulfur hexafluoride
UN1081	Tetrafluoroethylene, stabilized
UN1082	Trifluorochloroethylene, stabilized
UN1083	Trimethylamine, anhydrous
UN1085	Vinyl bromide, stabilized
UN1086	Vinyl chloride, stabilized
UN1087	Vinyl methyl ether, stabilized
UN1088	Acetal
UN1089	Acetaldehyde
UN1090	Acetone
UN1091	Acetone oils
UN1092	Acrolein, stabilized
UN1093	Acrylonitrile, stabilized
UN1098	Allyl alcohol
UN1099	Allyl bromide
UN1100	Allyl chloride
UN1104	Amyl acetates
UN1105	Pentanols
UN1106	Amylamines

ID Number	Description
UN1107	Amyl chlorides
UN1108	1-Pentene
UN1109	Amyl formates
UN1110	n-Amyl methyl ketone
UN1111	Amyl mercaptans
UN1112	Amyl nitrate
UN1113	Amyl nitrites
UN1114	Benzene
UN1120	Butanols
UN1123	Butyl acetates
UN1125	n-Butylamine
UN1126	1-Bromobutane
UN1127	Chlorobutanes
UN1128	n-Butyl formate
UN1129	Butyraldehyde
UN1130	Camphor oil
UN1131	Carbon disulfide
UN1133	Adhesives
UN1134	Chlorobenzene
UN1135	Ethylene chlorohydrin
UN1136	Coal tar distillates, flammable
UN1139	Coating solution
UN1143	Crotonaldehyde, stabilized
UN1144	Crotonylene
UN1145	Cyclohexane
UN1146	Cyclopentane
UN1147	Decahydronaphthalene
UN1148	Diacetone alcohol
UN1149	Dibutyl ethers
UN1150	1,2-Dichloroethylene
UN1152	Dichloropentanes
UN1153	Ethylene glycol diethyl ether
UN1154	Diethylamine
UN1155	Diethyl ether or Ethyl ether
UN1156	Diethyl ketone
UN1157	Diisobutyl ketone
UN1158	Diisopropylamine
UN1159	Diisopropyl ether
UN1160	Dimethylamine solution
UN1161	Dimethyl carbonate
UN1162	Dimethyldichlorosilane
UN1163	Dimethylhydrazine, unsymmetrical
UN1164	Dimethyl sulfide
UN1165	Dioxane

ID Number	Description
UN1166	Dioxolane
UN1167	Divinyl ether, stabilized
UN1169	Extracts, aromatic, liquid
UN1170	Ethanol or Ethyl alcohol or Ethanol solutions or Ethyl alcohol solutions
UN1171	Ethylene glycol monoethyl ether
UN1172	Ethylene glycol monoethyl ether acetate
UN1173	Ethyl acetate
UN1175	Ethylbenzene
UN1176	Ethyl borate
UN1177	2-Ethylbutyl acetate
UN1178	2-Ethylbutyraldehyde
UN1179	Ethyl butyl ether
UN1180	Ethyl butyrate
UN1181	Ethyl chloroacetate
UN1182	Ethyl chloroformate
UN1183	Ethyldichlorosilane
UN1184	Ethylene dichloride
UN1185	Ethyleneimine, stabilized
UN1188	Ethylene glycol monomethyl ether
UN1189	Ethylene glycol monomethyl ether acetate
UN1190	Ethyl formate
UN1191	Octyl aldehydes
UN1192	Ethyl lactate
UN1193	Ethyl methyl ketone or Methyl ethyl ketone
UN1194	Ethyl nitrite solutions
UN1195	Ethyl propionate
UN1196	Ethyltrichlorosilane
UN1197	Extracts, flavoring, liquid
UN1198	Formaldehyde, solutions, flammable
UN1199	Furaldehydes
UN1201	Fusel oil
UN1202	Gas oil or Diesel fuel or Heating oil, light
NA1203	Gasohol
UN1203	Gasoline
UN1204	Nitroglycerin solution in alcohol
UN1206	Heptanes
UN1207	Hexaldehyde
UN1208	Hexanes
UN1210	Printing ink or Printing ink related material
UN1212	Isobutanol or isobutyl alcohol
UN1213	Isobutyl acetate
UN1214	Isobutylamine
UN1216	Isooctenes

ID Number	Description
UN1218	Isoprene, stabilized
UN1219	Isopropanol or isopropyl alcohol
UN1220	Isopropyl acetate
UN1221	Isopropylamine
UN1222	Isopropyl nitrate
UN1223	Kerosene
UN1224	Ketones, liquid, n.o.s.
UN1228	Mercaptans, liquid, flammable, toxic, n.o.s. or Mercaptan mixtures, liquid, flammable, toxic, n.o.s.
UN1229	Mesityl oxide
UN1230	Methanol
UN1231	Methyl acetate
UN1233	Methylamyl acetate
UN1234	Methylal
UN1235	Methylamine, aqueous solution
UN1237	Methyl butyrate
UN1238	Methyl chloroformate
UN1239	Methyl chloromethyl ether
UN1242	Methyldichlorosilane
UN1243	Methyl formate
UN1244	Methylhydrazine
UN1245	Methyl isobutyl ketone
UN1246	Methyl isopropenyl ketone, stabilized
UN1247	Methyl methacrylate monomer, stabilized
UN1248	Methyl propionate
UN1249	Methyl propyl ketone
UN1250	Methyltrichlorosilane
UN1251	Methyl vinyl ketone, stabilized
UN1259	Nickel carbonyl
UN1261	Nitromethane
UN1262	Octanes
UN1263	Paint
UN1263	Paint related material
UN1264	Paraldehyde
UN1265	Pentanes
UN1266	Perfumery products
UN1267	Petroleum crude oil
UN1268	Petroleum distillates, n.o.s. or Petroleum products, n.o.s.
NA1270	Petroleum oil
UN1272	Pine oil
UN1274	n-Propanol or Propyl alcohol, normal
UN1275	Propionaldehyde
UN1276	n-Propyl acetate
UN1277	Propylamine

ID Number	Description
UN1278	1-Chloropropane
UN1278	Propyl chloride
UN1279	1,2-Dichloropropane
UN1280	Propylene oxide
UN1281	Propyl formates
UN1282	Pyridine
UN1286	Rosin oil
UN1287	Rubber solution
UN1288	Shale oil
UN1289	Sodium methylate solutions
UN1292	Tetraethyl silicate
UN1293	Tinctures, medicinal
UN1294	Toluene
UN1295	Trichlorosilane
UN1296	Triethylamine
UN1297	Trimethylamine, aqueous solutions
UN1298	Trimethylchlorosilane
UN1299	Turpentine
UN1300	Turpentine substitute
UN1301	Vinyl acetate, stabilized
UN1302	Vinyl ethyl ether, stabilized
UN1303	Vinylidene chloride, stabilized
UN1304	Vinyl isobutyl ether, stabilized
UN1305	Vinyltrichlorosilane, stabilized
UN1306	Wood preservatives, liquid
UN1307	Xylenes
UN1308	Zirconium suspended in a liquid
UN1309	Aluminum powder, coated
UN1310	Ammonium picrate, wetted
UN1312	Borneol
UN1313	Calcium resinate
UN1314	Calcium resinate, fused
UN1318	Cobalt resinate, precipitated
UN1320	Dinitrophenol, wetted
UN1321	Dinitrophenolates, wetted
UN1322	Dinitroresorcinol, wetted
UN1323	Ferrocerium
UN1324	Films, nitrocellulose base
NA1325	Fusee
UN1325	Flammable solids, organic, n.o.s.
UN1326	Hafnium powder, wetted
UN1328	Hexamethylenetetramine
UN1330	Manganese resinate
UN1331	Matches, strike anywhere

ID Number	Description
UN1332	Metaldehyde
UN1333	Cerium
UN1334	Naphthalene, crude or Naphthalene, refined
UN1336	Nitroguanidine, wetted or Picrite, wetted
UN1337	Nitrostarch, wetted
UN1338	Phosphorus, amorphous
UN1339	Phosphorus heptasulfide
UN1340	Phosphorus pentasulfide
UN1341	Phosphorus sesquisulfide
UN1343	Phosphorus trisulfide
UN1344	Trinitrophenol, wetted
UN1345	Rubber scrap or shoddy
UN1346	Silicon powder, amorphous
UN1347	Silver picrate, wetted
UN1348	Sodium dinitro-o-cresolate, wetted
UN1349	Sodium picramate, wetted
NA1350	Sulfur
UN1350	Sulfur
UN1352	Titanium powder, wetted
UN1353	Fibers or Fabrics inpregnated with weakly nitrated nitrocellulose, n.o.s.
UN1354	Trinitrobenzene, wetted
UN1355	Trinitrobenzoic acid, wetted
UN1356	Trinitrotoluene, wetted
UN1357	Urea nitrate, wetted
UN1358	Zirconium powder, wetted
UN1360	Calcium phosphide
NA1361	Charcoal
UN1361	Carbon
UN1362	Carbon, activated
UN1363	Copra
UN1364	Cotton waste, oily
NA1365	Cotton
UN1365	Cotton, wet
UN1366	Diethylzinc
UN1369	p-Nitrosodimethylaniline
UN1370	Dimethylzinc
UN1372	Fibers, animal or Fibers, vegetable
UN1373	Fibers or Fabrics, animal or vegetable or Synthetic, n.o.s.
UN1374	Fish meal, unstablized or Fish scrap, unstabilized
UN1376	Iron oxide, spent, or Iron sponge, spent
UN1378	Metal catalyst, wetted
UN1379	Paper, unsaturated oil treated
UN1380	Pentaborane

ID Number	Description
UN1381	Phosphorus, white dry or Phosphorus, white, under water or Phosphorus white, in solution or Phosphorus, yellow dry or Phosphorus, yellow, under water or Phosphorus, yellow, in solution
UN1382	Potassium sulfide, anhydrous or Potassium sulfide
UN1383	Pyrophoric metals, n.o.s., or Pyrophoric alloys, n.o.s.
UN1384	Sodium dithionite or Sodium hydrosulfite
UN1385	Sodium sulfide, anhydrous or Sodium sulfide
UN1386	Seed cake
UN1387	Wool waste, wet
UN1389	Alkali metal amalgam, liquid
UN1390	Alkali metal amides
UN1391	Alkali metal dispersions, or Alkaline earth metal dispersions
UN1392	Alkaline earth metal amalgams, liquid
UN1393	Alkaline earth metal alloys, n.o.s.
UN1394	Aluminum carbide
UN1395	Aluminum ferrosilicon powder
UN1396	Aluminum powder, uncoated
UN1397	Aluminum phosphide
UN1398	Aluminum silicon powder, uncoated
UN1400	Barium
UN1401	Calcium
UN1402	Calcium carbide
UN1403	Calcium cyanamide
UN1404	Calcium hydride
UN1405	Calcium silicide
UN1407	Cesium or Caesium
UN1408	Ferrosilicon
UN1409	Metal hydrides, water reactive, n.o.s.
UN1410	Lithium aluminum hydride
UN1411	Lithium aluminum hydride, ethereal
UN1413	Lithium borohydride
UN1414	Lithium hydride
UN1415	Lithium
UN1417	Lithium silicon
UN1418	Magnesium, powder or Magnesium alloys, powder
UN1419	Magnesium aluminum phosphide
UN1420	Potassium, metal alloys, liquid
UN1421	Alkali metal alloys, liquid, n.o.s.
UN1422	Potassium sodium alloys, liquid
UN1423	Rubidium
UN1426	Sodium borohydride
UN1427	Sodium hydride
UN1428	Sodium
UN1431	Sodium methylate

ID Number	Description
UN1432	Sodium phosphide
UN1433	Stannic phosphide
UN1435	Zinc ashes
UN1436	Zinc powder or Zinc dust
UN1437	Zirconium hydride
UN1438	Aluminum nitrate
UN1439	Ammonium dichromate
UN1442	Ammonium perchlorate
UN1444	Ammonium persulfate
UN1445	Barium chlorate, solid
UN1446	Barium nitrate
UN1447	Barium perchlorate, solid
UN1448	Barium permanganate
UN1449	Barium peroxide
UN1450	Bromates, inorganic, n.o.s.
UN1451	Cesium nitrate or Caesium nitrate
UN1452	Calcium chlorate
UN1453	Calcium chlorite
UN1454	Calcium nitrate
UN1455	Calcium perchlorate
UN1456	Calcium permanganate
UN1457	Calcium peroxide
UN1458	Chlorate and borate mixtures
UN1459	Chlorate and magnesium chloride mixture, solid
UN1461	Chlorates, inorganic, n.o.s.
UN1462	Chlorites, inorganic, n.o.s.
UN1463	Chromium trioxide, anhydrous
UN1465	Didymium nitrate
UN1466	Ferric nitrate
UN1467	Guanidine nitrate
UN1469	Lead nitrate
UN1470	Lead perchlorate, solid
UN1471	Lithium hypochlorite, dry or Lithium hypochlorite mixtures, dry
UN1472	Lithium peroxide
UN1473	Magnesium bromate
UN1474	Magnesium nitrate
UN1475	Magnesium perchlorate
UN1476	Magnesium peroxide
UN1477	Nitrates, inorganic, n.o.s.
UN1479	Oxidizing, solid, n.o.s.
UN1481	Perchlorates, inorganic, n.o.s.
UN1482	Permanganates, inorganic, n.o.s.
UN1483	Peroxides, inorganic, n.o.s.
UN1484	Potassium bromate

ID Number	Description
UN1485	Potassium chlorate
UN1486	Potassium nitrate
UN1487	Potassium nitrate and sodium nitrite mixtures
UN1488	Potassium nitrite
UN1489	Potassium perchlorate
UN1490	Potassium permanganate
UN1491	Potassium peroxide
UN1492	Potassium persulfate
UN1493	Silver nitrate
UN1494	Sodium bromate
UN1495	Sodium chlorate
UN1496	Sodium chlorite
UN1498	Sodium nitrate
UN1499	Sodium nitrate and potassium nitrate mixtures
UN1500	Sodium nitrite
UN1502	Sodium perchlorate
UN1503	Sodium permanganate
UN1504	Sodium peroxide
UN1505	Sodium persulfate
UN1506	Strontium chlorate
UN1507	Strontium nitrate
UN1508	Strontium perchlorate
UN1509	Strontium peroxide
UN1510	Tetranitromethane
UN1511	Urea hydrogen peroxide
UN1512	Zinc ammonium nitrite
UN1513	Zinc chlorate
UN1514	Zinc nitrate
UN1515	Zinc permanganate
UN1516	Zinc peroxide
UN1517	Zirconium picramate, wetted
UN1541	Acetone cyanohydrin, stabilized
UN1544	Alkaloids, solid, n.o.s. or Alkaloid salts, solid, n.o.s.
UN1545	Allyl isothiocyanate, stabilized
UN1546	Ammonium arsenate
UN1547	Aniline
UN1548	Aniline hydrochloride
UN1549	Antimony compounds, inorganic, solid, n.o.s.
UN1550	Antimony lactate
UN1551	Antimony potassium tartrate
UN1553	Arsenic acid, liquid
UN1554	Arsenic acid, solid
UN1555	Arsenic bromide
NA1556	Methyldichloroarsine

ID Number	Description
UN1556	Arsenic compounds, liquid, n.o.s.
UN1557	Arsenic compounds, solid, n.o.s.
UN1558	Arsenic
UN1559	Arsenic pentoxide
UN1560	Arsenic trichloride
UN1561	Arsenic trioxide
UN1562	Arsenical dust
UN1564	Barium compounds, n.o.s.
UN1565	Barium cyanide
UN1566	Beryllium compounds, n.o.s.
UN1567	Beryllium, powder
UN1569	Bromoacetone
UN1570	Brucine
UN1571	Barium azide, wetted
UN1572	Cacodylic acid
UN1573	Calcium arsenate
UN1574	Calcium arsenate and calcium arsenite, mixtures, solid
UN1575	Calcium cyanide
UN1577	Chlorodinitrobenzenes, liquid
UN1578	Chloronitrobenzenes, solid
UN1579	4-Chloro-o-toluidine hydrochloride, solid
UN1580	Chloropicrin
UN1581	Chloropicrin and methyl bromide mixtures
UN1582	Chloropicrin and methyl chloride mixtures
UN1583	Chloropicrin mixtures, n.o.s.
UN1585	Copper acetoarsenite
UN1586	Copper arsenite
UN1587	Copper cyanide
UN1588	Cyanides, inorganic, solid, n.o.s.
UN1589	Cyanogen chloride, stabilized
UN1590	Dichloroanilines, liquid
UN1591	o-Dichlorobenzene
UN1593	Dichloromethane
UN1594	Diethyl sulfate
UN1595	Dimethyl sulfate
UN1596	Dinitroanilines
UN1597	Dinitrobenzenes, liquid
UN1598	Dinitro-o-cresol
UN1599	Dinitrophenol solutions
UN1600	Dinitrotoluenes, molten
UN1601	Disinfectants, solid, toxic, n.o.s.
UN1602	Dyes, liquid, toxic, n.o.s. or Dye intermediates, liquid, toxic, n.o.s.
UN1603	Ethyl bromoacetate
UN1604	Ethylenediamine

ID Number	Description
UN1605	Ethylene dibromide
UN1606	Ferric arsenate
UN1607	Ferric arsenite
UN1608	Ferrous arsenate
UN1611	Hexaethyl tetraphosphate
UN1612	Hexaethyl tetraphosphate and compressed gas mixtures
NA1613	Hydrocyanic acid, aqueous solutions
UN1613	Hydrocyanic acid, aqueous solutions or Hydrogen cyanide, aqueous solutions
UN1614	Hydrogen cyanide, stabilized
UN1616	Lead acetate
UN1617	Lead arsenates
UN1618	Lead arsenites
UN1620	Lead cyanide
UN1621	London purple
UN1622	Magnesium arsenate
UN1623	Mercuric arsenate
UN1624	Mercuric chloride
UN1625	Mercuric nitrate
UN1626	Mercuric potassium cyanide
UN1627	Mercurous nitrate
UN1629	Mercury acetate
UN1630	Mercury ammonium chloride
UN1631	Mercury benzoate
UN1634	Mercury bromides
UN1636	Mercury cyanide
UN1637	Mercury gluconate
UN1638	Mercury iodide
UN1639	Mercury nucleate
UN1640	Mercury oleate
UN1641	Mercury oxide
UN1642	Mercury oxycyanide, desensitized
UN1643	Mercury potassium iodide
UN1644	Mercury salicylate
UN1645	Mercury sulfates
UN1646	Mercury thiocyanate
UN1647	Methyl bromide and ethylene dibromide mixtures, liquid
UN1648	Acetonitrile
UN1649	Motor fuel anti-knock mixtures
UN1650	beta-Naphthylamine, solid
UN1651	Naphthylthiourea
UN1652	Naphthylurea
UN1653	Nickel cyanide
UN1654	Nicotine

ID Number	Description
UN1655	Nicotine compounds, solid, n.o.s. or Nicotine preparations, solid, n.o.s.
UN1656	Nicotine hydrochloride liquid or solution
UN1657	Nicotine salicylate
UN1658	Nicotine sulfate solution
UN1659	Nicotine tartrate
UN1660	Nitric oxide, compressed
UN1661	Nitroanilines
UN1662	Nitrobenzene
UN1663	Nitrophenols
UN1664	Nitrotoluenes, liquid
UN1665	Nitroxylenes, liquid
UN1669	Pentachloroethane
UN1670	Perchloromethyl mercaptan
UN1671	Phenol, solid
UN1672	Phenylcarbylamine chloride
UN1673	Phenylenediamines
UN1674	Phenylmercuric acetate
UN1677	Potassium arsenate
UN1678	Potassium arsenite
UN1679	Potassium cuprocyanide
UN1680	Potassium cyanide, solid
UN1683	Silver arsenite
UN1684	Silver cyanide
UN1685	Sodium arsenate
UN1686	Sodium arsenite, aqueous solutions
UN1687	Sodium azide
UN1688	Sodium cacodylate
UN1689	Sodium cyanide, solid
UN1690	Sodium fluoride, solid
UN1691	Strontium arsenite
UN1692	Strychnine or Strychnine salts
NA1693	Tear gas devices
UN1693	Tear gas substances, liquid, n.o.s.
UN1694	Bromobenzyl cyanides, liquid
UN1695	Chloroacetone, stabilized
UN1697	Chloroacetophenone, solid
UN1698	Diphenylamine chloroarsine
UN1699	Diphenylchloroarsine, liquid
UN1700	Tear gas candles
UN1701	Xylyl bromide, liquid
UN1702	1,1,2,2-Tetrachloroethane
UN1704	Tetraethyl dithiopyrophosphate
UN1707	Thallium compounds, n.o.s.

ID Number	Description
UN1708	Toluidines, liquid
UN1709	2,4-Toluylenediamine, solid or 2,4-Toluenediamine, solid
UN1710	Trichloroethylene
UN1711	Xylidines, liquid
UN1712	Zinc arsenate or Zinc arsenite or Zinc arsenate and zinc arsenite mixtures
UN1713	Zinc cyanide
UN1714	Zinc phosphide
UN1715	Acetic anhydride
UN1716	Acetyl bromide
UN1717	Acetyl chloride
UN1718	Butyl acid phosphate
UN1719	Caustic alkali liquids, n.o.s.
UN1722	Allyl chloroformate
UN1723	Allyl iodide
UN1724	Allyltrichlorosilane, stabilized
UN1725	Aluminum bromide, anhydrous
UN1726	Aluminum chloride, anhydrous
UN1727	Ammonium hydrogendifluoride, solid
UN1728	Amyltrichlorosilane
UN1729	Anisoyl chloride
UN1730	Antimony pentachloride, liquid
UN1731	Antimony pentachloride, solutions
UN1732	Antimony pentafluoride
UN1733	Antimony trichloride, liquid
UN1733	Antimony trichloride, solid
UN1736	Benzoyl chloride
UN1737	Benzyl bromide
UN1738	Benzyl chloride
UN1739	Benzyl chloroformate
UN1740	Hydrogendifluorides, n.o.s.
UN1741	Boron trichloride
UN1742	Boron trifluoride acetic acid complex, liquid
UN1743	Boron trifluoride propionic acid complex, liquid
UN1744	Bromine or Bromine solutions
UN1745	Bromine pentafluoride
UN1746	Bromine trifluoride
UN1747	Butyltrichlorosilane
UN1748	Calcium hypochlorite, dry or Calcium hypochlorite mixtures, dry
UN1749	Chlorine trifluoride
UN1750	Chloroacetic acid, solution
UN1751	Chloroacetic acid, solid
UN1752	Chloroacetyl chloride
UN1753	Chlorophenyltrichlorosilane

ID Number	Description
UN1754	Chlorosulfonic acid
UN1755	Chromic acid solution
UN1756	Chromic fluoride, solid
UN1757	Chromic fluoride, solution
UN1758	Chromium oxychloride
NA1759	Ferrous chloride, solid
UN1759	Corrosive solids, n.o.s.
NA1760	Chemical kit
NA1760	Compounds, cleaning liquid
NA1760	Compounds, tree killing, liquid or Compounds, weed killing, liquid
NA1760	Ferrous chloride, solution
UN1760	Corrosive liquids, n.o.s.
UN1761	Cupriethylenediamine solution
UN1762	Cyclohexenyltrichlorosilane
UN1763	Cyclohexyltrichlorosilane
UN1764	Dichloroacetic acid
UN1765	Dichloroacetyl chloride
UN1766	Dichlorophenyltrichlorosilane
UN1767	Diethyldichlorosilane
UN1768	Difluorophosphoric acid, anhydrous
UN1769	Diphenyldichlorosilane
UN1770	Diphenylmethyl bromide
UN1771	Dodecyltrichlorosilane
UN1773	Ferric chloride, anhydrous
UN1774	Fire extinguisher charges
UN1775	Fluoroboric acid
UN1776	Fluorophosphoric acid anhydrous
UN1777	Fluorosulfonic acid
UN1778	Fluorosilicic acid
UN1779	Formic acid
UN1780	Fumaryl chloride
UN1781	Hexadecyltrichlorosilane
UN1782	Hexafluorophosphoric acid
UN1783	Hexamethylenediamine solution
UN1784	Hexyltrichlorosilane
UN1786	Hydrofluoric acid and Sulfuric acid mixtures
UN1787	Hydriodic acid
UN1788	Hydrobromic acid
UN1789	Hydrochloric acid
UN1790	Hydrofluoric acid
UN1791	Hypochlorite solutions
UN1792	Iodine monochloride
UN1793	Isopropyl acid phosphate

ID Number	Description
UN1794	Lead sulfate
UN1796	Nitrating acid mixtures
UN1798	Nitrohydrochloric acid
UN1799	Nonyltrichlorosilane
UN1800	Octadecyltrichlorosilane
UN1801	Octyltrichlorosilane
UN1802	Perchloric acid
UN1803	Phenolsulfonic acid, liquid
UN1804	Phenyltrichlorosilane
UN1805	Phosphoric acid solution
UN1806	Phosphorus pentachloride
UN1807	Phosphorus pentoxide
UN1808	Phosphorus tribromide
UN1809	Phosphorus trichloride
UN1810	Phosphorus oxychloride
UN1811	Potassium hydrogendifluoride solid
UN1812	Potassium fluoride, solid
UN1813	Potassium hydroxide, solid
UN1814	Potassium hydroxide, solution
UN1815	Propionyl chloride
UN1816	Propyltrichlorosilane
UN1817	Pyrosulfuryl chloride
UN1818	Silicon tetrachloride
UN1819	Sodium aluminate, solution
UN1823	Sodium hydroxide, solid
UN1824	Sodium hydroxide solution
UN1825	Sodium monoxide
UN1826	Nitrating acid mixtures spent
UN1826	Nitrating acid mixtures, spent
UN1827	Stannic chloride, anhydrous
UN1828	Sulfur chlorides
UN1829	Sulfur trioxide, stabilized
UN1830	Sulfuric acid
UN1831	Sulfuric acid, fuming
UN1832	Sulfuric acid, spent
UN1833	Sulfurous acid
UN1834	Sulfuryl chloride
UN1835	Tetramethylammonium hydroxide solution
UN1836	Thionyl chloride
UN1837	Thiophosphoryl chloride
UN1838	Titanium tetrachloride
UN1839	Trichloroacetic acid
UN1840	Zinc chloride, solution
UN1841	Acetaldehyde ammonia

ID Number	Description
UN1843	Ammonium dinitro-o-cresolate, solid
UN1845	Carbon dioxide, solid or Dry ice
UN1846	Carbon tetrachloride
UN1847	Potassium sulfide, hydrated
UN1848	Propionic acid
UN1849	Sodium sulfide, hydrated
UN1851	Medicine, liquid, toxic, n.o.s.
UN1854	Barium alloys, pyrophoric
UN1855	Calcium, pyrophoric or Calcium alloys, pyrophoric
UN1856	Rags, oily
UN1857	Textile waste, wet
UN1858	Hexafluoropropylene, compressed or Refrigerant gas R 1216
UN1859	Silicon tetrafluoride
UN1860	Vinyl fluoride, stabilized
UN1862	Ethyl crotonate
UN1863	Fuel, aviation, turbine engine
UN1865	n-Propyl nitrate
UN1866	Resin solution
UN1868	Decaborane
UN1869	Magnesium or Magnesium alloys
UN1870	Potassium borohydride
UN1871	Titanium hydride
UN1872	Lead dioxide
UN1873	Perchloric acid
UN1884	Barium oxide
UN1885	Benzidine
UN1886	Benzylidene chloride
UN1887	Bromochloromethane
UN1888	Chloroform
UN1889	Cyanogen bromide
UN1891	Ethyl bromide
UN1892	Ethyldichloroarsine
UN1894	Phenylmercuric hydroxide
UN1895	Phenylmercuric nitrate
UN1897	Tetrachloroethylene
UN1898	Acetyl iodide
UN1902	Diisooctyl acid phosphate
UN1903	Disinfectants, liquid, corrosive n.o.s.
UN1905	Selenic acid
UN1906	Sludge, acid
UN1907	Soda lime
UN1908	Chlorite solution
UN1910	Calcium oxide
NA1911	Diborane mixtures

ID Number	Description
UN1911	Diborane
UN1912	Methyl chloride and methylene chloride mixtures
UN1913	Neon, refrigerated liquid
UN1914	Butyl propionates
UN1915	Cyclohexanone
UN1916	2,2'-Dichlorodiethyl ether
UN1917	Ethyl acrylate, stabilized
UN1918	Isopropylbenzene
UN1919	Methyl acrylate, stabilized
UN1920	Nonanes
UN1921	Propyleneimine, stabilized
UN1922	Pyrrolidine
UN1923	Calcium dithionite or Calcium hydrosulfite
UN1928	Methyl magnesium bromide, in ethyl ether
UN1929	Potassium dithionite or Potassium hydrosulfite
UN1931	Zinc dithionite or Zinc hydrosulfite
UN1932	Zirconium scrap
UN1935	Cyanide solutions, n.o.s.
UN1938	Bromoacetic acid solution
UN1939	Phosphorus oxybromide
UN1940	Thioglycolic acid
UN1941	Dibromodifluoromethane
UN1942	Ammonium nitrate
UN1944	Matches, safety
UN1945	Matches, wax, Vesta
UN1950	Aerosols
UN1950	Aerosols, flammable, n.o.s.
UN1951	Argon, refrigerated liquid
UN1952	Ethylene oxide and carbon dioxide mixtures
UN1953	Compressed gas, toxic, flammable, n.o.s.
NA1954	Refrigerant gases, n.o.s. or Dispersant gases, n.o.s.
UN1954	Compressed gas, flammable, n.o.s.
NA1955	Organic phosphate, mixed with compressed gas or Organic phosphate compound, mixed with compressed gas or Organic phosphorus compound, mixed with compressed gas
UN1955	Compressed gas, toxic, n.o.s.
UN1956	Compressed gas, n.o.s.
UN1957	Deuterium, compressed
UN1958	1,2-Dichloro-1,1,2,2-tetrafluoroethane or Refrigerant gas R 114
UN1959	1,1-Difluoroethylene or Refrigerant gas R 1132a
NA1961	Ethane-Propane mixture, refrigerated liquid
UN1961	Ethane, refrigerated liquid
UN1962	Ethylene
UN1963	Helium, refrigerated liquid
UN1964	Hydrocarbon gas mixture, compressed, n.o.s.

ID Number	Description
UN1965	Hydrocarbon gas mixture, liquefied, n.o.s.
UN1966	Hydrogen, refrigerated liquid
NA1967	Parathion and compressed gas mixture
UN1967	Insecticide gases, toxic, n.o.s.
UN1968	Insecticide gases, n.o.s.
UN1969	Isobutane
UN1970	Krypton, refrigerated liquid
UN1971	Methane, compressed or Natural gas, compressed
UN1972	Methane, refrigerated liquid or Natural gas, refrigerated liquid
UN1973	Chlorodifluoromethane and chloropentafluoroethane mixture or Refrigerant gas R502
UN1974	Chlorodifluorobromomethane or Refrigerant gas R12B1
UN1975	Nitric oxide and dinitrogen tetroxide mixtures or Nitric oxide and nitrogen dioxide mixtures
UN1976	Octafluorocyclobutane or Refrigerant gas RC 318
UN1977	Nitrogen, refrigerated liquid
UN1978	Propane
UN1979	Rare gases, mixtures, compressed
UN1980	Rare gases and oxygen mixtures, compressed
UN1981	Rare gases and nitrogen mixtures, compressed
UN1982	Tetrafluoromethane or Refrigerant gas R 14
UN1983	1-Chloro-2,2,2-trifluoroethane or refrigerant gas R 133a
UN1984	Trifluoromethane or Refrigerant gas R 23
UN1986	Alcohols, flammable, toxic, n.o.s.
UN1987	Alcohols, n.o.s.
UN1988	Aldehydes, flammable, toxic, n.o.s.
UN1989	Aldehydes, n.o.s.
UN1990	Benzaldehyde
UN1991	Chloroprene, stabilized
UN1992	Flammable liquids, toxic, n.o.s.
NA1993	Combustible liquid, n.o.s.
NA1993	Compounds, cleaning liquid
NA1993	Compounds, tree killing, liquid or Compounds, weed killing, liquid
NA1993	Diesel fuel
NA1993	Fuel oil
UN1993	Flammable liquids, n.o.s.
UN1994	Iron pentacarbonyl
NA1999	Asphalt
UN1999	Tars, liquid
UN2000	Celluloid
UN2001	Cobalt naphthenates, powder
UN2002	Celluloid, scrap
UN2004	Magnesium diamide
UN2005	Magnesium diphenyl

ID Number	Description
UN2006	Plastics, nitrocellulose-based, self-heating, n.o.s.
UN2008	Zirconium powder, dry
UN2009	Zirconium, dry
UN2010	Magnesium hydride
UN2011	Magnesium phosphide
UN2012	Potassium phosphide
UN2013	Strontium phosphide
UN2014	Hydrogen peroxide, aqueous solutions
UN2015	Hydrogen peroxide, stabilized or Hydrogen peroxide aqueous solutions, stabilized
UN2016	Ammunition, toxic, non-explosive
UN2017	Ammunition, tear-producing, non-explosive
UN2018	Chloroanilines, solid
UN2019	Chloroanilines, liquid
UN2020	Chlorophenols, solid
UN2021	Chlorophenols, liquid
UN2022	Cresylic acid
UN2023	Epichlorohydrin
UN2024	Mercury compounds, liquid, n.o.s.
UN2025	Mercury compounds, solid, n.o.s.
UN2026	Phenylmercuric compounds, n.o.s.
UN2027	Sodium arsenite, solid
UN2028	Bombs, smoke, non-explosive
UN2029	Hydrazine, anhydrous
UN2030	Hydrazine aqueous solution
UN2031	Nitric acid
UN2032	Nitric acid, red fuming
UN2033	Potassium monoxide
UN2034	Hydrogen and Methane mixtures, compressed
UN2035	1,1,1,-Trifluoroethane or Refrigerant gas, R 143a
UN2036	Xenon
UN2037	Gas cartridges
UN2037	Receptacles, small, containing gas (gas cartridges)
UN2038	Dinitrotoluenes
UN2044	2,2-Dimethylpropane
UN2045	Isobutyraldehyde or isobutyl aldehyde
UN2046	Cymenes
UN2047	Dichloropropenes
UN2048	Dicyclopentadiene
UN2049	Diethylbenzene
UN2050	Diisobutylene, isomeric compounds
UN2051	2-Dimethylaminoethanol
UN2052	Dipentene
UN2053	Methyl isobutyl carbinol

ID Number	Description
UN2054	Morpholine
UN2055	Styrene monomer, stabilized
UN2056	Tetrahydrofuran
UN2057	Tripropylene
UN2058	Valeraldehyde
UN2059	Nitrocellulose, solution, flammable
UN2067	Ammonium nitrate based fertilizer
UN2071	Ammonium nitrate based fertilizer
UN2073	Ammonia solutions
UN2074	Acrylamide, solid
UN2075	Chloral, anhydrous, stabilized
UN2076	Cresols, liquid
UN2077	alpha-Naphthylamine
UN2078	Toluene diisocyanate
UN2079	Diethylenetriamine
UN2186	Hydrogen chloride, refrigerated liquid
UN2187	Carbon dioxide, refrigerated liquid
UN2188	Arsine
UN2189	Dichlorosilane
UN2190	Oxygen difluoride, compressed
UN2191	Sulfuryl fluoride
UN2192	Germane
UN2193	Hexafluoroethane or Refrigerant gas R 116
UN2194	Selenium hexafluoride
UN2195	Tellurium hexafluoride
UN2196	Tungsten hexafluoride
UN2197	Hydrogen iodide, anhydrous
UN2198	Phosphorus pentafluoride
UN2199	Phosphine
UN2200	Propadiene, stabilized
UN2201	Nitrous oxide, refrigerated liquid
UN2202	Hydrogen selenide, anhydrous
UN2203	Silane
UN2204	Carbonyl sulfide
UN2205	Adiponitrile
UN2206	Isocyanates, toxic, n.o.s. or Isocyanate, solutions, toxic, n.o.s.
UN2208	Calcium hypochlorite mixtures, dry
UN2209	Formaldehyde, solutions
UN2210	Maneb or Maneb preparations
UN2211	Polymeric beads, expandable
NA2212	Asbestos
UN2212	Blue Asbestos or Brown Asbestos
UN2213	Paraformaldehyde
UN2214	Phthalic anhydride

ID Number	Description
UN2215	Maleic anhydride
UN2215	Maleic anhydride, molten
UN2216	Fish meal, stabilized or Fish scrap, stabilized
UN2217	Seed cake
UN2218	Acrylic acid, stabilized
UN2219	Allyl glycidyl ether
UN2222	Anisole
UN2224	Benzonitrile
UN2225	Benzene sulfonyl chloride
UN2226	Benzotrichloride
UN2227	n-Butyl methacrylate, stabilized
UN2232	2-Chloroethanal
UN2233	Chloroanisidines
UN2234	Chlorobenzotrifluorides
UN2235	Chlorobenzyl chlorides, liquid
UN2236	3-Chloro-4-methylphenyl isocyanate, liquid
UN2237	Chloronitroanilines
UN2238	Chlorotoluenes
UN2239	Chlorotoluidines, solid
UN2240	Chromosulfuric acid
UN2241	Cycloheptane
UN2242	Cycloheptene
UN2243	Cyclohexyl acetate
UN2244	Cyclopentanol
UN2245	Cyclopentanone
UN2246	Cyclopentene
UN2247	n-Decane
UN2248	Di-n-butylamine
UN2249	Dichlorodimethyl ether, symmetrical
UN2250	Dichlorophenyl isocyanates
UN2251	Bicyclo[2,2,1]hepta-2,5-diene, stabilized or 2,5-Norbornadiene, stabilized
UN2252	1,2-Dimethoxyethane
UN2253	N,N-Dimethylaniline
UN2254	Matches, fusee
UN2256	Cyclohexene
UN2257	Potassium
UN2258	1,2-Propylenediamine
UN2259	Triethylenetetramine
UN2260	Tripropylamine
UN2261	Xylenols, solid
UN2262	Dimethylcarbamoyl chloride
UN2263	Dimethylcyclohexanes
UN2264	N,N-Dimethylcyclohexylamine

ID Number	Description
UN2265	N,N-Dimethylformamide
UN2266	Dimethyl-N-propylamine
UN2267	Dimethyl thiophosphoryl chloride
UN2269	3,3'-Iminodipropylamine
UN2270	Ethylamine, aqueous solution
UN2271	Ethyl amyl ketone
UN2272	N-Ethylaniline
UN2273	2-Ethylaniline
UN2274	N-Ethyl-N-benzylaniline
UN2275	2-Ethylbutanol
UN2276	2-Ethylhexylamine
UN2277	Ethyl methacrylate, stabilized
UN2278	n-Heptene
UN2279	Hexachlorobutadiene
UN2280	Hexamethylenediamine, solid
UN2281	Hexamethylene diisocyanate
UN2282	Hexanols
UN2283	Isobutyl methacrylate, stabilized
UN2284	Isobutyronitrile
UN2285	Isocyanatobenzotrifluorides
UN2286	Pentamethylheptane
UN2287	Isoheptenes
UN2288	Isohexenes
UN2289	Isophoronediamine
UN2290	Isophorone diisocyanate
UN2291	Lead compounds, soluble, n.o.s.
UN2293	4-Methoxy-4-methylpentan-2-one
UN2294	N-Methylaniline
UN2295	Methyl chloroacetate
UN2296	Methylcyclohexane
UN2297	Methylcyclohexanone
UN2298	Methylcyclopentane
UN2299	Methyl dichloroacetate
UN2300	2-Methyl-5-ethylpyridine
UN2301	2-Methylfuran
UN2302	5-Methylhexan-2-one
UN2303	Isopropenylbenzene
UN2304	Naphthalene, molten
UN2305	Nitrobenzenesulfonic acid
UN2306	Nitrobenzotrifluorides, liquid
UN2307	3-Nitro-4-chlorobenzotrifluoride
UN2308	Nitrosylsulfuric acid, liquid
UN2309	Octadiene
UN2310	Pentane-2,4-dione

ID Number	Description
UN2311	Phenetidines
UN2312	Phenol, molten
UN2313	Picolines
UN2315	Polychlorinated biphenyls, liquid
UN2316	Sodium cuprocyanide, solid
UN2317	Sodium cuprocyanide, solution
UN2318	Sodium hydrosulfide
UN2319	Terpene hydrocarbons, n.o.s.
UN2320	Tetraethylenepentamine
UN2321	Trichlorobenzenes, liquid
UN2322	Trichlorobutene
UN2323	Triethyl phosphite
UN2324	Triisobutylene
UN2325	1,3,5-Trimethylbenzene
UN2326	Trimethylcyclohexylamine
UN2327	Trimethylhexamethylenediamines
UN2328	Trimethylhexamethylene diisocyanate
UN2329	Trimethyl phosphite
UN2330	Undecane
UN2331	Zinc chloride, anhydrous
UN2332	Acetaldehyde oxime
UN2333	Allyl acetate
UN2334	Allylamine
UN2335	Allyl ethyl ether
UN2336	Allyl formate
UN2337	Phenyl mercaptan
UN2338	Benzotrifluoride
UN2339	2-Bromobutane
UN2340	2-Bromoethyl ethyl ether
UN2341	1-Bromo-3-methylbutane
UN2342	Bromomethylpropanes
UN2343	2-Bromopentane
UN2344	Bromopropanes
UN2345	3-Bromopropyne
UN2346	Butanedione
UN2347	Butyl mercaptans
UN2348	Butyl acrylates, stabilized
UN2350	Butyl methyl ether
UN2351	Butyl nitrites
UN2352	Butyl vinyl ether, stabilized
UN2353	Butyryl chloride
UN2354	Chloromethyl ethyl ether
UN2356	2-Chloropropane
UN2357	Cyclohexylamine

ID Number	Description
UN2358	Cyclooctatetraene
UN2359	Diallylamine
UN2360	Diallylether
UN2361	Diisobutylamine
UN2362	1,1-Dichloroethane
UN2363	Ethyl mercaptan
UN2364	n-Propyl benzene
UN2366	Diethyl carbonate
UN2367	alpha-Methylvaleraldehyde
UN2368	alpha-Pinene
UN2370	1-Hexene
UN2371	Isopentenes
UN2372	1,2-Di-(dimethylamino)ethane
UN2373	Diethoxymethane
UN2374	3,3-Diethoxypropene
UN2375	Diethyl sulfide
UN2376	2,3-Dihydropyran
UN2377	1,1-Dimethoxyethane
UN2378	2-Dimethylaminoacetonitrile
UN2379	1,3-Dimethylbutylamine
UN2380	Dimethyldiethoxysilane
UN2381	Dimethyl disulfide
UN2382	Dimethylhydrazine, symmetrical
UN2383	Dipropylamine
UN2384	Di-n-propyl ether
UN2385	Ethyl isobutyrate
UN2386	1-Ethylpiperidine
UN2387	Fluorobenzene
UN2388	Fluorotoluenes
UN2389	Furan
UN2390	2-Iodobutane
UN2391	Iodomethylpropanes
UN2392	Iodopropanes
UN2393	Isobutyl formate
UN2394	Isobutyl propionate
UN2395	Isobutyryl chloride
UN2396	Methacrylaldehyde, stabilized
UN2397	3-Methylbutan-2-one
UN2398	Methyl tert-butyl ether
UN2399	1-Methylpiperidine
UN2400	Methyl isovalerate
UN2401	Piperidine
UN2402	Propanethiols
UN2403	Isopropenyl acetate

ID Number	Description
UN2404	Propionitrile
UN2405	Isopropyl butyrate
UN2406	Isopropyl isobutyrate
UN2407	Isopropyl chloroformate
UN2409	Isopropyl propionate
UN2410	1,2,3,6-Tetrahydropyridine
UN2411	Butyronitrile
UN2412	Tetrahydrothiophene
UN2413	Tetrapropylorthotitanate
UN2414	Thiophene
UN2416	Trimethyl borate
UN2417	Carbonyl fluoride
UN2418	Sulfur tetrafluoride
UN2419	Bromotrifluoroethylene
UN2420	Hexafluoroacetone
UN2421	Nitrogen trioxide
UN2422	Octafluorobut-2-ene or Refrigerant gas R 1318
UN2424	Octafluoropropane or Refrigerant gas R 218
UN2426	Ammonium nitrate, liquid
UN2427	Potassium chlorate, aqueous solution
UN2428	Sodium chlorate, aqueous solution
UN2429	Calcium chlorate aqueous solution
UN2430	Alkylphenols, solid, n.o.s.
UN2431	Anisidines
UN2432	N,N-Diethylaniline
UN2433	Chloronitrotoluenes, liquid
UN2434	Dibenzyldichlorosilane
UN2435	Ethylphenyldichlorosilane
UN2436	Thioacetic acid
UN2437	Methylphenyldichlorosilane
UN2438	Trimethylacetyl chloride
UN2439	Sodium hydrogendifluoride
UN2440	Stannic chloride pentahydrate
UN2441	Titanium trichloride, pyrophoric or Titanium trichloride mixtures, pyrophoric
UN2442	Trichloroacetyl chloride
UN2443	Vanadium oxytrichloride
UN2444	Vanadium tetrachloride
UN2445	Lithium alkyls, liquid
UN2446	Nitrocresols, solid
UN2447	Phosphorus white, molten
NA2448	Sulfur, molten
UN2448	Sulfur, molten
UN2451	Nitrogen trifluoride

ID Number	Description
UN2452	Ethylacetylene, stabilized
UN2453	Ethyl fluoride or Refrigerant gas R161
UN2454	Methyl fluoride or Refrigerant gas R 41
UN2456	2-Chloropropene
UN2457	2,3-Dimethylbutane
UN2458	Hexadiene
UN2459	2-Methyl-1-butene
UN2460	2-Methyl-2-butene
UN2461	Methylpentadienes
UN2463	Aluminum hydride
UN2464	Beryllium nitrate
UN2465	Dichloroisocyanuric acid, dry or Dichloroisocyanuric acid salts
UN2466	Potassium superoxide
UN2468	Trichloroisocyanuric acid, dry
UN2469	Zinc bromate
UN2470	Phenylacetonitrile, liquid
UN2471	Osmium tetroxide
UN2473	Sodium arsanilate
UN2474	Thiophosgene
UN2475	Vanadium trichloride
UN2477	Methyl isothiocyanate
UN2478	Isocyanates, flammable, toxic, n.o.s. or Isocyanate solutions, flammable, toxic, n.o.s.
UN2480	Methyl isocyanate
UN2481	Ethyl isocyanate
UN2482	n-Propyl isocyanate
UN2483	Isopropyl isocyanate
UN2484	tert-Butyl isocyanate
UN2485	n-Butyl isocyanate
UN2486	Isobutyl isocyanate
UN2487	Phenyl isocyanate
UN2488	Cyclohexyl isocyanate
UN2490	Dichloroisopropyl ether
UN2491	Ethanolamine or Ethanolamine solutions
UN2493	Hexamethyleneimine
UN2495	Iodine pentafluoride
UN2496	Propionic anhydride
UN2498	1,2,3,6-Tetrahydrobenzaldehyde
UN2501	Tris-(1-aziridinyl)phosphine oxide, solution
UN2502	Valeryl chloride
UN2503	Zirconium tetrachloride
UN2504	Tetrabromoethane
UN2505	Ammonium fluoride
UN2506	Ammonium hydrogen sulfate

ID Number	Description
UN2507	Chloroplatinic acid, solid
UN2508	Molybdenum pentachloride
UN2509	Potassium hydrogen sulfate
UN2511	2-Chloropropionic acid
UN2512	Aminophenols
UN2513	Bromoacetyl bromide
UN2514	Bromobenzene
UN2515	Bromoform
UN2516	Carbon tetrabromide
UN2517	1-Chloro-1,1-difluoroethane or Refrigerant gas R 142b
UN2518	1,5,9-Cyclododecatriene
UN2520	Cyclooctadienes
UN2521	Diketene, stabilized
UN2522	2-Dimethylaminoethyl methacrylate
UN2524	Ethyl orthoformate
UN2525	Ethyl oxalate
UN2526	Furfurylamine
UN2527	Isobutyl acrylate, inhibited
UN2528	Isobutyl isobutyrate
UN2529	Isobutyric acid
UN2531	Methacrylic acid, stabilized
UN2533	Methyl trichloroacetate
UN2534	Methylchlorosilane
UN2535	4-Methylmorpholine or n-methlymorpholine
UN2536	Methyltetrahydrofuran
UN2538	Nitronaphthalene
UN2541	Terpinolene
UN2542	Tributylamine
UN2545	Hafnium powder, dry
UN2546	Titanium powder, dry
UN2547	Sodium superoxide
UN2548	Chlorine pentafluoride
UN2552	Hexafluoroacetone hydrate, liquid
UN2554	Methyl allyl chloride
UN2555	Nitrocellulose with water
UN2556	Nitrocellulose with alcohol
UN2557	Nitrocellulose, or Nitrocellulose mixture with pigment or Nitrocellulose mixture with plasticizer or Nitrocellulose mixture with pigment and plasticizer
UN2558	Epibromohydrin
UN2560	2-Methylpentan-2-ol
UN2561	3-Methyl-1-butene
UN2564	Trichloroacetic acid, solution
UN2565	Dicyclohexylamine
UN2567	Sodium pentachlorophenate

ID Number	Description
UN2570	Cadmium compounds
UN2571	Alkylsulfuric acids
UN2572	Phenylhydrazine
UN2573	Thallium chlorate
UN2574	Tricresyl phosphate
UN2576	Phosphorus oxybromide, molten
UN2577	Phenylacetyl chloride
UN2578	Phosphorus trioxide
UN2579	Piperazine
UN2580	Aluminum bromide, solution
UN2581	Aluminum chloride, solution
UN2582	Ferric chloride, solution
UN2583	Alkyl sulfonic acids, solid or Aryl sulfonic acids, solid
UN2584	Alkyl sulfonic acids, liquid or Aryl sulfonic acids, liquid
UN2585	Alkyl sulfonic acids, solid or Aryl sulfonic acids, solid
UN2586	Alkyl sulfonic acids, liquid or Aryl sulfonic acids, liquid
UN2587	Benzoquinone
UN2588	Pesticides, solid, toxic, n.o.s.
UN2589	Vinyl chloroacetate
UN2590	White asbestos
UN2591	Xenon, refrigerated liquid
UN2599	Chlorotrifluoromethane and trifluoromethane azeotropic mixture or Refrigerant gas R 503
UN2600	Carbon monoxide and hydrogen mixture, compressed
UN2601	Cyclobutane
UN2602	Dichlorodifluoromethane and difluoroethane azeotropic mixture or Refrigerant gas R 500
UN2603	Cycloheptatriene
UN2604	Boron trifluoride diethyl etherate
UN2605	Methoxymethyl isocyanate
UN2606	Methyl orthosilicate
UN2607	Acrolein dimer, stabilized
UN2608	Nitropropanes
UN2609	Triallyl borate
UN2610	Triallylamine
UN2611	Propylene chlorohydrin
UN2612	Methyl propyl ether
UN2614	Methallyl alcohol
UN2615	Ethyl propyl ether
UN2616	Triisopropyl borate
UN2617	Methylcyclohexanols
UN2618	Vinyl toluenes, stabilized
UN2619	Benzyldimethylamine
UN2620	Amyl butyrates
UN2621	Acetyl methyl carbinol

ID Number	Description
UN2622	Glycidaldehyde
UN2623	Firelighters, solid
UN2624	Magnesium silicide
UN2626	Chloric acid aqueous solution
UN2627	Nitrites, inorganic, n.o.s.
UN2628	Potassium fluoroacetate
UN2629	Sodium fluoroacetate
UN2630	Selenates or Selenites
UN2642	Fluoroacetic acid
UN2643	Methyl bromoacetate
UN2644	Methyl iodide
UN2645	Phenacyl bromide
UN2646	Hexachlorocyclopentadiene
UN2647	Malononitrile
UN2648	1,2-Dibromobutan-3-one
UN2649	1,3-Dichloroacetone
UN2650	1,1-Dichloro-1-nitroethane
UN2651	4,4'-Diaminodiphenyl methane
UN2653	Benzyl iodide
UN2655	Potassium fluorosilicate
UN2656	Quinoline
UN2657	Selenium disulfide
UN2659	Sodium chloroacetate
UN2660	Nitrotoluidines (mono)
UN2661	Hexachloroacetone
UN2662	Hydroquinone, solid
UN2664	Dibromomethane
UN2667	Butyltoluenes
UN2668	Chloroacetonitrile
UN2669	Chlorocresols solution
UN2670	Cyanuric chloride
UN2671	Aminopyridines
UN2672	Ammonia solutions
UN2673	2-Amino-4-chlorophenol
UN2674	Sodium fluorosilicate
UN2676	Stibine
UN2677	Rubidium hydroxide solution
UN2678	Rubidium hydroxide
UN2679	Lithium hydroxide, solution
UN2680	Lithium hydroxide
UN2681	Caesium hydroxide solution
UN2682	Caesium hydroxide
UN2683	Ammonium sulfide solution
UN2684	3-Diethylamino-propylamine

ID Number	Description
UN2685	N,N-Diethylethylenediamine
UN2686	2-Diethylaminoethanol
UN2687	Dicyclohexylammonium nitrite
UN2688	1-Bromo-3-chloropropane
UN2689	Glycerol alpha-monochlorohydrin
UN2690	N-n-Butyl imidazole
UN2691	Phosphorus pentabromide
UN2692	Boron tribromide
UN2693	Bisulfites, aqueous solutions, n.o.s.
UN2698	Tetrahydrophthalic anhydrides
UN2699	Trifluoroacetic acid
UN2705	1-Pentol
UN2707	Dimethyldioxanes
UN2709	Butyl benzenes
UN2710	Dipropyl ketone
UN2713	Acridine
UN2714	Zinc resinate
UN2715	Aluminum resinate
UN2716	1,4-Butynediol
UN2717	Camphor
UN2719	Barium bromate
UN2720	Chromium nitrate
UN2721	Copper chlorate
UN2722	Lithium nitrate
UN2723	Magnesium chlorate
UN2724	Manganese nitrate
UN2725	Nickel nitrate
UN2726	Nickel nitrite
UN2727	Thallium nitrate
UN2728	Zirconium nitrate
UN2729	Hexachlorobenzene
UN2730	Nitroanisole, liquid
UN2732	Nitrobromobenzenes, liquid
UN2733	Amines, flammable, corrosive, n.o.s. or Polyamines, flammable, corrosive, n.o.s.
UN2734	Amines, liquid, corrosive, flammable, n.o.s. or Polyamines, liquid, corrosive, flammable, n.o.s.
UN2735	Amines, liquid, corrosive, n.o.s. or Polyamines, liquid, corrosive, n.o.s.
UN2738	N-Butylaniline
UN2739	Butyric anhydride
UN2740	n-Propyl chloroformate
UN2741	Barium hypochlorite
NA2742	Isobutyl chloroformate
NA2742	sec-Butyl chloroformate

ID Number	Description
UN2742	Chloroformates, toxic, corrosive, flammable, n.o.s.
UN2743	n-Butyl chloroformate
UN2744	Cyclobutyl chloroformate
UN2745	Chloromethyl chloroformate
UN2746	Phenyl chloroformate
UN2747	tert-Butylcyclohexylchloroformate
UN2748	2-Ethylhexyl chloroformate
UN2749	Tetramethylsilane
UN2750	1,3-Dichloropropanol-2
UN2751	Diethylthiophosphoryl chloride
UN2752	1,2-Epoxy-3-ethoxypropane
UN2753	N-Ethylbenzyltoluidines liquid
UN2754	N-Ethyltoluidines
UN2757	Carbamate pesticides, solid, toxic
UN2758	Carbamate pesticides, liquid, flammable, toxic
UN2759	Arsenical pesticides, solid, toxic
UN2760	Arsenical pesticides, liquid, flammable, toxic
UN2761	Organochlorine, pesticides, solid, toxic
UN2762	Organochlorine pesticides liquid, flammable, toxic
UN2763	Triazine pesticides, solid, toxic
UN2764	Triazine pesticides, liquid, flammable, toxic
UN2771	Thiocarbamate pesticides, solid, toxic
UN2772	Thiocarbamate pesticide, liquid, flammable, toxic
UN2775	Copper based pesticides, solid, toxic
UN2776	Copper based pesticides, liquid, flammable, toxic
UN2777	Mercury based pesticides, solid, toxic
UN2778	Mercury based pesticides, liquid, flammable, toxic
UN2779	Substituted nitrophenol pesticides, solid, toxic
UN2780	Substituted nitrophenol pesticides, liquid, flammable, toxic
UN2781	Bipyridilium pesticides, solid, toxic
UN2782	Bipyridilium pesticides, liquid, flammable, toxic
UN2783	Organophosphorus pesticides, solid, toxic
UN2784	Organophosphorus pesticides, liquid, flammable, toxic
UN2785	4-Thiapentanal
UN2786	Organotin pesticides, solid, toxic
UN2787	Organotin pesticides, liquid, flammable, toxic
UN2788	Organotin compounds, liquid, n.o.s.
UN2789	Acetic acid, glacial or Acetic acid solution
UN2790	Acetic acid solution
UN2793	Ferrous metal borings or Ferrous metal shavings or Ferrous metal turnings or Ferrous metal cuttings
UN2794	Batteries, wet, filled with acid
UN2795	Batteries, wet, filled with alkali
UN2796	Battery fluid, acid

ID Number	Description
UN2796	Sulfuric acid
UN2797	Battery fluid, alkali
UN2798	Phenyl phosphorus dichloride
UN2799	Phenyl phosphorus thiodichloride
UN2800	Batteries, wet, non-spillable
UN2801	Dyes, liquid, corrosive n.o.s. or Dye intermediates, liquid, corrosive, n.o.s.
UN2802	Copper chloride
UN2803	Gallium
UN2805	Lithium hydride, fused solid
UN2806	Lithium nitride
UN2809	Mercury
NA2810	Compounds, tree killing, liquid or Compounds, weed killing, liquid
UN2810	Toxic, liquids, organic, n.o.s.
UN2811	Toxic, solids, organic, n.o.s.
UN2812	Sodium aluminate, solid
UN2813	Water-reactive solid, n.o.s.
UN2814	Infectious substances, affecting humans
UN2815	N-Aminoethylpiperazine
UN2817	Ammonium hydrogendifluoride, solution
UN2818	Ammonium polysulfide, solution
UN2819	Amyl acid phosphate
UN2820	Butyric acid
UN2821	Phenol solutions
UN2822	2-Chloropyridine
UN2823	Crotonic acid
UN2826	Ethyl chlorothioformate
UN2829	Caproic acid
UN2830	Lithium ferrosilicon
UN2831	1,1,1-Trichloroethane
UN2834	Phosphorous acid
UN2835	Sodium aluminum hydride
UN2837	Bisulfate, aqueous solution
UN2838	Vinyl butyrate, stabilized
UN2839	Aldol
UN2840	Butyraldoxime
UN2841	Di-n-amylamine
UN2842	Nitroethane
UN2844	Calcium manganese silicon
NA2845	Ethyl phosphonous dichloride, anhydrous
NA2845	Methyl phosphonous dichloride
UN2845	Pyrophoric liquids, organic, n.o.s.
UN2846	Pyrophoric solids, organic, n.o.s.
UN2849	3-Chloropropanol-1

ID Number	Description
UN2850	Propylene tetramer
UN2851	Boron trifluoride dihydrate
UN2852	Dipicryl sulfide, wetted
UN2853	Magnesium fluorosilicate
UN2854	Ammonium fluorosilicate
UN2855	Zinc fluorosilicate
UN2856	Fluorosilicates, n.o.s.
UN2857	Refrigerating machines
UN2858	Zirconium, dry
UN2859	Ammonium metavanadate
UN2861	Ammonium polyvanadate
UN2862	Vanadium pentoxide
UN2863	Sodium ammonium vanadate
UN2864	Potassium metavanadate
UN2865	Hydroxylamine sulfate
UN2869	Titanium trichloride mixtures
UN2870	Aluminum borohydride or Aluminum borohydride in devices
UN2871	Antimony powder
UN2872	Dibromochloropropane
UN2873	Dibutylaminoethanol
UN2874	Furfuryl alcohol
UN2875	Hexachlorophene
UN2876	Resorcinol
UN2878	Titanium sponge granules or Titanium sponge powders
UN2879	Selenium oxychloride
UN2880	Calcium hypochlorite, hydrated or Calcium hypochlorite, hydrated mixtures
UN2881	Metal catalyst, dry
UN2900	Infectious substances, affecting animals
UN2901	Bromine chloride
UN2902	Pesticides, liquid, toxic, n.o.s.
UN2903	Pesticides, liquid, toxic, flammable, n.o.s.
UN2904	Chlorophenolates, liquid or Phenolates, liquid
UN2905	Chlorophenolates, solid or Phenolates, solid
UN2907	Isosorbide dinitrate mixture
UN2908	Radioactive material, excepted package-empty packaging
UN2909	Radioactive material, excepted package-articles manufactured from natural uranium or depleted uranium or natural thorium
UN2910	Radioactive material, excepted package-limited quantity of material
UN2911	Radioactive material, excepted package-instruments or articles
UN2912	Radioactive material, low specific activity (LSA-I)
UN2913	Radioactive material, surface contaminated objects (SCO-I or SCO-II)
UN2915	Radioactive material, Type A package

ID Number	Description
UN2916	Radioactive material, Type B(U) package
UN2917	Radioactive material, Type B(M) package
UN2919	Radioactive material, transported under special arrangement
UN2920	Corrosive liquids, flammable, n.o.s.
UN2921	Corrosive solids, flammable, n.o.s.
UN2922	Corrosive liquids, toxic, n.o.s.
UN2923	Corrosive solids, toxic, n.o.s.
UN2924	Flammable liquids, corrosive, n.o.s.
UN2925	Flammable solids, corrosive, organic, n.o.s.
UN2926	Flammable solids, toxic, organic, n.o.s.
NA2927	Ethyl phosphonothioic dichloride, anhydrous
NA2927	Ethyl phosphorodichloridate
UN2927	Toxic liquids, corrosive, organic, n.o.s.
UN2928	Toxic solids, corrosive, organic n.o.s.
UN2929	Toxic liquids, flammable, organic, n.o.s.
UN2930	Toxic solids, flammable, organic, n.o.s.
UN2931	Vanadyl sulfate
UN2933	Methyl 2-chloropropionate
UN2934	Isopropyl 2-chloropropionate
UN2935	Ethyl 2-chloropropionate
UN2936	Thiolactic acid
UN2937	alpha-Methylbenzyl alcohol, liquid
UN2940	9-Phosphabicyclononanes or Cyclooctadiene phosphines
UN2941	Fluoroanilines
UN2942	2-Trifluoromethylaniline
UN2943	Tetrahydrofurfurylamine
UN2945	N-Methylbutylamine
UN2946	2-Amino-5-diethylaminopentane
UN2947	Isopropyl chloroacetate
UN2948	3-Trifluoromethylaniline
UN2949	Sodium hydrosulfide
UN2950	Magnesium granules, coated
UN2956	5-tert-Butyl-2,4,6-trinitro-m-xylene or Musk xylene
UN2965	Boron trifluoride dimethyl etherate
UN2966	Thioglycol
UN2967	Sulfamic acid
UN2968	Maneb stabilized or Maneb preparations, stabilized
UN2969	Castor beans or Castor meal or Castor pomace or Castor flake
UN2977	Radioactive material, uranium hexafluoride, fissile
UN2978	Radioactive material, uranium hexafluoride
UN2983	Ethylene oxide and propylene oxide mixtures
UN2984	Hydrogen peroxide, aqueous solutions
UN2985	Chlorosilanes, flammable, corrosive, n.o.s.
UN2986	Chlorosilanes, corrosive, flammable, n.o.s.

ID Number	Description
UN2987	Chlorosilanes, corrosive, n.o.s.
UN2988	Chlorosilanes, water-reactive, flammable, corrosive, n.o.s.
UN2989	Lead phosphite, dibasic
UN2990	Life-saving appliances, self inflating
UN2991	Carbamate pesticides, liquid, toxic, flammable
UN2992	Carbamate pesticides, liquid, toxic
UN2993	Arsenical pesticides, liquid, toxic, flammable
UN2994	Arsenical pesticides, liquid, toxic
UN2995	Organochlorine pesticides, liquid, toxic, flammable.
UN2996	Organochlorine pesticides, liquid, toxic
UN2997	Triazine pesticides, liquid, toxic, flammable
UN2998	Triazine pesticides, liquid, toxic
UN3002	Phenyl urea pesticides, liquid, toxic
UN3005	Thiocarbamate pesticide, liquid, toxic, flammable
UN3006	Thiocarbamate pesticide, liquid, toxic
UN3009	Copper based pesticides, liquid, toxic, flammable
UN3010	Copper based pesticides, liquid, toxic
UN3011	Mercury based pesticides, liquid, toxic, flammable
UN3012	Mercury based pesticides, liquid, toxic
UN3013	Substituted nitrophenol pesticides, liquid, toxic, flammable
UN3014	Substituted nitrophenol pesticides, liquid, toxic
UN3015	Bipyridilium pesticides, liquid, toxic, flammable
UN3016	Bipyridilium pesticides, liquid, toxic
UN3017	Organophosphorus pesticides, liquid, toxic, flammable
UN3018	Organophosphorus pesticides, liquid, toxic
UN3019	Organotin pesticides, liquid, toxic, flammable
UN3020	Organotin pesticides, liquid, toxic
UN3021	Pesticides, liquid, flammable, toxic
UN3022	1,2-Butylene oxide, stabilized
UN3023	2-Methly-2-heptanethiol
UN3024	Coumarin derivative pesticides, liquid, flammable, toxic
UN3025	Coumarin derivative pesticides, liquid, toxic, flammable
UN3026	Coumarin derivative pesticides, liquid, toxic
UN3027	Coumarin derivative pesticides, solid, toxic
UN3028	Batteries, dry, containing potassium hydroxide solid
UN3048	Aluminum phosphide pesticides
UN3051	Aluminum alkyls
UN3052	Aluminum alkyl halides, liquid
UN3053	Magnesium alkyls
UN3054	Cyclohexyl mercaptan
UN3055	2-(2-Aminoethoxy) ethanol
UN3056	n-Heptaldehyde
UN3057	Trifluoroacetyl chloride
UN3064	Nitroglycerin, solution in alcohol

ID Number	Description
UN3065	Alcoholic beverages
UN3066	Paint or Paint related material
UN3070	Ethylene oxide and dichlorodifluoromethane mixture
UN3071	Mercaptans, liquid, toxic, flammable, n.o.s. or Mercaptan mixtures, liquid, toxic, flammable, n.o.s.
UN3072	Life-saving appliances, not self inflating
UN3073	Vinylpyridines, stabilized
UN3076	Aluminum alkyl hydrides
NA3077	Hazardous waste, solid, n.o.s.
NA3077	Other regulated substances, solid, n.o.s.
UN3077	Environmentally hazardous substances, solid, n.o.s.
UN3078	Cerium
UN3079	Methacrylonitrile, stabilized
UN3080	Isocyanates, toxic, flammable, n.o.s. or Isocyanate solutions, toxic, flammable, n.o.s.
NA3082	Hazardous waste, liquid, n.o.s.
NA3082	Other regulated substances, liquid, n.o.s.
UN3082	Environmentally hazardous substances, liquid, n.o.s.
UN3083	Perchloryl fluoride
UN3084	Corrosive solids, oxidizing, n.o.s.
UN3085	Oxidizing solid, corrosive, n.o.s.
UN3086	Toxic solids, oxidizing, n.o.s.
UN3087	Oxidizing solid, toxic, n.o.s.
UN3088	Self-heating, solid, organic, n.o.s.
UN3089	Metal powders, flammable, n.o.s.
UN3090	Lithium battery
UN3091	Lithium batteries, contained in equipment
UN3091	Lithium batteries, packed with equipment
UN3092	1-Methoxy-2-proponal
UN3093	Corrosive liquids, oxidizing, n.o.s.
UN3094	Corrosive liquids, water-reactive, n.o.s.
UN3095	Corrosive solids, self-heating, n.o.s.
UN3096	Corrosive solids, water-reactive, n.o.s.
UN3097	Flammable solid, oxidizing, n.o.s.
UN3098	Oxidizing liquid, corrosive, n.o.s.
UN3099	Oxidizing liquid, toxic, n.o.s.
UN3100	Oxidizing solid, self-heating, n.o.s.
UN3101	Organic peroxide type B, liquid
UN3102	Organic peroxide type B, solid
UN3103	Organic peroxide type C, liquid
UN3104	Organic peroxide type C, solid
UN3105	Organic peroxide type D, liquid
UN3106	Organic peroxide type D, solid
UN3107	Organic peroxide type E, liquid
UN3108	Organic peroxide type E, solid

ID Number	Description
UN3109	Organic peroxide type F, liquid
UN3110	Organic peroxide type F, solid
UN3111	Organic peroxide type B, liquid, temperature controlled
UN3112	Organic peroxide type B, solid, temperature controlled
UN3113	Organic peroxide type C, liquid, temperature controlled
UN3114	Organic peroxide type C, solid, temperature controlled
UN3115	Organic peroxide type D, liquid, temperature controlled
UN3116	Organic peroxide type D, solid, temperature controlled
UN3117	Organic peroxide type E, liquid, temperature controlled
UN3118	Organic peroxide type E, solid, temperature controlled
UN3119	Organic peroxide type F, liquid, temperature controlled
UN3120	Organic peroxide type F, solid, temperature controlled
UN3121	Oxidizing solid, water-reactive, n.o.s.
UN3122	Toxic liquids, oxidizing, n.o.s.
UN3123	Toxic liquids, water-reactive, n.o.s.
UN3124	Toxic solids, self-heating, n.o.s.
UN3125	Toxic solids, water-reactive, n.o.s.
UN3126	Self-heating, solid, corrosive, organic, n.o.s.
UN3127	Self-heating, solid, oxidizing, n.o.s.
UN3128	Self-heating, solid, toxic, organic, n.o.s.
UN3129	Water-reactive liquid, corrosive, n.o.s.
UN3130	Water-reactive liquid, toxic, n.o.s.
UN3131	Water-reactive solid, corrosive, n.o.s.
UN3132	Water-reactive solid, flammable, n.o.s.
UN3133	Water-reactive solid, oxidizing, n.o.s.
UN3134	Water-reactive solid, toxic, n.o.s.
UN3135	Water-reactive solid, self-heating, n.o.s.
UN3136	Trifluoromethane, refrigerated liquid
UN3137	Oxidizing, solid, flammable, n.o.s.
UN3138	Ethylene, acetylene and propylene in mixture, refrigerated liquid
UN3139	Oxidizing, liquid, n.o.s.
UN3140	Alkaloids, liquid, n.o.s. or Alkaloid salts, liquid, n.o.s.
UN3141	Antimony compounds, inorganic, liquid, n.o.s.
UN3142	Disinfectants, liquid, toxic, n.o.s
UN3143	Dyes, solid, toxic, n.o.s. or Dye intermediates, solid, toxic, n.o.s.
UN3144	Nicotine compounds, liquid, n.o.s. or Nicotine preparations, liquid, n.o.s.
UN3145	Alkylphenols, liquid, n.o.s.
UN3146	Organotin compounds, solid, n.o.s.
UN3147	Dyes, solid, corrosive, n.o.s. or Dye intermediates, solid, corrosive, n.o.s.
UN3148	Water-reactive, liquid, n.o.s.
UN3149	Hydrogen peroxide and peroxyacetic acid mixtures, stabilized
UN3150	Devices, small, hydrocarbon gas powered or Hydrocarbon gas refills for small devices

ID Number	Description
UN3151	Polyhalogenated biphenyls, liquid or Polyhalogenated terphenyls liquid
UN3152	Polyhalogenated biphenyls, solid or Polyhalogenated terphenyls, solid
UN3153	Perfluoro(methyl vinyl ether)
UN3154	Perfluoro(ethyl vinyl ether)
UN3155	Pentachlorophenol
UN3156	Compressed gas, oxidizing, n.o.s.
UN3157	Liquefied gas, oxidizing, n.o.s.
UN3158	Gas, refrigerated liquid, n.o.s.
UN3159	1,1,1,2-Tetrafluoroethane or Refrigerant gas R 134a
UN3160	Liquefied gas, toxic, flammable, n.o.s.
UN3161	Liquefied gas, flammable, n.o.s.
UN3162	Liquefied gas, toxic, n.o.s.
UN3163	Liquefied gas, n.o.s.
UN3164	Articles, pressurized pneumatic or hydraulic
UN3165	Aircraft hydraulic power unit fuel tank
UN3166	Engines, internal combustion
UN3166	Vehicle, flammable gas powered
UN3166	Vehicle, flammable liquid powered
UN3167	Gas sample, non-pressurized, flammable, n.o.s.
UN3168	Gas sample, non-pressurized, toxic, flammable, n.o.s.
UN3169	Gas sample, non-pressurized, toxic, n.o.s.
UN3170	Aluminum smelting by-products or Aluminum remelting by-products
UN3171	Battery-powered vehicle or Battery-powered equipment
UN3172	Toxins, extracted from living sources, liquid, n.o.s.
UN3174	Titanium disulphide
UN3175	Solids containing flammable liquid, n.o.s.
UN3176	Flammable solid, organic, molten, n.o.s.
NA3178	Smokeless powder for small arms
UN3178	Flammable solid, inorganic, n.o.s.
UN3179	Flammable solid, toxic, inorganic, n.o.s.
UN3180	Flammable solid, corrosive, inorganic, n.o.s.
UN3181	Metal salts of organic compounds, flammable, n.o.s.
UN3182	Metal hydrides, flammable, n.o.s.
UN3183	Self-heating liquid, organic, n.o.s.
UN3184	Self-heating liquid, toxic, organic, n.o.s.
UN3185	Self-heating liquid, corrosive, organic, n.o.s.
UN3186	Self-heating liquid, inorganic, n.o.s.
UN3187	Self-heating liquid, toxic, inorganic, n.o.s.
UN3188	Self-heating liquid, corrosive, inorganic, n.o.s.
UN3189	Metal powder, self-heating, n.o.s.
UN3190	Self-heating solid, inorganic, n.o.s.
UN3191	Self-heating solid, toxic, inorganic, n.o.s.

ID Number	Description
UN3192	Self-heating solid, corrosive, inorganic, n.o.s.
UN3194	Pyrophoric liquid, inorganic, n.o.s.
UN3200	Pyrophoric solid, inorganic, n.o.s.
UN3205	Alkaline earth metal alcoholates, n.o.s.
UN3206	Alkali metal alcoholates, self-heating, corrosive, n.o.s.
UN3208	Metallic substance, water-reactive, n.o.s.
UN3209	Metallic substance, water-reactive, self-heating, n.o.s.
UN3210	Chlorates, inorganic, aqueous solution, n.o.s.
UN3211	Perchlorates, inorganic, aqueous solution, n.o.s.
UN3212	Hypochlorites, inorganic, n.o.s.
UN3213	Bromates, inorganic, aqueous solution, n.o.s.
UN3214	Permanganates, inorganic, aqueous solution, n.o.s.
UN3215	Persulfates, inorganic, n.o.s.
UN3216	Persulfates, inorganic, aqueous solution, n.o.s.
UN3218	Nitrates, inorganic, aqueous solution, n.o.s.
UN3219	Nitrites, inorganic, aqueous solution, n.o.s.
UN3220	Pentafluoroethane or Refrigerant gas R 125
UN3221	Self-reactive liquid type B
UN3222	Self-reactive solid type B
UN3223	Self-reactive liquid type C
UN3224	Self-reactive solid type C
UN3225	Self-reactive liquid type D
UN3226	Self-reactive solid type D
UN3227	Self-reactive liquid type E
UN3228	Self-reactive solid type E
UN3229	Self-reactive liquid type F
UN3230	Self-reactive solid type F
UN3231	Self-reactive liquid type B, temperature controlled
UN3232	Self-reactive solid type B, temperature controlled
UN3233	Self-reactive liquid type C, temperature controlled
UN3234	Self-reactive solid type C, temperature controlled
UN3235	Self-reactive liquid type D, temperature controlled
UN3236	Self-reactive solid type D, temperature controlled
UN3237	Self-reactive liquid type E, temperature controlled
UN3238	Self-reactive solid type E, temperature controlled
UN3239	Self-reactive liquid type F, temperature controlled
UN3240	Self-reactive solid type F, temperature controlled
UN3241	2-Bromo-2-nitropropane-1,3-diol
UN3242	Azodicarbonamide
UN3243	Solids containing toxic liquid, n.o.s.
UN3244	Solids containing corrosive liquid, n.o.s.
UN3246	Methanesulfonyl chloride
UN3247	Sodium peroxoborate, anhydrous
UN3248	Medicine, liquid, flammable, toxic, n.o.s.

ID Number	Description
UN3249	Medicine, solid, toxic, n.o.s.
UN3250	Chloroacetic acid, molten
UN3251	Isosorbide-5-mononitrate
UN3252	Difluoromethane or Refrigerant gas R 32
UN3253	Disodium trioxosilicate
UN3254	Tributylphosphane
UN3255	tert-Butyl hypochlorite
UN3256	Elevated temperature liquid, flammable, n.o.s.
UN3257	Elevated temperature liquid, n.o.s.
UN3258	Elevated temperature solid, n.o.s.
UN3259	Amines, solid, corrosive, n.o.s. or, Polyamines, solid, corrosive n.o.s.
UN3260	Corrosive solid, acidic, inorganic, n.o.s.
UN3261	Corrosive solid, acidic, organic, n.o.s.
UN3262	Corrosive solid, basic, inorganic, n.o.s.
UN3263	Corrosive solid, basic, organic, n.o.s.
UN3264	Corrosive liquid, acidic, inorganic, n.o.s.
UN3265	Corrosive liquid, acidic, organic, n.o.s.
UN3266	Corrosive liquid, basic, inorganic, n.o.s.
UN3267	Corrosive liquid, basic, organic, n.o.s.
UN3268	Air bag inflators or Air bag modules or Seat-belt pre-tensioners
UN3269	Polyester resin kit
UN3270	Nitrocellulose membrane filters
UN3271	Ethers, n.o.s.
UN3272	Esters, n.o.s.
UN3273	Nitriles, flammable, toxic, n.o.s.
UN3274	Alcoholates solution, n.o.s.
UN3275	Nitriles, toxic, flammable, n.o.s.
UN3276	Nitriles, toxic, liquid, n.o.s.
UN3277	Chloroformates, toxic, corrosive, n.o.s.
UN3278	Organophosphorus compound, toxic, liquid, n.o.s.
UN3279	Organophosphorus compound, toxic, flammable, n.o.s.
UN3280	Organoarsenic compound, liquid, n.o.s.
UN3281	Metal carbonyls, liquid, n.o.s.
UN3282	Organometallic compound, toxic, liquid, n.o.s.
UN3283	Selenium compound, solid, n.o.s.
UN3284	Tellurium compound, n.o.s.
UN3285	Vanadium compound, n.o.s.
UN3286	Flammable liquid, toxic, corrosive, n.o.s.
UN3287	Toxic liquid, inorganic, n.o.s.
UN3288	Toxic solid, inorganic, n.o.s.
UN3289	Toxic liquid, corrosive, inorganic, n.o.s.
UN3290	Toxic solid, corrosive, inorganic, n.o.s.
UN3291	Regulated medical waste

ID Number	Description
UN3292	Batteries, containing sodium
UN3292	Cells, containing sodium
UN3293	Hydrazine, aqueous solution
UN3294	Hydrogen cyanide, solution in alcohol
UN3295	Hydrocarbons, liquid, n.o.s.
UN3296	Heptafluoropropane or Refrigerant gas R 227
UN3297	Ethylene oxide and chlorotetra-fluoroethane mixture
UN3298	Ethylene oxide and pentafluoroethane mixture
UN3299	Ethylene oxide and tetrafluorethane mixture
UN3300	Ethylene oxide and carbon dioxide mixture
UN3301	Corrosive liquid, self-heating, n.o.s.
UN3302	2-Dimethylaminoethyl acrylate
UN3303	Compressed gas, toxic, oxidizing, n.o.s.
UN3304	Compressed gas, toxic, corrosive, n.o.s.
UN3305	Compressed gas, toxic, flammable, corrosive, n.o.s.
UN3306	Compressed gas, toxic, oxidizing, corrosive, n.o.s.
UN3307	Liquified gas, toxic, oxidizing, n.o.s.
UN3308	Liquified gas, toxic, corrosive, n.o.s.
UN3309	Liquified gas, toxic, flammable, corrosive, n.o.s.
UN3310	Liquified gas, toxic, oxidizing, corrosive, n.o.s.
UN3311	Gas, refrigerated liquid, oxidizing, n.o.s.
UN3312	Gas, refrigerated liguid, flammable, n.o.s.
UN3313	Organic pigments, self-heating
UN3314	Plastic molding compound
UN3316	Chemical kits
UN3316	First aid kits
UN3317	2-Amino-4,6-Dinitrophenol, wetted
UN3318	Ammonia solution
UN3319	Nitroglycerin mixture, desensitized, solid, n.o.s.
UN3320	Sodium borohydride and sodium hydroxide solution
UN3321	Radioactive material, low specific activity (LSA-II)
UN3322	Radioactive material, low specific activity (LSA-III)
UN3327	Radioactive material, Type A package, fissile
UN3328	Radioactive material, Type B(U) package, fissile
UN3329	Radioactive material, Type B(M) package, fissile
UN3331	Radioactive material, transported under special arrangement, fissile
UN3332	Radioactive material, Type A package, special form
UN3333	Radioactive material, Type A package, special form, fissile
NA3334	Self-defense spray, non-pressurized
UN3334	Aviation regulated liquid, n.o.s.
UN3335	Aviation regulated solid, n.o.s.
UN3336	Mercaptans, liquid, flammable, n.o.s. or Mercaptan mixture, liquid, flammable, n.o.s.
UN3337	Refrigerant gas R404A

ID Number	Description
UN3338	Refrigerant gas R407A
UN3339	Refrigerant gas R407B
UN3340	Refrigerant gas R407C
UN3341	Thiourea dioxide
UN3342	Xanthates
UN3343	Nitroglycerin mixture, desensitized, liquid, flammable, n.o.s.
UN3344	Pentaerythrit tetranitrate mixture, desensitized solid, n.o.s.
UN3345	Phenoxyacetic acid derivative pesticide, solid, toxic
UN3346	Phenoxyacetic acid derivative pesticide, liquid, flammable, toxic
UN3347	Phenoxyacetic acid derivative pesticide, liquid, toxic, flammable
UN3348	Phenoxyacetic acid derivative pesticide, liquid, toxic
UN3349	Pyrethroid pesticide, solid, toxic
UN3350	Pyrethroid pesticide, liquid, flammable, toxic
UN3351	Pyrethroid pesticide, liquid, toxic, flammable
UN3352	Pyrethroid pesticide, liquid, toxic
UN3353	Air bag inflators, compressed gas or Air bag modules, compressed gas or seat-belt pretensioners, compressed gas
UN3354	Insecticide gases, flammable, n.o.s.
UN3355	Insecticide gases toxic, flammable, n.o.s.
NA3356	Oxygen generator, chemical, spent
UN3356	Oxygen generator, chemical
UN3357	Nitroglycerin mixture, desensitized, liquid, n.o.s.
UN3358	Refrigerating machines
UN3360	Fibers, vegetable, dry
UN3361	Chlorosilanes, toxic, corrosive, n.o.s.
UN3362	Chlorosilanes, toxic, corrosive, flammable, n.o.s.
UN3363	Dangerous goods in machinery or Dangerous goods in apparatus
UN3364	Trinitrophenol (picric acid), wetted
UN3365	Trinitrochlorobenzene (picryl chloride), wetted
UN3366	Trinitrotoluene (TNT), wetted
UN3367	Trinitrobenzene, wetted
UN3368	Trinitrobenzoic acid, wetted
UN3369	Sodium dinitro-o-cresolate, wetted
UN3370	Urea nitrate, wetted
UN3371	2-Methylbutanal
UN3375	Ammonium nitrate emulsion or Ammonium nitrate suspension or Ammonium nitrate gel
UN3376	4-Nitrophenylhydrazine
UN3377	Sodium perborate monohydrate
UN3378	Sodium carbonate peroxyhydrate
UN3379	Desensitized explosive, liquid, n.o.s.
UN3380	Desensitized explosive, solid, n.o.s.
UN3381	Toxic by inhalation liquid, n.o.s.
UN3382	Toxic by inhalation liquid, n.o.s.

ID Number	Description
UN3383	Toxic by inhalation liquid, flammable, n.o.s.
UN3384	Toxic by inhalation liquid, flammable, n.o.s.
UN3385	Toxic by inhalation liquid, water-reactive, n.o.s.
UN3386	Toxic by inhalation liquid, water-reactive, n.o.s.
UN3387	Toxic by inhalation liquid, oxidizing, n.o.s.
UN3388	Toxic by inhalation liquid, oxidizing, n.o.s.
UN3389	Toxic by inhalation liquid, corrosive, n.o.s.
UN3390	Toxic by inhalation liquid, corrosive, n.o.s.
UN3391	Organometallic substance, solid, pyrophoric
UN3392	Organometallic substance, liquid, pyrophoric
UN3393	Organometallic substance, solid, pyrophoric, water-reactive
UN3394	Organometallic substance, liquid, pyrophoric, water-reactive
UN3395	Organometallic substance, solid, water-reactive
UN3396	Organometallic substance, solid, water-reactive, flammable
UN3397	Organometallic substance, solid, water-reactive, self-heating
UN3398	Organometallic substance, liquid, water-reactive
UN3399	Organometallic substance, liquid, water-reactive, flammable
UN3400	Organometallic substance, solid, self-heating
UN3401	Alkali metal amalgam, solid
UN3402	Alkaline earth metal amalgams, solid
UN3403	Potassium, metal alloys, solid
UN3404	Potassium sodium alloys, solid
UN3405	Barium chlorate, solution
UN3406	Barium perchlorate, solution
UN3407	Chlorate and magnesium chloride mixture solution
UN3408	Lead perchlorate, solution
UN3409	Chloronitrobenzene, liquid
UN3410	4-Chloro-o-toluidine hydrochloride, solution
UN3411	beta-Naphthylamine solution
UN3413	Potassium cyanide solution
UN3414	Sodium cyanide solution
UN3415	Sodium fluoride solution
UN3416	Chloroacetophenone, liquid
UN3417	Xylyl bromide, solid
UN3418	2,4-Toluylenediamine solution or 2,4-Toluenediamine solution
UN3419	Boron trifluoride acetic acid complex, solid
UN3420	Boron trifluoride propionic acid complex, solid
UN3421	Potassium hydrogendifluoride solution
UN3422	Potassium fluoride solution
UN3423	Tetramethylammonium hydroxide, solid
UN3424	Ammonium dinitro-o-cresolate solution
UN3425	Bromoacetic acid solid
UN3426	Acrylamide solution
UN3427	Chlorobenzyl chlorides, solid

ID Number	Description
UN3428	3-Chloro-4-methylphenyl isocyanate, solid
UN3429	Chlorotoluidines, liquid
UN3430	Xylenols, liquid
UN3431	Nitrobenzotrifluorides, solid
UN3432	Polychlorinated biphenyls, solid
UN3433	Lithium alkyls, solid
UN3434	Nitrocresols, liquid
UN3435	Hydroquinone solution
UN3436	Hexafluoroacetone hydrate, solid
UN3437	Chlorocresols, solid
UN3438	alpha-Methylbenzyl alcohol, solid
UN3439	Nitriles, toxic, solid, n.o.s.
UN3440	Selenium compound, liquid, n.o.s.
UN3441	Chlorodinitro-benzenes, solid
UN3442	Dichloroanilines, solid
UN3443	Dinitrobenzenes, solid
UN3444	Nicotine hydrochloride, solid
UN3445	Nicotine sulphate, solid
UN3446	Nitrotoluenes, solid
UN3447	Nitroxylenes, solid
UN3448	Tear gas substance, solid, n.o.s.
UN3449	Bromobenzyl cyanides, solid
UN3450	Diphenyl-chloroarsine, solid
UN3451	Toluidines, solid
UN3452	Xylidines, solid
UN3453	Phosphoric acid, solid
UN3454	Dinitrotoluenes, solid
UN3455	Cresols, solid
UN3456	Nitrosylsulphuric acid, solid
UN3457	Chloronitrotoluenes, solid
UN3458	Nitroanisoles, solid
UN3459	Nitrobromobenzenes, solid
UN3460	N-Ethylbenzyltoluidines, solid
UN3461	Aluminum alkyl halides, solid
UN3462	Toxins, extracted from living sources, solid, n.o.s.
UN3464	Organophosphorus compound, toxic, solid, n.o.s.
UN3465	Organoarsenic compound, solid, n.o.s.
UN3466	Metal carbonyls, solid, n.o.s.
UN3467	Organometallic compound, toxic, solid, n.o.s.
UN3468	Hydrogen in a metal hydride storage system
NA9035	Gas identification set
NA9191	Chlorine dioxide, hydrate, frozen
NA9202	Carbon monoxide, refrigerated liquid
NA9206	Methyl phosphonic dichloride

ID Number	Description
NA9260	Aluminum, molten
NA9263	Chloropivaloyl chloride
NA9264	3,5-Dichloro-2,4,6-trifluoropyridine
NA9269	Trimethoxysilane

Hazardous Materials Table

PUBLISHER'S NOTE: Space limitations preclude our using the entire §172.101 Hazardous Materials Table. We are including the first seven columns of the table. We are also including a ERG Guide No. column and a placard column, which directly relate to drivers of vehicles transporting hazardous materials.

§172.101 Purpose and use of hazardous materials table.

(a) The Hazardous Materials Table (Table) in this section designates the materials listed therein as hazardous materials for the purpose of transportation of those materials. For each listed material, the Table identifies the hazard class or specifies that the material is forbidden in transportation, and gives the proper shipping name or directs the user to the preferred proper shipping name. In addition, the Table specifies or references requirements in this subchapter pertaining to labeling, packaging, quantity limits aboard aircraft and stowage of hazardous materials aboard vessels.

(b) ***Column 1: Symbols.*** Column 1 of the Table contains six symbols ("+", "A", "D", "G", "I", and "W"), as follows:

(1) The plus (+) sign fixes the proper shipping name, hazard class and packing group for that entry without regard to whether the material meets the definition of that class, packing group or any other hazard class definition. When the plus sign is assigned to a proper shipping name in Column (1) of the §172.101 Table, it means that the material is known to pose a risk to humans. When a plus sign is assigned to mixtures or solutions containing a material where the hazard to humans is significantly different from that of the pure material or where no hazard to humans is posed, the material may be described using an alternative shipping name that represents the hazards posed by the material. An appropriate alternate proper shipping name and hazard class may be authorized by the Associate Administrator.

(2) The letter "A" restricts the application of requirements of this subchapter to materials offered or intended for transportation by aircraft, unless the material is a hazardous substance or a hazardous waste.

(3) The letter "D" identifies proper shipping names which are appropriate for describing materials for domestic transportation but may be inappropriate for international transportation under the provisions of international regulations (e.g., IMO, ICAO). An alternate proper shipping name may be selected when either domestic or international transportation is involved.

(4) The letter "G" identifies proper shipping names for which one or more technical names of the hazardous material must be entered in parentheses, in association with the basic description. (See §172.203(k).)

(5) The letter "I" identifies proper shipping names which are appropriate for describing materials in international transportation. An alternate proper shipping name may be selected when only domestic transportation is involved.

(6) The letter "W" restricts the application of requirements of this subchapter to materials offered or intended for transportation by vessel, unless the material is a hazardous substance or a hazardous waste.

(c) ***Column 2: Hazardous materials descriptions and proper shipping names.*** Column 2 lists the hazardous materials descriptions and proper shipping names of materials designated as hazardous materials. Modification of a proper shipping name may otherwise be required or authorized by this section. Proper shipping names are limited to those shown in Roman type (not italics).

(1) Proper shipping names may be used in the singular or plural and in either capital or lower case letters. Words may be alternatively spelled in the same manner as they appear in the ICAO Technical Instructions or the IMDG Code. For example "aluminum" may be spelled "aluminium" and "sulfur" may be spelled "sulphur". However, the word "inflammable" may not be used in place of the word "flammable".

(2) Punctuation marks and words in italics are not part of the proper shipping name, but may be used in addition to the proper shipping name. The word "or" in italics indicates that terms in the sequence may be used as the proper shipping name, as appropriate.

(3) The word "poison" or "poisonous" may be used interchangeably with the word "toxic" when only domestic transpor-

tation is involved. The abbreviation "n.o.i." or "n.o.i.b.n." may be used interchangeably with "n.o.s.".

(4) Except for hazardous wastes, when qualifying words are used as part of the proper shipping name, their sequence in the package markings and shipping paper description is optional. However, the entry in the Table reflects the preferred sequence.

(5) When one entry references another entry by use of the word "see", if both names are in Roman type, either name may be used as the proper shipping name (e.g., Ethyl alcohol, *see* Ethanol).

(6) When a proper shipping name includes a concentration range as part of the shipping description, the actual concentration, if it is within the range stated, may be used in place of the concentration range. For example, an aqueous solution of hydrogen peroxide containing 30 percent peroxide may be described as "Hydrogen peroxide, aqueous solution *with not less than 20 percent but not more than 40 percent hydrogen peroxide*" or "Hydrogen peroxide, aqueous solution *with 30 percent hydrogen peroxide*".

(7) Use of the prefix "mono" is optional in any shipping name, when appropriate. Thus, Iodine monochloride may be used interchangeably with Iodine chloride. In "Glycerol alpha-monochlorohydrin" the term "mono" is considered a prefix to the term "chlorohydrin" and may be deleted.

(8) Use of the word "liquid" or "solid". The word "liquid" or "solid" may be added to a proper shipping name when a hazardous material specifically listed by name may, due to differing physical states, be a liquid or solid. When the packaging specified in Column 8 is inappropriate for the physical state of the material, the table provided in paragraph (i)(4) of this section should be used to determine the appropriate packaging section.

(9) *Hazardous wastes.* If the word "waste" is not included in the hazardous material description in Column 2 of the Table, the proper shipping name for a hazardous waste (as defined in §171.8 of this subchapter), shall include the word "Waste" preceding the proper shipping name of the material. For example: Waste acetone.

(10) *Mixtures and solutions.* (i) A mixture or solution not identified specifically by name, comprised of a hazardous mate-

rial identified in the Table by technical name and non-hazardous material, shall be described using the proper shipping name of the hazardous material and the qualifying word “mixture” or “solution”, as appropriate, unless–

(A) Except as provided in §172.101(i)(4) the packaging specified in Column 8 is inappropriate to the physical state of the material;

(B) The shipping description indicates that the proper shipping name applies only to the pure or technically pure hazardous material;

(C) The hazard class, packing group, or subsidiary hazard of the mixture or solution is different from that specified for the entry;

(D) There is a significant change in the measures to be taken in emergencies;

(E) The material is identified by special provision in Column 7 of the §172.101 Table as a material poisonous by inhalation; however, it no longer meets the definition of poisonous by inhalation or it falls within a different hazard zone than that specified in the special provision; or

(F) The material can be appropriately described by a shipping name that describes its intended application, such as “Coating solution", “Extracts, flavoring" or “Compound, cleaning liquid".

(ii) If one or more of the conditions specified in paragraph (c)(10)(i) of this section is satisfied then a proper shipping name shall be selected as prescribed in paragraph (c)(12)(ii) of this section.

(iii) A mixture or solution not identified in the Table specifically by name, comprised of two or more hazardous materials in the same hazard class, shall be described using an appropriate shipping description (e.g., “Flammable liquid, n.o.s.”). The name that most appropriately describes the material shall be used; e.g., an alcohol not listed by its technical name in the Table shall be described as “Alcohol, n.o.s.” rather than “Flammable liquid, n.o.s.”. Some mixtures may be more appropriately described according to their application, such as “Coating solution” or “Extracts, flavoring liquid” rather than by an n.o.s. entry. Under the provisions of subparts C and D of this part, the technical names of at least two components most predominately contributing to the hazards of the mixture or solution may be required in association with the proper shipping name.

(11) Except for a material subject to or prohibited by §§173.21, 173.54, 173.56(d), 173.56(e), 173.224(c) or 173.225(b) of this subchapter, a material that is considered to be a hazardous waste or a sample of a material for which the hazard class is uncertain and must be determined by testing may be assigned a tentative proper shipping name, hazard class, identification number and packing group, if applicable, based on the shipper's tentative determination according to:

(i) Defining criteria in this subchapter;

(ii) The hazard precedence prescribed in §173.2a of this subchapter;

(iii) The shippers knowledge of the material;

(iv) In addition to paragraphs (c)(11)(i) through (iii) of this section, for a sample of a material other than a waste, the following must be met:

(A) Except when the word "Sample" already appears in the proper shipping name, the word "Sample" must appear as part of the proper shipping name or in association with the basic description on the shipping paper;

(B) When the proper shipping description for a sample is assigned a "G" in Column (1) of the §172.101 Table, and the primary constituent(s) for which the tentative classification is based are not known, the provisions requiring a technical name for the constituent(s) do not apply; and

(C) A sample must be transported in a combination packaging which conforms to the requirements of this subchapter that are applicable to the tentative packing group assigned, and may not exceed a net mass of 2.5 kg. (5.5 pounds) per package.

Note to Paragraph (c)(11): For the transportation of self-reactive, organic peroxide and explosive samples, see §§173.224(c)(3), 173.225(b)(2) and 173.56(d) of this subchapter, respectively.

(12) Except when the proper shipping name in the Table is preceded by a plus (+)—

(i) If it is specifically determined that a material meets the definition of a hazard class or packing group, other than the class or packing group shown in association with the proper shipping name, or does not meet the defining criteria for a subsidiary hazard shown in Column 6 of the Table, the material shall be described by an appropriate proper shipping name listed in association with the correct hazard class, packing group, or subsidiary hazard for the material.

(ii) *Generic or n.o.s. descriptions.* If an appropriate technical name is not shown in the Table, selection of a proper shipping name shall be made from the generic or n.o.s. descriptions corresponding to the specific hazard class, packing group, or subsidiary hazard, if any, for the material. The name that most appropriately describes the material shall be used; e.g, an alcohol not listed by its technical name in the Table shall be described as "Alcohol, n.o.s." rather than "Flammable liquid, n.o.s.". Some mixtures may be more appropriately described according to their application, such as "Coating solution" or "Extracts, flavoring, liquid", rather than by an n.o.s. entry, such as "Flammable liquid, n.o.s." It should be noted, however, that an n.o.s. description as a proper shipping name may not provide sufficient information for shipping papers and package marking. Under the provisions of subparts C and D of this part, the technical name of one or more constituents which makes the product a hazardous material may be required in association with the proper shipping name.

(iii) *Multiple hazard materials.* If a material meets the definition of more than one hazard class, and is not identified in the Table specifically by name (e.g., acetyl chloride), the hazard class of the material shall be determined by using the precedence specified in §173.2a of this subchapter, and an appropriate shipping description (e.g., "Flammable liquid, corrosive n.o.s.") shall be selected as described in paragraph (c)(12)(ii) of this section.

(iv) If it is specifically determined that a material is not a forbidden material and does not meet the definition of any hazard class, the material is not a hazardous material.

(13) *Self-reactive materials and organic peroxides.* A generic proper shipping name for a self-reactive material or an organic peroxide, as listed in Column 2 of the Table, must be selected based on the material's technical name and concentration, in accordance with the provisions of §§173.224 or 173.225 of this subchapter, respectively.

(14) A proper shipping name that describes all isomers of a material may be used to identify any isomer of that material if the isomer meets criteria for the same hazard class or division, subsidiary risk(s) and packing group, unless the isomer is specifically identified in the Table.

(15) Unless a hydrate is specifically listed in the Table, a proper shipping name for the equivalent anhydrous substance may be used, if the hydrate meets the same hazard class or division, subsidiary risk(s) and packing group.

(16) Unless it is already included in the proper shipping name in the §172.101 Table, the qualifying words "liquid" or "solid" may be added in association with the proper shipping name when a hazardous material specifically listed by name in the §172.101 Table may, due to the differing physical states of the various isomers of the material, be either a liquid or a solid (for example "Dinitrotoluenes, liquid" and "Dinitrotoluenes, solid"). Use of the words "liquid" or "solid" is subject to the limitations specified for the use of the words "mixture" or "solution" in paragraph (c)(10) of this section. The qualifying word "molten" may be added in association with the proper shipping name when a hazardous material, which is a solid in accordance with the definition in §171.8 of this subchapter, is offered for transportation in the molten state (for example, "Alkylphenols, solid, n.o.s., molten").

(d) ***Column 3: Hazard class or Division.*** Column 3 contains a designation of the hazard class or division corresponding to each proper shipping name, or the word "Forbidden".

(1) A material for which the entry in this column is "Forbidden" may not be offered for transportation or transported. This prohibition does not apply if the material is diluted, stabilized or incorporated in a device and it is classed in accordance with the definitions of hazardous materials contained in part 173 of this subchapter.

(2) When a reevaluation of test data or new data indicates a need to modify the "Forbidden" designation or the hazard class or packing group specified for a material specifically identified in the Table, this data should be submitted to the Associate Administrator.

(3) A basic description of each hazard class and the section reference for class definitions appear in §173.2 of this subchapter.

(4) When an entry in this column reads "Comb liq", the material is assigned to the hazard class "Combustible liquid." Additionally, each reference to a Class 3 material is modified to read "Combustible liquid" when that material is reclassified in accordance with §173.150(e) or (f) of this subchapter or has a flash point above 60.5°C (141°F) but below 93°C (200°F).

(e) ***Column 4: Identification number.*** Column 4 lists the identification number assigned to each proper shipping name. Those preceded by the letter "UN" are associated with proper shipping names considered appropriate for international transportation as well as domestic transportation. Those preceded by the letters "NA" are associated with proper shipping names not recognized for international transportation, except to and from Canada. Identification numbers in the "NA9000" series are associated with proper shipping names not appropriately covered by international hazardous materials (dangerous goods) transportation standards, or not appropriately addressed by the international transportation standards for emergency response information purposes, except for transportation between the United States and Canada.

(f) ***Column 5: Packing group.*** Column 5 specifies one or more packing groups assigned to a material corresponding to the proper shipping name and hazard class for that material. Class 2, Class 7, Division 6.2 (other than regulated medical wastes), and ORM–D materials, do not have packing groups, Packing Groups I, II, and III indicate the degree of danger presented by the material is either great, medium or minor, respectively. If more than one packing group is indicated for an entry, the packing group for the hazardous material is determined using the criteria for assignment of packing groups specified in subpart D of part 173. When a reevaluation of test data or new data indicates a need to modify the specified packing group(s), the data should be submitted to the Associate Administrator. Each reference in this column to a material which is a hazardous waste or a hazardous substance, and whose proper shipping name is preceded in Column 1 of the Table by the letter "A" or "W", is modified to read "III" on those occasions when the material is offered for transportation or transported by a mode in which its transportation is not otherwise subject to requirements of this subchapter.

(g) ***Column 6: Labels.*** Column 6 specifies codes which represent the hazard warning labels required for a package filled with a material conforming to the associated hazard class and proper shipping name, unless the package is otherwise excepted from labeling by a provision in subpart E of this part, or part 173 of this subchapter. The first code is indicative of the primary hazard of the material.

Additional label codes are indicative of subsidiary hazards. Provisions in §172.402 may require that a label other than that specified in Column 6 be affixed to the package in addition to that specified in Column 6. No label is required for a material classed as a combustible liquid or for a Class 3 material that is reclassed as a combustible liquid. The codes contained in Column 6 are defined according to the following table:

LABEL SUBSTITUTION TABLE

Label code	Label name
1	Explosive.
1.1[1]	Explosive 1.1.[1]
1.2[1]	Explosive 1.2.[1]
1.3[1]	Explosive 1.3.[1]
1.4[1]	Explosive 1.4.[1]
1.5[1]	Explosive 1.5.[1]
1.6[1]	Explosive 1.6.[1]
2.1	Flammable Gas.
2.2	Non-Flammable Gas.
2.3	Poison Gas.
3	Flammable Liquid.
4.1	Flammable Solid.
4.2	Spontaneously Combustible.
4.3	Dangerous When Wet.
5.1	Oxidizer.
5.2	Organic Peroxide.
6.1 (inhalation hazard, Zone A or B)	Poison Inhalation Hazard.
6.1 (other than inhalation hazard, Zone A or B)[2]	Poison.
6.2	Infectious Substance.
7	Radioactive.
8	Corrosive.
9	Class 9.

[1] Refers to the appropriate compatibility group letter.
[2] The packing group for a material is indicated in column 5 of the table.

(h) ***Column 7: Special provisions.*** Column 7 specifies codes for special provisions applicable to hazardous materials. When Column 7 refers to a special provision for a hazardous material, the meaning and requirements of that special provision are as set forth in §172.102 of this subpart.

ERG Guide No. The ERG Guide No. column is not part of the §172.101 Table in the Hazardous Materials Regulations. This column has been added for your convenience. This column provides the three-digit emergency response guide page number assigned to the name of the material in the 2004 Emergency Response Guidebook.

The letter "P" following some guide numbers indicates that the material may undergo violent polymerization if subjected to heat or contamination.

ERG Guide numbers that are shaded indicate that the Table of Initial Isolation and Protective Action Distances (the green pages of the ERG) should be consulted. These materials are either TIH (Toxic Inhalation Hazard) material, or a chemical warfare agent, or a Dangerous Water Reactive Material (produces toxic gas upon contact with water).

Placard Advisory. The placard advisory column is not part of the §172.101 Table in the Hazardous Materials Regulations. This column has been added for your convenience. It provides a quick indication of the placard required for the shipping description, based only on the information in the other columns of the §172.101 Table. To determine the actual placards required for a specific shipment, consult the Hazardous Materials Regulations (§172.504 & §172.505).

* - An asterisk after the placard name indicates that placarding is required for any quantity of material being transported. If multiple placards are listed, all placards are required for any quantity.

Sym-bols	Hazardous materials descriptions and proper shipping names	Hazard class or Division	Identification Numbers	PG	Label Codes	Special provisions (§172.102)	ERG Guide No.	Placard Advisory Consult §172.504 & §172.505 *Placard any quantity
(1)	(2)	(3)	(4)	(5)	(6)	(7)		
	Accellerene, see **p-Nitrosodimethylaniline**							
	Accumulators, electric, see **Batteries, wet** *etc.*							
	Accumulators, pressurized, pneumatic or hydraulic (containing non-flammable gas) see **Articles pressurized, pneumatic** *or* **hydraulic** *(containing non-flammable gas)*							
	Acetal	3	UN1088	II	3	IB2, T4, TP1	127	FLAMMABLE
	Acetaldehyde	3	UN1089	I	3	A3, B16, T11, TP2, TP7	129	FLAMMABLE
A	**Acetaldehyde ammonia**	9	UN1841	III	9	IB8, IP3, IP7, T1, TP33	171	CLASS 9
	Acetaldehyde oxime	3	UN2332	III	3	B1, IB3, T4, TP1	129	FLAMMABLE
	Acetic acid, glacial *or* **Acetic acid solution,** *with more than 80 percent acid, by mass*	8	UN2789	II	8, 3	A3, A6, A7, A10, B2, IB2, T7, TP2	132	CORROSIVE
	Acetic acid solution, *not less than 50 percent but not more than 80 percent acid, by mass*	8	UN2790	II	8	A3, A6, A7, A10, B2, IB2, T7, TP2	153	CORROSIVE
	Acetic acid solution, *with more than 10 percent and less than 50 percent acid, by mass*	8	UN2790	III	8	IB3, T4, TP1	153	CORROSIVE

Sym-bols	Hazardous materials descriptions and proper shipping names	Hazard class or Division	Identification Numbers	PG	Label Codes	Special provisions (§172.102)	ERG Guide No.	Placard Advisory Consult §172.504 & §172.505 *Placard any quantity
(1)	(2)	(3)	(4)	(5)	(6)	(7)		
	Acetic anhydride	8	UN1715	II	8, 3	A3, A6, A7, A10, B2, IB2, T7, TP2	137	CORROSIVE
	Acetone	3	UN1090	II	3	IB2, T4, TP1	127	FLAMMABLE
	Acetone cyanohydrin, stabilized	6.1	UN1541	I	6.1	2, B9, B14, B32, B76, B77, N34, T20, TP2, TP13, TP38, TP45	155	POISON INHALATION HAZARD*
	Acetone oils	3	UN1091	II	3	IB2, T4, TP1, TP8	127	FLAMMABLE
	Acetonitrile	3	UN1648	II	3	IB2, T7, TP2	127	FLAMMABLE
	Acetyl acetone peroxide with more than 9 percent by mass active oxygen	Forbidden						
	Acetyl benzoyl peroxide, solid, or with more than 40 percent in solution	Forbidden						
	Acetyl bromide	8	UN1716	II	8	B2, IB2, T8, TP2, TP12	156	CORROSIVE
	Acetyl chloride	3	UN1717	II	3, 8	A3, A6, A7, IB1, N34, T8, TP2, TP12	155	FLAMMABLE
	Acetyl cyclohexanesulfonyl peroxide, with more than 82 percent wetted with less than 12 percent water	Forbidden						
	Acetyl iodide	8	UN1898	II	8	B2, IB2, T7, TP2, TP13	156	CORROSIVE
	Acetyl methyl carbinol	3	UN2621	III	3	B1, IB3, T2, TP1	127	FLAMMABLE

Symbols	Hazardous materials descriptions and proper shipping names	Hazard class or Division	Identification Numbers	PG	Label Codes	Special provisions (§172.102)	ERG Guide No.	Placard Advisory Consult §172.504 & §172.505 *Placard any quantity
(1)	(2)	(3)	(4)	(5)	(6)	(7)		
	Acetyl peroxide, solid, or with more than 25 percent in solution	Forbidden						
	Acetylene, dissolved	2.1	UN1001		2.1		116	FLAMMABLE GAS
	Acetylene (liquefied)	Forbidden						
	Acetylene silver nitrate	Forbidden						
	Acetylene tetrabromide, see **Tetrabromoethane**							
	Acid butyl phosphate, see **Butyl acid phosphate**							
	Acid, sludge, *see* **Sludge acid**							
	Acridine	6.1	UN2713	III	6.1	IB8, IP3, T1, TP33	153	POISON
	Acrolein dimer, stabilized	3	UN2607	III	3	B1, IB3, T2, TP1	129P	FLAMMABLE
	Acrolein, stabilized	6.1	UN1092	I	6.1, 3	1, B9, B14, B30, B42, B72, B77, T22, TP2, TP7, TP13, TP38, TP44	131P	POISON INHALATION HAZARD*
	Acrylamide, solid	6.1	UN2074	III	6.1	IB8, IP3, T1, TP33	153P	POISON
	Acrylamide solution	6.1	UN3426	III	6.1	IB3, T4, TP1	153P	POISON
	Acrylic acid, stabilized	8	UN2218	II	8, 3	B2, IB2, T7, TP2	132P	CORROSIVE
	Acrylonitrile, stabilized	3	UN1093	I	3, 6.1	B9, T14, TP2, TP13	131P	FLAMMABLE

Sym-bols	Hazardous materials descriptions and proper shipping names	Hazard class or Division	Identification Numbers	PG	Label Codes	Special provisions (§172.102)	ERG Guide No.	Placard Advisory Consult §172.504 & §172.505 *Placard any quantity
(1)	(2)	(3)	(4)	(5)	(6)	(7)		
	Actuating cartridge, explosive, see **Cartridges, power device**							
	Adhesives, *containing a flammable liquid*	3	UN1133	I	3	B42, T11, TP1, TP8, TP27	128	FLAMMABLE
				II	3	149, B52, IB2, T4, TP1, TP8	128	FLAMMABLE
				III	3	B1, B52, IB3, T2, TP1	128	FLAMMABLE
	Adiponitrile	6.1	UN2205	III	6.1	IB3, T3, TP1	153	POISON
	Aerosols, *corrosive, Packing Group II or III, (each not exceeding 1 L capacity)*	2.2	UN1950		2.2, 8	A34	126	NONFLAMMABLE GAS
	Aerosols, *flammable, (each not exceeding 1 L capacity)*	2.1	UN1950		2.1	N82	126	FLAMMABLE GAS
	Aerosols, flammable, n.o.s. *(engine starting fluid) (each not exceeding 1 L capacity)*	2.1	UN1950		2.1	N82	126	FLAMMABLE GAS
	Aerosols, *non-flammable, (each not exceeding 1 L capacity)*	2.2	UN1950		2.2		126	NONFLAMMABLE GAS
	Aerosols, *poison, each not exceeding 1 L capacity*	2.2	UN1950		2.2, 6.1		126	NONFLAMMABLE GAS

Symbols	Hazardous materials descriptions and proper shipping names	Hazard class or Division	Identification Numbers	PG	Label Codes	Special provisions (§172.102)	ERG Guide No.	Placard Advisory Consult §172.504 & §172.505 *Placard any quantity
(1)	(2)	(3)	(4)	(5)	(6)	(7)		
	Air bag inflators, compressed gas *or* **Air bag modules, compressed gas** *or* **Seat-belt pretensioners, compressed gas**	2.2	UN3353		2.2	133	126	NONFLAMMABLE GAS
I	**Air bag inflators,** *or* **Air bag modules,** *or* **Seat-belt pretensioners**	1.4G	UN0503	II	1.4G	161	114	EXPLOSIVES 1.4
	Air bag inflators, *or* **Air bag modules,** *or* **Seat-belt pretensioners**	9	UN3268	III	9	160	171	CLASS 9
	Air, compressed	2.2	UN1002		2.2	78	122	NONFLAMMABLE GAS
	Air, refrigerated liquid, *(cryogenic liquid)*	2.2	UN1003		2.2, 5.1	T75, TP5, TP22	122	NONFLAMMABLE GAS
	Air, refrigerated liquid, *(cryogenic liquid) non-pressurized*	2.2	UN1003		2.2, 5.1	T75, TP5, TP22	122	NONFLAMMABLE GAS
	Aircraft engines (including turbines), see **Engines, internal combustion**							
	Aircraft evacuation slides, see **Life saving appliances** *etc.*							
	Aircraft hydraulic power unit fuel tank *(containing a mixture of anhydrous hydrazine and monomethyl hydrazine) (M86 fuel)*	3	UN3165	I	3, 6.1, 8		131	FLAMMABLE
	Aircraft survival kits, see **Life saving appliances** *etc.*							

Symbols	Hazardous materials descriptions and proper shipping names	Hazard class or Division	Identification Numbers	PG	Label Codes	Special provisions (§172.102)	ERG Guide No.	Placard Advisory Consult §172.504 & §172.505 *Placard any quantity
(1)	(2)	(3)	(4)	(5)	(6)	(7)		
G	**Alcoholates solution, n.o.s.,** *in alcohol*	3	UN3274	II	3, 8	IB2	132	FLAMMABLE
	Alcoholic beverages	3	UN3065	II	3	24, 149, B1, IB2, T4, TP1	127	FLAMMABLE
				III	3	24, B1, IB3, N11, T2, TP1	127	FLAMMABLE
	Alcohols, n.o.s	3	UN1987	I	3	172, T11, TP1, TP8, TP27	127	FLAMMABLE
				II	3	172, IB2, T7, TP1, TP8, TP28	127	FLAMMABLE
				III	3	172, B1, IB3, T4, TP1, TP29	127	FLAMMABLE
G	**Alcohols, flammable, toxic, n.o.s.**	3	UN1986	I	3, 6.1	T14, TP2, TP13, TP27	131	FLAMMABLE
				II	3, 6.1	IB2, T11, TP2, TP27	131	FLAMMABLE
				III	3, 6.1	B1, IB3, T7, TP1, TP28	131	FLAMMABLE
	Aldehydes, n.o.s.	3	UN1989	I	3	T11, TP1, TP27	129	FLAMMABLE
				II	3	IB2, T7, TP1, TP8, TP28	129	FLAMMABLE
				III	3	B1, IB3, T4, TP1, TP29	129	FLAMMABLE

Symbols (1)	Hazardous materials descriptions and proper shipping names (2)	Hazard class or Division (3)	Identification Numbers (4)	PG (5)	Label Codes (6)	Special provisions (§172.102) (7)	ERG Guide No.	Placard Advisory Consult §172.504 & §172.505 *Placard any quantity
G	**Aldehydes, flammable, toxic, n.o.s.**	3	UN1988	I	3, 6.1	T14, TP2, TP13, TP27	131	FLAMMABLE
				II	3, 6.1	IB2, T11, TP2, TP27	131	FLAMMABLE
				III	3, 6.1	B1, IB3, T7, TP1, TP28	131	FLAMMABLE
	Aldol	6.1	UN2839	II	6.1	IB2, T7, TP2	153	POISON
G	**Alkali metal alcoholates, self-heating, corrosive, n.o.s.**	4.2	UN3206	II	4.2, 8	64, A7, IB5, IP2, T3, TP33	136	SPONTANEOUSLY COMBUSTIBLE
				III	4.2, 8	64, A7, IB8, IP3, T1, TP33	136	SPONTANEOUSLY COMBUSTIBLE
	Alkali metal alloys, liquid, n.o.s.	4.3	UN1421	I	4.3	A2, A3, A7, B48, N34	138	DANGEROUS WHEN WET*
	Alkali metal amalgam, liquid	4.3	UN1389	I	4.3	A2, A3, A7, N34	138	DANGEROUS WHEN WET*
	Alkali metal amalgam, solid	4.3	UN3401	I	4.3	IB4, IP1, N40, T9, TP7, TP33	138	DANGEROUS WHEN WET*
	Alkali metal amides	4.3	UN1390	II	4.3	A6, A7, A8, A19, A20, IB7, IP2	139	DANGEROUS WHEN WET*
	Alkali metal dispersions, *or* **Alkaline earth metal dispersions**	4.3	UN1391	I	4.3	A2, A3, A7	138	DANGEROUS WHEN WET*
	Alkaline corrosive liquids, n.o.s., see **Caustic alkali liquids, n.o.s.**							

Sym-bols	Hazardous materials descriptions and proper shipping names	Hazard class or Division	Identification Numbers	PG	Label Codes	Special provisions (§172.102)	ERG Guide No.	Placard Advisory Consult §172.504 & §172.505 *Placard any quantity
(1)	(2)	(3)	(4)	(5)	(6)	(7)		
G	**Alkaline earth metal alcoholates, n.o.s.**	4.2	UN3205	II	4.2	65, A7, IB6, IP2, T3, TP33	135	SPONTANEOUSLY COMBUSTIBLE
				III	4.2	65, A7, IB8, IP3, T1, TP33	135	SPONTANEOUSLY COMBUSTIBLE
	Alkaline earth metal alloys, n.o.s.	4.3	UN1393	II	4.3	A19, IB7, IP2, T3, TP33	138	DANGEROUS WHEN WET*
	Alkaline earth metal amalgams, liquid	4.3	UN1392	I	4.3	A19, N34, N40	138	DANGEROUS WHEN WET*
	Alkaline earth metal amalgams, solid	4.3	UN3402	I	4.3	A19, N34, N40, T9, TP7, TP33	138	DANGEROUS WHEN WET*
G	**Alkaloids, liquid, n.o.s.,** *or* **Alkaloid salts, liquid, n.o.s.**	6.1	UN3140	I	6.1	A4, T14, TP2, TP27	151	POISON
				II	6.1	IB2, T11, TP2, TP27	151	POISON
				III	6.1	IB3, T7, TP1, TP28	151	POISON
G	**Alkaloids, solid, n.o.s.** *or* **Alkaloid salts, solid, n.o.s. poisonous**	6.1	UN1544	I	6.1	IB7, IP1, T6, TP33	151	POISON
				II	6.1	IB8, IP2, IP4, T3, TP33	151	POISON
				III	6.1	IB8, IP3, T1, TP33	151	POISON
	Alkyl sulfonic acids, liquid *or* **Aryl sulfonic acids, liquid** *with more than 5 percent free sulfuric acid*	8	UN2584	II	8	B2, IB2, T8, TP2, TP12, TP13	153	CORROSIVE

Sym-bols	Hazardous materials descriptions and proper shipping names	Hazard class or Division	Identifica-tion Numbers	PG	Label Codes	Special provisions (§172.102)	ERG Guide No.	Placard Advisory Consult §172.504 & §172.505 *Placard any quantity
(1)	(2)	(3)	(4)	(5)	(6)	(7)		
	Alkyl sulfonic acids, liquid *or* **Aryl sulfonic acids, liquid** *with not more than 5 percent free sulfuric acid*	8	UN2586	III	8	IB3, T4, TP1	153	CORROSIVE
	Alkyl sulfonic acids, solid *or* **Aryl sulfonic acids, solid,** *with more than 5 percent free sulfuric acid*	8	UN2583	II	8	IB8, IP2, IP4, T3, TP33	153	CORROSIVE
	Alkyl sulfonic acids, solid *or* **Aryl sulfonic acids, solid** *with not more than 5 percent free sulfuric acid*	8	UN2585	III	8	IB8, IP3, T1, TP33	153	CORROSIVE
	Alkylphenols, liquid, n.o.s. *(including C2-C12 homologues)*	8	UN3145	I	8	A6, T14, TP2	153	CORROSIVE
				II	8	IB2, T11, TP2, TP27	153	CORROSIVE
				III	8	IB3, T7, TP1, TP28	153	CORROSIVE
	Alkylphenols, solid, n.o.s. *(including C2-C12 homologues)*	8	UN2430	I	8	IB7, IP1, T6, TP33	153	CORROSIVE
				II	8	IB8, IP2, IP4, T3, TP33	153	CORROSIVE
				III	8	IB8, IP3, T1, TP33	153	CORROSIVE
	Alkylsulfuric acids	8	UN2571	II	8	B2, IB2, T8, TP2, TP12, TP13, TP28	156	CORROSIVE
	Allethrin, see **Pesticides, liquid, toxic, n.o.s.**							
	Allyl acetate	3	UN2333	II	3, 6.1	IB2, T7, TP1, TP13	131	FLAMMABLE

Symbols	Hazardous materials descriptions and proper shipping names	Hazard class or Division	Identification Numbers	PG	Label Codes	Special provisions (§172.102)	ERG Guide No.	Placard Advisory Consult §172.504 & §172.505 *Placard any quantity
(1)	(2)	(3)	(4)	(5)	(6)	(7)		
	Allyl alcohol	6.1	UN1098	I	6.1, 3	2, B9, B14, B32, B74, B77, T20, TP2, TP13, TP38, TP45	131	POISON INHALATION HAZARD*
	Allyl bromide	3	UN1099	I	3, 6.1	T14, TP2, TP13	131	FLAMMABLE
	Allyl chloride	3	UN1100	I	3, 6.1	T14, TP2, TP13	131	FLAMMABLE
	Allyl chlorocarbonate, see **Allyl chloroformate**							
	Allyl chloroformate	6.1	UN1722	I	6.1, 3, 8	2, B9, B14, B32, B74, N41, T20, TP2, TP13, TP38, TP45	155	POISON INHALATION HAZARD*
	Allyl ethyl ether	3	UN2335	II	3, 6.1	IB2, T7, TP1, TP13	131	FLAMMABLE
	Allyl formate	3	UN2336	I	3, 6.1	T14, TP2, TP13	131	FLAMMABLE
	Allyl glycidyl ether	3	UN2219	III	3	B1, IB3, T2, TP1	129	FLAMMABLE
	Allyl iodide	3	UN1723	II	3, 8	A3, A6, IB1, N34, T7, TP2, TP13	132	FLAMMABLE
	Allyl isothiocyanate, stabilized	6.1	UN1545	II	6.1, 3	A3, A7, IB2, T7, TP2	155	POISON
	Allylamine	6.1	UN2334	I	6.1, 3	2, B9, B14, B32, B74, T20, TP2, TP13, TP38, TP45	131	POISON INHALATION HAZARD*

Sym-bols	Hazardous materials descriptions and proper shipping names	Hazard class or Division	Identifica-tion Numbers	PG	Label Codes	Special provisions (§172.102)	ERG Guide No.	Placard Advisory Consult §172.504 & §172.505 *Placard any quantity
(1)	(2)	(3)	(4)	(5)	(6)	(7)		
	Allyltrichlorosilane, stabilized	8	UN1724	II	8, 3	A7, B2, B6, IB2, N34, T7, TP2, TP13	155	CORROSIVE
	Aluminum alkyl halides, liquid	4.2	UN3052	I	4.2, 4.3	173, B9, B11, T21, TP2, TP7	135	SPONTANEOUSLY COMBUSTIBLE, DANGEROUS WHEN WET*
	Aluminum alkyl halides, solid	4.2	UN3461	I	4.2, 4.3	173, T21, TP7, TP33	135	SPONTANEOUSLY COMBUSTIBLE, DANGEROUS WHEN WET*
	Aluminum alkyl hydrides	4.2	UN3076	I	4.2, 4.3	173, B9, B11, T21, TP2, TP7	138	SPONTANEOUSLY COMBUSTIBLE, DANGEROUS WHEN WET*
	Aluminum alkyls	4.2	UN3051	I	4.2, 4.3	173, B9, B11, T21, TP2, TP7	135	SPONTANEOUSLY COMBUSTIBLE, DANGEROUS WHEN WET*
	Aluminum borohydride *or* **Aluminum borohydride in devices**	4.2	UN2870	I	4.2, 4.3	B11, T21, TP7, TP33	135	SPONTANEOUSLY COMBUSTIBLE, DANGEROUS WHEN WET*
	Aluminum bromide, anhydrous	8	UN1725	II	8	IB8, IP2, IP4, T3, TP33	137	CORROSIVE
	Aluminum bromide, solution	8	UN2580	III	8	IB3, T4, TP1	154	CORROSIVE

Sym-bols	Hazardous materials descriptions and proper shipping names	Hazard class or Division	Identification Numbers	PG	Label Codes	Special provisions (§172.102)	ERG Guide No.	Placard Advisory Consult §172.504 & §172.505 *Placard any quantity
(1)	(2)	(3)	(4)	(5)	(6)	(7)		
	Aluminum carbide	4.3	UN1394	II	4.3	A20, IB7, IP2, N41, T3, TP33	138	DANGEROUS WHEN WET*
	Aluminum chloride, anhydrous	8	UN1726	II	8	IB8, IP2, IP4, T3, TP33	137	CORROSIVE
	Aluminum chloride, solution	8	UN2581	III	8	IB3, T4, TP1	154	CORROSIVE
	Aluminum dross, wet or hot	Forbidden						
	Aluminum ferrosilicon powder	4.3	UN1395	II	4.3, 6.1	A19, IB5, IP2, T3, TP33	139	DANGEROUS WHEN WET*
				III	4.3, 6.1	A19, A20, IB4	139	DANGEROUS WHEN WET*
	Aluminum hydride	4.3	UN2463	I	4.3	A19, N40	138	DANGEROUS WHEN WET*
D	**Aluminum, molten**	9	NA9260	III	9	IB3, T1, TP3	169	CLASS 9
	Aluminum nitrate	5.1	UN1438	III	5.1	A1, A29, IB8, IP3, T1, TP33	140	OXIDIZER
	Aluminum phosphate solution, see **Corrosive liquids,** *etc.*							
	Aluminum phosphide	4.3	UN1397	I	4.3, 6.1	A8, A19, N40	139	DANGEROUS WHEN WET*
	Aluminum phosphide pesticides	6.1	UN3048	I	6.1	A8, IB7, IP1, T6, TP33	157	POISON
	Aluminum powder, coated	4.1	UN1309	II	4.1	IB8, IP2, IP4, T3, TP33	170	FLAMMABLE SOLID

Symbols	Hazardous materials descriptions and proper shipping names	Hazard class or Division	Identification Numbers	PG	Label Codes	Special provisions (§172.102)	ERG Guide No.	Placard Advisory Consult §172.504 & §172.505 *Placard any quantity
(1)	(2)	(3)	(4)	(5)	(6)	(7)		
				III	4.1	IB8, IP3, T1, TP33	170	FLAMMABLE SOLID
	Aluminum powder, uncoated	4.3	UN1396	II	4.3	A19, A20, IB7, IP2, T3, TP33	138	DANGEROUS WHEN WET*
				III	4.3	A19, A20, IB8, IP4, T1, TP33	138	DANGEROUS WHEN WET*
	Aluminum resinate	4.1	UN2715	III	4.1	IB6, T1, TP33	133	FLAMMABLE SOLID
	Aluminum silicon powder, uncoated	4.3	UN1398	III	4.3	A1, A19, IB8, IP4, T1, TP33	138	DANGEROUS WHEN WET*
	Aluminum smelting by-products *or* **Aluminum remelting by-products**	4.3	UN3170	II	4.3	128, B115, IB7, IP2, T3, TP33	138	DANGEROUS WHEN WET*
				III	4.3	128, B115, IB8, IP4, T1, TP33	138	DANGEROUS WHEN WET*
	Amatols, see **Explosives, blasting, type B**							
G	**Amines, flammable, corrosive, n.o.s.** *or* **Polyamines, flammable, corrosive, n.o.s.**	3	UN2733	I	3, 8	T14, TP1, TP27	132	FLAMMABLE
				II	3, 8	IB2, T11, TP1, TP27	132	FLAMMABLE
				III	3, 8	B1, IB3, T7, TP1, TP28	132	FLAMMABLE

Sym-bols	Hazardous materials descriptions and proper shipping names	Hazard class or Division	Identifica-tion Numbers	PG	Label Codes	Special provisions (§172.102)	ERG Guide No.	Placard Advisory Consult §172.504 & §172.505 *Placard any quantity
(1)	(2)	(3)	(4)	(5)	(6)	(7)		
G	**Amines, liquid, corrosive, flammable, n.o.s.** *or* **Polyamines, liquid, corrosive, flammable, n.o.s.**	8	UN2734	I	8, 3	A3, A6, N34, T14, TP2, TP27	132	CORROSIVE
				II	8, 3	IB2, T11, TP2, TP27	132	CORROSIVE
G	**Amines, liquid, corrosive, n.o.s,** *or* **Polyamines, liquid, corrosive, n.o.s.**	8	UN2735	I	8	A3, A6, B10, N34, T14, TP2, TP27	153	CORROSIVE
				II	8	B2, IB2, T11, TP1, TP27	153	CORROSIVE
				III	8	IB3, T7, TP1, TP28	153	CORROSIVE
G	**Amines, solid, corrosive, n.o.s.,** *or* **Polyamines, solid, corrosive n.o.s.**	8	UN3259	I	8	IB7, IP1, T6, TP33	154	CORROSIVE
				II	8	IB8, IP2, IP4, T3, TP33	154	CORROSIVE
				III	8	IB8, IP3, T1, TP33	154	CORROSIVE
	2-Amino-4-chlorophenol	6.1	UN2673	II	6.1	IB8, IP2, IP4, T3, TP33	151	POISON
	2-Amino-5-diethylaminopentane	6.1	UN2946	III	6.1	IB3, T4, TP1	153	POISON
	2-Amino-4,6-Dinitrophenol, wetted *with not less than 20 percent water by mass*	4.1	UN3317	I	4.1	23, A8, A19, A20, N41	113	FLAMMABLE SOLID
	2-(2-Aminoethoxy) ethanol	8	UN3055	III	8	IB3, T4, TP1	154	CORROSIVE
	N-Aminoethylpiperazine	8	UN2815	III	8	IB3, T4, TP1	153	CORROSIVE

Symbols	Hazardous materials descriptions and proper shipping names	Hazard class or Division	Identification Numbers	PG	Label Codes	Special provisions (§172.102)	ERG Guide No.	Placard Advisory Consult §172.504 & §172.505 *Placard any quantity
(1)	(2)	(3)	(4)	(5)	(6)	(7)		
+	**Aminophenols (o-; m-; p-)**	6.1	UN2512	III	6.1	IB8, IP3, T1, TP33	152	POISON
	Aminopropyldiethanolamine, see **Amines,** *etc.*							
	n-Aminopropylmorpholine, see **Amines,** *etc.*							
	Aminopyridines *(o-; m-; p-)*	6.1	UN2671	II	6.1	IB8, IP2, IP4, T3, TP33	153	POISON
I	**Ammonia, anhydrous**	2.3	UN1005		2.3, 8	4, T50	125	POISON GAS*
D	**Ammonia, anhydrous**	2.2	UN1005		2.2	13, T50	125	NONFLAMMABLE GAS
D	**Ammonia solution,** *relative density less than 0.880 at 15 degrees C in water, with more than 50 percent ammonia*	2.2	UN3318		2.2	13, T50	125	NONFLAMMABLE GAS
I	**Ammonia solution,** *relative density less than 0.880 at 15 degrees C in water, with more than 50 percent ammonia*	2.3	UN3318		2.3, 8	4, T50	125	POISON GAS*
	Ammonia solutions, *relative density between 0.880 and 0.957 at 15 degrees C in water, with more than 10 percent but not more than 35 percent ammonia*	8	UN2672	III	8	IB3, IP8, T7, TP1	154	CORROSIVE

Symbols	Hazardous materials descriptions and proper shipping names	Hazard class or Division	Identification Numbers	PG	Label Codes	Special provisions (§172.102)	ERG Guide No.	Placard Advisory Consult §172.504 & §172.505 *Placard any quantity
(1)	(2)	(3)	(4)	(5)	(6)	(7)		
	Ammonia solutions, *relative density less than 0.880 at 15 degrees C in water, with more than 35 percent but not more than 50 percent ammonia*	2.2	UN2073		2.2		125	NONFLAMMABLE GAS
	Ammonium arsenate	6.1	UN1546	II	6.1	IB8, IP2, IP4, T3, TP33	151	POISON
	Ammonium azide	Forbidden						
	Ammonium bifluoride, solid, see **Ammonium hydrogen difluoride, solid**							
	Ammonium bifluoride solution, see **Ammonium hydrogen difluoride, solution**							
	Ammonium bromate	Forbidden						
	Ammonium chlorate	Forbidden						
	Ammonium dichromate	5.1	UN1439	II	5.1	IB8, IP2, IP4, T3, TP33	141	OXIDIZER
	Ammonium dinitro-o-cresolate, solid	6.1	UN1843	II	6.1	IB8, IP2, IP4, T3, TP33	141	POISON
	Ammonium dinitro-o-cresolate solution	6.1	UN3424	II	6.1	IB2, T7, TP2	141	POISON
				III	6.1	IB2, T7, TP2	141	POISON
	Ammonium fluoride	6.1	UN2505	III	6.1	IB8, IP3, T1, TP33	154	POISON

Symbols	Hazardous materials descriptions and proper shipping names	Hazard class or Division	Identification Numbers	PG	Label Codes	Special provisions (§172.102)	ERG Guide No.	Placard Advisory Consult §172.504 & §172.505 *Placard any quantity
(1)	(2)	(3)	(4)	(5)	(6)	(7)		
	Ammonium fluorosilicate	6.1	UN2854	III	6.1	IB8, IP3, T1, TP33	151	POISON
	Ammonium fulminate	Forbidden						
	Ammonium hydrogen sulfate	8	UN2506	II	8	IB8, IP2, IP4, T3, TP33	154	CORROSIVE
	Ammonium hydrogendifluoride, solid	8	UN1727	II	8	IB8, IP2, IP4, N34, T3, TP33	154	CORROSIVE
	Ammonium hydrogendifluoride, solution	8	UN2817	II	8, 6.1	IB2, N34, T8, TP2, TP12, TP13	154	CORROSIVE
				III	8, 6.1	IB3, N3, T4, TP1, TP12, TP13	154	CORROSIVE
	Ammonium hydrosulfide, solution, see **Ammonium sulfide solution**							
D	**Ammonium hydroxide,** *see* **Ammonia solutions,** *etc.*							
	Ammonium metavanadate	6.1	UN2859	II	6.1	IB8, IP2, IP4, T3, TP33	154	POISON
	Ammonium nitrate based fertilizer	5.1	UN2067	III	5.1	52, 150, IB8, IP3, T1, TP33	140	OXIDIZER
A W	**Ammonium nitrate based fertilizer**	9	UN2071	III	9	132, IB8, IP3	140	CLASS 9
	Ammonium nitrate emulsion *or* **Ammonium nitrate suspension** *or* **Ammonium nitrate gel,** *intermediate for blasting explosives*	5.1	UN3375	II	5.1	147, 163	140	OXIDIZER

Symbols	Hazardous materials descriptions and proper shipping names	Hazard class or Division	Identification Numbers	PG	Label Codes	Special provisions (§172.102)	ERG Guide No.	Placard Advisory Consult §172.504 & §172.505 *Placard any quantity
(1)	(2)	(3)	(4)	(5)	(6)	(7)		
D	**Ammonium nitrate-fuel oil mixture** *containing only prilled ammonium nitrate and fuel oil*	1.5D	NA0331	II	1.5D		112	EXPLOSIVES 1.5
	Ammonium nitrate, liquid *(hot concentrated solution)*	5.1	UN2426		5.1	B5, T7	140	OXIDIZER
	Ammonium nitrate, *with more than 0.2 percent combustible substances, including any organic substance calculated as carbon, to the exclusion of any other added substance*	1.1D	UN0222	II	1.1D		112	EXPLOSIVES 1.1*
	Ammonium nitrate, *with not more than 0.2% total combustible material, including any organic substance, calculated as carbon to the exclusion of any other added substance*	5.1	UN1942	III	5.1	A1, A29, IB8, IP3, T1, TP33	140	OXIDIZER
	Ammonium nitrite	Forbidden						
	Ammonium perchlorate	1.1D	UN0402	II	1.1D	107	112	EXPLOSIVES 1.1*
	Ammonium perchlorate	5.1	UN1442	II	5.1	107, A9, IB6, IP2, T3, TP33	143	OXIDIZER
	Ammonium permanganate	Forbidden						
	Ammonium persulfate	5.1	UN1444	III	5.1	A1, A29, IB8, IP3, T1, TP33	140	OXIDIZER
	Ammonium picrate, *dry or wetted with less than 10 percent water, by mass*	1.1D	UN0004	II	1.1D		112	EXPLOSIVES 1.1*

Symbols	Hazardous materials descriptions and proper shipping names	Hazard class or Division	Identification Numbers	PG	Label Codes	Special provisions (§172.102)	ERG Guide No.	Placard Advisory Consult §172.504 & §172.505 *Placard any quantity
(1)	(2)	(3)	(4)	(5)	(6)	(7)		
	Ammonium picrate, wetted *with not less than 10 percent water, by mass*	4.1	UN1310	I	4.1	23, A2, N41	113	FLAMMABLE SOLID
	Ammonium polysulfide, solution	8	UN2818	II	8, 6.1	IB2, T7, TP2, TP13	154	CORROSIVE
				III	8, 6.1	IB3, T4, TP1, TP13	154	CORROSIVE
	Ammonium polyvanadate	6.1	UN2861	II	6.1	IB8, IP2, IP4, T3, TP33	151	POISON
	Ammonium silicofluoride, see **Ammonium fluorosilicate**							
	Ammonium sulfide solution	8	UN2683	II	8, 6.1, 3	IB1, T7, TP2, TP13	132	CORROSIVE
	Ammunition, blank, see **Cartridges for weapons, blank**							
	Ammunition, illuminating *with or without burster, expelling charge or propelling charge*	1.2G	UN0171	II	1.2G		112	EXPLOSIVES 1.2*
	Ammunition, illuminating *with or without burster, expelling charge or propelling charge*	1.3G	UN0254	II	1.3G		112	EXPLOSIVES 1.3*
	Ammunition, illuminating *with or without burster, expelling charge or propelling charge*	1.4G	UN0297	II	1.4G		114	EXPLOSIVES 1.4
	Ammunition, incendiary *liquid or gel, with burster, expelling charge or propelling charge*	1.3J	UN0247	II	1.3J		112	EXPLOSIVES 1.3*

Symbols	Hazardous materials descriptions and proper shipping names	Hazard class or Division	Identification Numbers	PG	Label Codes	Special provisions (§172.102)	ERG Guide No.	Placard Advisory Consult §172.504 & §172.505 *Placard any quantity
(1)	(2)	(3)	(4)	(5)	(6)	(7)		
	Ammunition, incendiary *(water-activated contrivances)* **with burster,** *expelling charge or propelling charge, see* **Contrivances, water-activated, etc.**							
	Ammunition, incendiary, white phosphorus, *with burster, expelling charge or propelling charge*	1.2H	UN0243	II	1.2H		112	EXPLOSIVES 1.2*
	Ammunition, incendiary, white phosphorus, *with burster, expelling charge or propelling charge*	1.3H	UN0244	II	1.3H		112	EXPLOSIVES 1.3*
	Ammunition, incendiary *with or without burster, expelling charge, or propelling charge*	1.2G	UN0009	II	1.2G		112	EXPLOSIVES 1.2*
	Ammunition, incendiary *with or without burster, expelling charge, or propelling charge*	1.3G	UN0010	II	1.3G		112	EXPLOSIVES 1.3*
	Ammunition, incendiary *with or without burster, expelling charge or propelling charge*	1.4G	UN0300	II	1.4G		114	EXPLOSIVES 1.4
	Ammunition, practice	1.4G	UN0362	II	1.4G		114	EXPLOSIVES 1.4
	Ammunition, practice	1.3G	UN0488	II	1.3G		112	EXPLOSIVES 1.3*
	Ammunition, proof	1.4G	UN0363	II	1.4G		114	EXPLOSIVES 1.4
	Ammunition, rocket, see **Warheads, rocket** *etc.*							

Symbols	Hazardous materials descriptions and proper shipping names	Hazard class or Division	Identification Numbers	PG	Label Codes	Special provisions (§172.102)	ERG Guide No.	Placard Advisory Consult §172.504 & §172.505 *Placard any quantity
(1)	(2)	(3)	(4)	(5)	(6)	(7)		
	Ammunition, SA (small arms), see **Cartridges for weapons,** *etc.*							
	Ammunition, smoke (water-activated contrivances), white phosphorus, with burster, expelling charge or propelling charge, see **Contrivances, water-activated,** *etc. (UN 0248)*							
	Ammunition, smoke (water-activated contrivances), without white phosphorus or phosphides, with burster, expelling charge or propelling charge, see **Contrivances, water-activated,** *etc. (UN 0249)*							
	Ammunition smoke, white phosphorus *with burster,expelling charge, or propelling charge*	1.2H	UN0245	II	1.2H		112	EXPLOSIVES 1.2*
	Ammunition, smoke, white phosphorus *with burster, expelling charge, or propelling charge*	1.3H	UN0246	II	1.3H		112	EXPLOSIVES 1.3*
	Ammunition, smoke *with or without burster, expelling charge or propelling charge*	1.2G	UN0015	II	1.2G		112	EXPLOSIVES 1.2*
	Ammunition, smoke *with or without burster, expelling charge or propelling charge*	1.3G	UN0016	II	1.3G		112	EXPLOSIVES 1.3*

Sym-bols	Hazardous materials descriptions and proper shipping names	Hazard class or Division	Identifica-tion Numbers	PG	Label Codes	Special provisions (§172.102)	ERG Guide No.	Placard Advisory Consult §172.504 & §172.505 *Placard any quantity
(1)	(2)	(3)	(4)	(5)	(6)	(7)		
	Ammunition, smoke *with or without burster, expelling charge or propelling charge*	1.4G	UN0303	II	1.4G		114	EXPLOSIVES 1.4
	Ammunition, sporting, see **Cartridges for weapons,** *etc. (UN 0012; UN 0328; UN 0339)*							
	Ammunition, tear-producing, non-explosive, *without burster or expelling charge, non-fuzed*	6.1	UN2017	II	6.1, 8		159	POISON
	Ammunition, tear-producing *with burster, expelling charge or propelling charge*	1.2G	UN0018	II	1.2G, 8, 6.1		112	EXPLOSIVES 1.2*
	Ammunition, tear-producing *with burster, expelling charge or propelling charge*	1.3G	UN0019	II	1.3G, 8, 6.1		112	EXPLOSIVES 1.3*
	Ammunition, tear-producing *with burster, expelling charge or propelling charge*	1.4G	UN0301	II	1.4G, 8, 6.1		114	EXPLOSIVES 1.4
	Ammunition, toxic, non-explosive, *without burster or expelling charge, non-fuzed*	6.1	UN2016	II	6.1		151	POISON
	Ammunition, toxic (water-activated contrivances), with burster, expelling charge or propelling charge, see **Contrivances, water-activated,** *etc.*							

Symbols	Hazardous materials descriptions and proper shipping names	Hazard class or Division	Identification Numbers	PG	Label Codes	Special provisions (§172.102)	ERG Guide No.	Placard Advisory Consult §172.504 & §172.505 *Placard any quantity
(1)	(2)	(3)	(4)	(5)	(6)	(7)		
G	**Ammunition, toxic** *with burster, expelling charge, or propelling charge*	1.2K	UN0020	II	1.2K, 6.1		112	EXPLOSIVES 1.2*
G	**Ammunition, toxic** *with burster, expelling charge, or propelling charge*	1.3K	UN0021	II	1.3K, 6.1		112	EXPLOSIVES 1.3*
	Amyl acetates	3	UN1104	III	3	B1, IB3, T2, TP1	129	FLAMMABLE
	Amyl acid phosphate	8	UN2819	III	8	IB3, T4, TP1	153	CORROSIVE
	Amyl butyrates	3	UN2620	III	3	B1, IB3, T2, TP1	130	FLAMMABLE
	Amyl chlorides	3	UN1107	II	3	IB2, T4, TP1	129	FLAMMABLE
	Amyl formates	3	UN1109	III	3	B1, IB3, T2, TP1	129	FLAMMABLE
	Amyl mercaptans	3	UN1111	II	3	A3, A6, IB2, T4, TP1	130	FLAMMABLE
	n-Amyl methyl ketone	3	UN1110	III	3	B1, IB3, T2, TP1	127	FLAMMABLE
	Amyl nitrate	3	UN1112	III	3	B1, IB3, T2, TP1	140	FLAMMABLE
	Amyl nitrites	3	UN1113	II	3	IB2, T4, TP1	129	FLAMMABLE
	Amylamines	3	UN1106	II	3, 8	IB2, T7, TP1	132	FLAMMABLE
				III	3, 8	B1, IB3, T4, TP1	132	FLAMMABLE
	Amyltrichlorosilane	8	UN1728	II	8	A7, B2, B6, IB2, N34, T7, TP2, TP13	155	CORROSIVE
	Anhydrous ammonia, *see* **Ammonia, anhydrous**							

Sym-bols	Hazardous materials descriptions and proper shipping names	Hazard class or Division	Identification Numbers	PG	Label Codes	Special provisions (§172.102)	ERG Guide No.	Placard Advisory Consult §172.504 & §172.505 *Placard any quantity
(1)	(2)	(3)	(4)	(5)	(6)	(7)		
	Anhydrous hydrofluoric acid, see **Hydrogen fluoride, anhydrous**							
+	**Aniline**	6.1	UN1547	II	6.1	IB2, T7, TP2	153	POISON
	Aniline hydrochloride	6.1	UN1548	III	6.1	IB8, IP3, T1, TP33	153	POISON
	Aniline oil, see **Aniline**							
	Anisidines	6.1	UN2431	III	6.1	IB3, T4, TP1	153	POISON
	Anisole	3	UN2222	III	3	B1, IB3, T2, TP1	128	FLAMMABLE
	Anisoyl chloride	8	UN1729	II	8	B2, B4, IB8, IP2, IP4, T3, TP33	156	CORROSIVE
	Anti-freeze, liquid, see **Flammable liquids, n.o.s.**							
	Antimonous chloride, see **Antimony trichloride**							
	Antimony compounds, inorganic, liquid, n.o.s.	6.1	UN3141	III	6.1	35, IB3, T7, TP1, TP28	157	POISON
	Antimony compounds, inorganic, solid, n.o.s.	6.1	UN1549	III	6.1	35, IB8, IP3, T1, TP33	157	POISON
	Antimony lactate	6.1	UN1550	III	6.1	IB8, IP3, T1, TP33	151	POISON
	Antimony pentachloride, liquid	8	UN1730	II	8	B2, IB2, T7, TP2	157	CORROSIVE
	Antimony pentachloride, solutions	8	UN1731	II	8	B2, IB2, T7, TP2	157	CORROSIVE
				III	8	IB3, T4, TP1	157	CORROSIVE

Symbols	Hazardous materials descriptions and proper shipping names	Hazard class or Division	Identification Numbers	PG	Label Codes	Special provisions (§172.102)	ERG Guide No.	Placard Advisory Consult §172.504 & §172.505 *Placard any quantity
(1)	(2)	(3)	(4)	(5)	(6)	(7)		
	Antimony pentafluoride	8	UN1732	II	8, 6.1	A3, A6, A7, A10, IB2, N3, N36, T7, TP2	157	CORROSIVE
	Antimony potassium tartrate	6.1	UN1551	III	6.1	IB8, IP3, T1, TP33	151	POISON
	Antimony powder	6.1	UN2871	III	6.1	IB8, IP3, T1, TP33	170	POISON
	Antimony sulfide and a chlorate, mixtures of	Forbidden						
	Antimony sulfide, solid, see **Antimony compounds, inorganic, n.o.s.**							
	Antimony trichloride, liquid	8	UN1733	II	8	B2, IB2	157	CORROSIVE
	Antimony trichloride, solid	8	UN1733	II	8	IB8, IP2, IP4	157	CORROSIVE
	Aqua ammonia, see **Ammonia solution,** *etc.*							
	Argon, compressed	2.2	UN1006		2.2		121	NONFLAMMABLE GAS
	Argon, refrigerated liquid *(cryogenic liquid)*	2.2	UN1951		2.2	T75, TP5	120	NONFLAMMABLE GAS
	Arsenic	6.1	UN1558	II	6.1	IB8, IP2, IP4, T3, TP33	152	POISON
	Arsenic acid, liquid	6.1	UN1553	I	6.1	T20, TP2, TP7, TP13	154	POISON
	Arsenic acid, solid	6.1	UN1554	II	6.1	IB8, IP2, IP4, T3, TP33	154	POISON

Symbols	Hazardous materials descriptions and proper shipping names	Hazard class or Division	Identification Numbers	PG	Label Codes	Special provisions (§172.102)	ERG Guide No.	Placard Advisory Consult §172.504 & §172.505 *Placard any quantity
(1)	(2)	(3)	(4)	(5)	(6)	(7)		
	Arsenic bromide	6.1	UN1555	II	6.1	IB8, IP2, IP4, T3, TP33	151	POISON
	Arsenic chloride, see **Arsenic trichloride**							
	Arsenic compounds, liquid, n.o.s. *inorganic, including arsenates, n.o.s.; arsenites, n.o.s.; arsenic sulfides, n.o.s.; and organic compounds of arsenic, n.o.s.*	6.1	UN1556	I	6.1	T14, TP2, TP13, TP27	152	POISON
				II	6.1	IB2, T11, TP2, TP13, TP27	152	POISON
				III	6.1	IB3, T7, TP2, TP28	152	POISON
	Arsenic compounds, solid, n.o.s. *inorganic, including arsenates, n.o.s.; arsenites, n.o.s.; arsenic sulfides, n.o.s.; and organic compounds of arsenic, n.o.s.*	6.1	UN1557	I	6.1	IB7, IP1, T6, TP33	152	POISON
				II	6.1	IB8, IP2, IP4, T3, TP33	152	POISON
				III	6.1	IB8, IP3, T1, TP33	152	POISON
	Arsenic pentoxide	6.1	UN1559	II	6.1	IB8, IP2, IP4, T3, TP33	151	POISON
	Arsenic sulfide and a chlorate, mixtures of	Forbidden						

Symbols	Hazardous materials descriptions and proper shipping names	Hazard class or Division	Identification Numbers	PG	Label Codes	Special provisions (§172.102)	ERG Guide No.	Placard Advisory Consult §172.504 & §172.505 *Placard any quantity
(1)	(2)	(3)	(4)	(5)	(6)	(7)		
	Arsenic trichloride	6.1	UN1560	I	6.1	2, B9, B14, B32, B74, T20, TP2, TP13, TP38, TP45	157	POISON INHALATION HAZARD*
	Arsenic trioxide	6.1	UN1561	II	6.1	IB8, IP2, IP4, T3, TP33	151	POISON
	Arsenic, white, solid, see **Arsenic trioxide**							
	Arsenical dust	6.1	UN1562	II	6.1	IB8, IP2, IP4, T3, TP33	152	POISON
	Arsenical pesticides, liquid, flammable, toxic, *flash point less than 23 degrees C*	3	UN2760	I	3, 6.1	T14, TP2, TP13, TP27	131	FLAMMABLE
				II	3, 6.1	IB2, T11, TP2, TP13, TP27	131	FLAMMABLE
	Arsenical pesticides, liquid, toxic	6.1	UN2994	I	6.1	T14, TP2, TP13, TP27	151	POISON
				II	6.1	IB2, T11, TP2, TP13, TP27	151	POISON
				III	6.1	IB3, T7, TP2, TP28	151	POISON
	Arsenical pesticides, liquid, toxic, flammable, *flash point not less than 23 degrees C*	6.1	UN2993	I	6.1, 3	T14, TP2, TP13, TP27	131	POISON
				II	6.1, 3	IB2, T11, TP2, TP13, TP27	131	POISON

Symbols	Hazardous materials descriptions and proper shipping names	Hazard class or Division	Identification Numbers	PG	Label Codes	Special provisions (§172.102)	ERG Guide No.	Placard Advisory Consult §172.504 & §172.505 *Placard any quantity
(1)	(2)	(3)	(4)	(5)	(6)	(7)		
				III	6.1, 3	B1, IB3, T7, TP2, TP28	131	POISON
	Arsenical pesticides, solid, toxic	6.1	UN2759	I	6.1	IB7, IP1, T6, TP33	151	POISON
				II	6.1	IB8, IP2, IP4, T3, TP33	151	POISON
				III	6.1	IB8, IP3, T1, TP33	151	POISON
	Arsenious acid, solid, see **Arsenic trioxide**							
	Arsenious and mercuric iodide solution, see **Arsenic compounds, liquid, n.o.s.**							
	Arsine	2.3	UN2188		2.3, 2.1	1	119	POISON GAS*
	Articles, explosive, extremely insensitive *or* **Articles, EEI**	1.6N	UN0486	II	1.6N	101	112	EXPLOSIVES 1.6
G	**Articles, explosive, n.o.s.**	1.4S	UN0349	II	1.4S	101	114	EXPLOSIVES 1.4
G	**Articles, explosive, n.o.s.**	1.4B	UN0350	II	1.4B	101	114	EXPLOSIVES 1.4
G	**Articles, explosive, n.o.s.**	1.4C	UN0351	II	1.4C	101	114	EXPLOSIVES 1.4
G	**Articles, explosive, n.o.s.**	1.4D	UN0352	II	1.4D	101	114	EXPLOSIVES 1.4
G	**Articles, explosive, n.o.s.**	1.4G	UN0353	II	1.4G	101	114	EXPLOSIVES 1.4
G	**Articles, explosive, n.o.s.**	1.1L	UN0354	II	1.1L	101	112	EXPLOSIVES 1.1*
G	**Articles, explosive, n.o.s.**	1.2L	UN0355	II	1.2L	101	112	EXPLOSIVES 1.2*

Symbols	Hazardous materials descriptions and proper shipping names	Hazard class or Division	Identification Numbers	PG	Label Codes	Special provisions (§172.102)	ERG Guide No.	Placard Advisory Consult §172.504 & §172.505 *Placard any quantity
(1)	(2)	(3)	(4)	(5)	(6)	(7)		
G	**Articles, explosive, n.o.s.**	1.3L	UN0356	II	1.3L	101	112	EXPLOSIVES 1.3*
G	**Articles, explosive, n.o.s.**	1.1C	UN0462	II	1.1C	101	112	EXPLOSIVES 1.1*
G	**Articles, explosive, n.o.s.**	1.1D	UN0463	II	1.1D	101	112	EXPLOSIVES 1.1*
G	**Articles, explosive, n.o.s.**	1.1E	UN0464	II	1.1E	101	112	EXPLOSIVES 1.1*
G	**Articles, explosive, n.o.s.**	1.1F	UN0465	II	1.1F	101	112	EXPLOSIVES 1.1*
G	**Articles, explosive, n.o.s.**	1.2C	UN0466	II	1.2C	101	112	EXPLOSIVES 1.2*
G	**Articles, explosive, n.o.s.**	1.2D	UN0467	II	1.2D	101	112	EXPLOSIVES 1.2*
G	**Articles, explosive, n.o.s.**	1.2E	UN0468	II	1.2E	101	112	EXPLOSIVES 1.2*
G	**Articles, explosive, n.o.s.**	1.2F	UN0469	II	1.2F	101	112	EXPLOSIVES 1.2*
G	**Articles, explosive, n.o.s.**	1.3C	UN0470	II	1.3C	101	112	EXPLOSIVES 1.3*
G	**Articles, explosive, n.o.s.**	1.4E	UN0471	II	1.4E	101	114	EXPLOSIVES 1.4
G	**Articles, explosive, n.o.s.**	1.4F	UN0472	II	1.4F	101	114	EXPLOSIVES 1.4
	Articles, pressurized pneumatic *or* **hydraulic** *containing non-flammable gas*	2.2	UN3164		2.2		126	NONFLAMMABLE GAS
	Articles, pyrophoric	1.2L	UN0380	II	1.2L		112	EXPLOSIVES 1.2*
	Articles, pyrotechnic *for technical purposes*	1.1G	UN0428	II	1.1G		112	EXPLOSIVES 1.1*
	Articles, pyrotechnic *for technical purposes*	1.2G	UN0429	II	1.2G		112	EXPLOSIVES 1.2*

Sym-bols	Hazardous materials descriptions and proper shipping names	Hazard class or Division	Identification Numbers	PG	Label Codes	Special provisions (§172.102)	ERG Guide No.	Placard Advisory Consult §172.504 & §172.505 *Placard any quantity
(1)	(2)	(3)	(4)	(5)	(6)	(7)		
	Articles, pyrotechnic *for technical purposes*	1.3G	UN0430	II	1.3G		112	EXPLOSIVES 1.3*
	Articles, pyrotechnic *for technical purposes*	1.4G	UN0431	II	1.4G		114	EXPLOSIVES 1.4
	Articles, pyrotechnic *for technical purposes*	1.4S	UN0432	II	1.4S		114	EXPLOSIVES 1.4
D	**Asbestos**	9	NA2212	III	9	156, IB8, IP2, IP4	171	CLASS 9
	Ascaridole (organic peroxide)	Forbidden						
D	**Asphalt,** *at or above its flashpoint*	3	NA1999	III	3	IB3, T1, TP3	130	FLAMMABLE
D	**Asphalt, cut back,** *see* **Tars, liquid,** *etc.*							
	Automobile, motorcycle, tractor, other self-propelled vehicle, engine, or other mechanical apparatus, see **Vehicles** *or* **Battery** *etc.*							
A G	**Aviation regulated liquid, n.o.s.**	9	UN3334		9	A35	171	CLASS 9
A G	**Aviation regulated solid, n.o.s.**	9	UN3335		9	A35	171	CLASS 9
	Azaurolic acid (salt of) (dry)	Forbidden						
	Azido guanidine picrate (dry)	Forbidden						
	5-Azido-1-hydroxy tetrazole	Forbidden						
	Azido hydroxy tetrazole (mercury and silver salts)	Forbidden						

Symbols	Hazardous materials descriptions and proper shipping names	Hazard class or Division	Identification Numbers	PG	Label Codes	Special provisions (§172.102)	ERG Guide No.	Placard Advisory Consult §172.504 & §172.505 *Placard any quantity
(1)	(2)	(3)	(4)	(5)	(6)	(7)		
	3-Azido-1,2-Propylene glycol dinitrate	Forbidden						
	Azidodithiocarbonic acid	Forbidden						
	Azidoethyl nitrate	Forbidden						
	1-Aziridinylphosphine oxide-(tris), see **Tris-(1-aziridinyl) phosphine oxide, solution**							
	Azodicarbonamide	4.1	UN3242	II	4.1	38, IB8, T3, TP33	149	FLAMMABLE SOLID
	Azotetrazole (dry)	Forbidden						
	Barium	4.3	UN1400	II	4.3	A19, IB7, IP2, T3, TP33	138	DANGEROUS WHEN WET*
	Barium alloys, pyrophoric	4.2	UN1854	I	4.2	T21, TP7, TP33	135	SPONTANEOUSLY COMBUSTIBLE
	Barium azide, *dry or wetted with less than 50 percent water, by mass*	1.1A	UN0224	II	1.1A, 6.1	111, 117	112	EXPLOSIVES 1.1*
	Barium azide, wetted *with not less than 50 percent water, by mass*	4.1	UN1571	I	4.1, 6.1	162, A2	113	FLAMMABLE SOLID
	Barium bromate	5.1	UN2719	II	5.1, 6.1	IB8, IP2, IP4, T3, TP33	141	OXIDIZER
	Barium chlorate, solid	5.1	UN1445	II	5.1, 6.1	A9, IB6, IP2, N34, T3, TP33	141	OXIDIZER
	Barium chlorate, solution	5.1	UN3405	II	5.1, 6.1	A9, IB2, N34, T4, TP1	141	OXIDIZER

Sym-bols	Hazardous materials descriptions and proper shipping names	Hazard class or Division	Identifica-tion Numbers	PG	Label Codes	Special provisions (§172.102)	ERG Guide No.	Placard Advisory Consult §172.504 & §172.505 *Placard any quantity
(1)	(2)	(3)	(4)	(5)	(6)	(7)		
				III	5.1, 6.1	A9, IB2, N34, T4, TP1	141	OXIDIZER
	Barium compounds, n.o.s.	6.1	UN1564	II	6.1	IB8, IP2, IP4, T3, TP33	154	POISON
				III	6.1	IB8, IP3, T1, TP33	154	POISON
	Barium cyanide	6.1	UN1565	I	6.1	IB7, IP1, N74, N75, T6, TP33	157	POISON
	Barium hypochlorite *with more than 22 percent available chlorine*	5.1	UN2741	II	5.1, 6.1	A7, A9, IB8, IP2, IP4, N34, T3, TP33	141	OXIDIZER
	Barium nitrate	5.1	UN1446	II	5.1, 6.1	IB8, IP2, IP4, T3, TP33	141	OXIDIZER
	Barium oxide	6.1	UN1884	III	6.1	IB8, IP3, T1, TP33	157	POISON
	Barium perchlorate, solid	5.1	UN1447	II	5.1, 6.1	IB6, IP2, T3, TP33	141	OXIDIZER
	Barium perchlorate, solution	5.1	UN3406	II	5.1, 6.1	IB2, T4, TP1	141	OXIDIZER
				III	5.1, 6.1	IB2, T4, TP1	141	OXIDIZER
	Barium permanganate	5.1	UN1448	II	5.1, 6.1	IB6, IP2, T3, TP33	141	OXIDIZER
	Barium peroxide	5.1	UN1449	II	5.1, 6.1	A9, IB6, IP2, T3, TP33	141	OXIDIZER

Symbols	Hazardous materials descriptions and proper shipping names	Hazard class or Division	Identification Numbers	PG	Label Codes	Special provisions (§172.102)	ERG Guide No.	Placard Advisory Consult §172.504 & §172.505 *Placard any quantity
(1)	(2)	(3)	(4)	(5)	(6)	(7)		
	Barium selenate, see **Selenates** *or* **Selenites**							
	Barium selenite, see **Selenates** *or* **Selenites**							
	Batteries, containing sodium	4.3	UN3292	II	4.3		138	DANGEROUS WHEN WET*
	Batteries, dry, containing potassium hydroxide solid, *electric, storage*	8	UN3028	III	8		154	CORROSIVE
	Batteries, wet, filled with acid, *electric storage*	8	UN2794	III	8		154	CORROSIVE
	Batteries, wet, filled with alkali, *electric storage*	8	UN2795	III	8		154	CORROSIVE
	Batteries, wet, filled with alkali, *electric storage*	8	UN2795	III	8		154	CORROSIVE
	Batteries, wet, non-spillable, *electric storage*	8	UN2800	III	8		154	CORROSIVE
	Battery, dry, *not subject to the requirements of this subchapter*					130		
	Battery fluid, acid	8	UN2796	II	8	A3, A7, B2, B15, IB2, N6, N34, T8, TP2, TP12	157	CORROSIVE
	Battery fluid, alkali	8	UN2797	II	8	B2, IB2, N6, T7, TP2, TP28	154	CORROSIVE

Symbols	Hazardous materials descriptions and proper shipping names	Hazard class or Division	Identification Numbers	PG	Label Codes	Special provisions (§172.102)	ERG Guide No.	Placard Advisory Consult §172.504 & §172.505 *Placard any quantity
(1)	(2)	(3)	(4)	(5)	(6)	(7)		
	Battery lithium type, see **Lithium batteries** *etc.*							
	Battery-powered vehicle *or* **Battery-powered equipment**	9	UN3171		9	134	154	CLASS 9
	Battery, wet, filled with acid or alkali with vehicle or mechanical equipment containing an internal combustion engine, see **Vehicle,** *etc. or* **Engines, Internal combustion,** *etc.*							
+	**Benzaldehyde**	9	UN1990	III	9	IB3, T2, TP1	129	CLASS 9
	Benzene	3	UN1114	II	3	IB2, T4, TP1	130	FLAMMABLE
	Benzene diazonium chloride (dry)	Forbidden						
	Benzene diazonium nitrate (dry)	Forbidden						
	Benzene phosphorus dichloride, see **Phenyl phosphorus dichloride**							
	Benzene phosphorus thiodichloride, see **Phenyl phosphorus thiodichloride**							
	Benzene sulfonyl chloride	8	UN2225	III	8	IB3, T4, TP1	156	CORROSIVE
	Benzene triozonide	Forbidden						
	Benzenethiol, see **Phenyl mercaptan**							
	Benzidine	6.1	UN1885	II	6.1	IB8, IP2, IP4, T3, TP33	153	POISON
	Benzol, see **Benzene**							

Sym-bols	Hazardous materials descriptions and proper shipping names	Hazard class or Division	Identification Numbers	PG	Label Codes	Special provisions (§172.102)	ERG Guide No.	Placard Advisory Consult §172.504 & §172.505 *Placard any quantity
(1)	(2)	(3)	(4)	(5)	(6)	(7)		
	Benzonitrile	6.1	UN2224	II	6.1	IB2, T7, TP2	152	POISON
	Benzoquinone	6.1	UN2587	II	6.1	IB8, IP2, IP4, T3, TP33	153	POISON
	Benzotrichloride	8	UN2226	II	8	B2, IB2, T7, TP2	156	CORROSIVE
	Benzotrifluoride	3	UN2338	II	3	IB2, T4, TP1	127	FLAMMABLE
	Benzoxidiazoles (dry)	Forbidden						
	Benzoyl azide	Forbidden						
	Benzoyl chloride	8	UN1736	II	8	B2, IB2, T8, TP2, TP12, TP13	137	CORROSIVE
	Benzyl bromide	6.1	UN1737	II	6.1, 8	A3, A7, IB2, N33, N34, T8, TP2, TP12, TP13	156	POISON
	Benzyl chloride	6.1	UN1738	II	6.1, 8	A3, A7, B70, IB2, N33, N42, T8, TP2, TP12, TP13	156	POISON
	Benzyl chloride *unstabilized*	6.1	UN1738	II	6.1, 8	A3, A7, B8, B11, IB2, N33, N34, N43, T8, TP2, TP12, TP13	156	POISON
	Benzyl chloroformate	8	UN1739	I	8	A3, A6, B4, N41, T10, TP2, TP12, TP13	137	CORROSIVE
	Benzyl iodide	6.1	UN2653	II	6.1	IB2, T7, TP2	156	POISON

Symbols	Hazardous materials descriptions and proper shipping names	Hazard class or Division	Identification Numbers	PG	Label Codes	Special provisions (§172.102)	ERG Guide No.	Placard Advisory Consult §172.504 & §172.505 *Placard any quantity
(1)	(2)	(3)	(4)	(5)	(6)	(7)		
	Benzyldimethylamine	8	UN2619	II	8, 3	B2, IB2, T7, TP2	132	CORROSIVE
	Benzylidene chloride	6.1	UN1886	II	6.1	IB2, T7, TP2	156	POISON
	Beryllium compounds, n.o.s.	6.1	UN1566	II	6.1	IB8, IP2, IP4, T3, TP33	154	POISON
				III	6.1	IB8, IP3, T1, TP33	154	POISON
	Beryllium nitrate	5.1	UN2464	II	5.1, 6.1	IB8, IP2, IP4, T3, TP33	141	OXIDIZER
	Beryllium, powder	6.1	UN1567	II	6.1, 4.1	IB8, IP2, IP4, T3, TP33	134	POISON
	Bicyclo [2,2,1] hepta-2,5-diene, stabilized *or* **2,5-Norbornadiene, stabilized**	3	UN2251	II	3	IB2, T7, TP2	128P	FLAMMABLE
	Biphenyl triozonide	Forbidden						
	Bipyridilium pesticides, liquid, flammable, toxic, *flash point less than 23 degrees C*	3	UN2782	I	3, 6.1	T14, TP2, TP13, TP27	131	FLAMMABLE
				II	3, 6.1	IB2, T11, TP2, TP13, TP27	131	FLAMMABLE
	Bipyridilium pesticides, liquid, toxic	6.1	UN3016	I	6.1	T14, TP2, TP13, TP27	151	POISON
				II	6.1	IB2, T11, TP2, TP13, TP27	151	POISON
				III	6.1	IB3, T7, TP2, TP28	151	POISON

Sym-bols	Hazardous materials descriptions and proper shipping names	Hazard class or Division	Identifica-tion Numbers	PG	Label Codes	Special provisions (§172.102)	ERG Guide No.	Placard Advisory Consult §172.504 & §172.505 *Placard any quantity
(1)	(2)	(3)	(4)	(5)	(6)	(7)		
	Bipyridilium pesticides, liquid, toxic, flammable, *flash point not less than 23 degrees C*	6.1	UN3015	I	6.1, 3	T14, TP2, TP13, TP27	131	POISON
				II	6.1, 3	IB2, T11, TP2, TP13, TP27	131	POISON
				III	6.1, 3	B1, IB3, T7, TP2, TP28	131	POISON
	Bipyridilium pesticides, solid, toxic	6.1	UN2781	I	6.1	IB7, IP1, T6, TP33	151	POISON
				II	6.1	IB8, IP2, IP4, T3, TP33	151	POISON
				III	6.1	IB8, IP3, T1, TP33	151	POISON
	Bis (Aminopropyl) piperazine, see **Corrosive liquid, n.o.s.**							
	Bisulfate, aqueous solution	8	UN2837	II	8	A7, B2, IB2, N34, T7, TP2	154	CORROSIVE
				III	8	A7, IB3, N34, T4, TP1	154	CORROSIVE
	Bisulfites, aqueous solutions, n.o.s.	8	UN2693	III	8	IB3, T7, TP1, TP28	154	CORROSIVE
	Black powder, compressed *or* **Gunpowder, compressed** *or* **Black powder, in pellets** *or* **Gunpowder, in pellets**	1.1D	UN0028	II	1.1D		112	EXPLOSIVES 1.1*
	Black powder *or* **Gunpowder,** *granular or as a meal*	1.1D	UN0027	II	1.1D		112	EXPLOSIVES 1.1*

Sym-bols	Hazardous materials descriptions and proper shipping names	Hazard class or Division	Identification Numbers	PG	Label Codes	Special provisions (§172.102)	ERG Guide No.	Placard Advisory Consult §172.504 & §172.505 *Placard any quantity
(1)	(2)	(3)	(4)	(5)	(6)	(7)		
D	**Black powder for small arms**	4.1	NA0027	I	4.1	70	—	FLAMMABLE SOLID
	Blasting agent, n.o.s., see **Explosives, blasting** *etc.*							
	Blasting cap assemblies, see **Detonator assemblies, non-electric,** *for blasting*							
	Blasting caps, electric, see **Detonators, electric** *for blasting*							
	Blasting caps, non-electric, see **Detonators, non-electric,** *for blasting*							
	Bleaching powder, see **Calcium hypochlorite mixtures,** *etc.*							
I	**Blue asbestos** *(Crocidolite) or* **Brown asbestos** *(amosite, mysorite)*	9	UN2212	II	9	156, IB8, IP2, IP4, T3, TP33	171	CLASS 9
	Bombs, photo-flash	1.1F	UN0037	II	1.1F		112	EXPLOSIVES 1.1*
	Bombs, photo-flash	1.1D	UN0038	II	1.1D		112	EXPLOSIVES 1.1*
	Bombs, photo-flash	1.2G	UN0039	II	1.2G		112	EXPLOSIVES 1.2*
	Bombs, photo-flash	1.3G	UN0299	II	1.3G		112	EXPLOSIVES 1.3*
	Bombs, smoke, non-explosive, *with corrosive liquid, without initiating device*	8	UN2028	II	8		153	CORROSIVE
	Bombs, *with bursting charge*	1.1F	UN0033	II	1.1F		112	EXPLOSIVES 1.1*
	Bombs, *with bursting charge*	1.1D	UN0034	II	1.1D		112	EXPLOSIVES 1.1*

Sym-bols	Hazardous materials descriptions and proper shipping names	Hazard class or Division	Identifica-tion Numbers	PG	Label Codes	Special provisions (§172.102)	ERG Guide No.	Placard Advisory Consult §172.504 & §172.505 *Placard any quantity
(1)	(2)	(3)	(4)	(5)	(6)	(7)		
	Bombs, *with bursting charge*	1.2D	UN0035	II	1.2D		112	EXPLOSIVES 1.2*
	Bombs, *with bursting charge*	1.2F	UN0291	II	1.2F		112	EXPLOSIVES 1.2*
	Bombs with flammable liquid, *with bursting charge*	1.1J	UN0399	II	1.1J		112	EXPLOSIVES 1.1*
	Bombs with flammable liquid, *with bursting charge*	1.2J	UN0400	II	1.2J		112	EXPLOSIVES 1.2*
	Boosters with detonator	1.1B	UN0225	II	1.1B		112	EXPLOSIVES 1.1*
	Boosters with detonator	1.2B	UN0268	II	1.2B		112	EXPLOSIVES 1.2*
	Boosters, *without detonator*	1.1D	UN0042	II	1.1D		112	EXPLOSIVES 1.1*
	Boosters, *without detonator*	1.2D	UN0283	II	1.2D		112	EXPLOSIVES 1.2*
	Borate and chlorate mixtures, see **Chlorate and borate mixtures**							
	Borneol	4.1	UN1312	III	4.1	A1, IB8, IP3, T1, TP33	133	FLAMMABLE SOLID
+	**Boron tribromide**	8	UN2692	I	8, 6.1	2, B9, B14, B32, B74, N34, T20, TP2, TP12, TP13, TP38, TP45	157	CORROSIVE, POISON INHALATION HAZARD*
	Boron trichloride	2.3	UN1741		2.3, 8	3, B9, B14	125	POISON GAS*
	Boron trifluoride	2.3	UN1008		2.3	2, B9, B14	125	POISON GAS*
	Boron trifluoride acetic acid complex, liquid	8	UN1742	II	8	B2, B6, IB2, T8, TP2, TP12	157	CORROSIVE
	Boron trifluoride acetic acid complex, solid	8	UN3419	II	8	B2, B6, IB8, IP2, IP4, T3, TP33	157	CORROSIVE

Symbols	Hazardous materials descriptions and proper shipping names	Hazard class or Division	Identification Numbers	PG	Label Codes	Special provisions (§172.102)	ERG Guide No.	Placard Advisory Consult §172.504 & §172.505 *Placard any quantity
(1)	(2)	(3)	(4)	(5)	(6)	(7)		
	Boron trifluoride diethyl etherate	8	UN2604	I	8, 3	A3, A19, T10, TP2	132	CORROSIVE
	Boron trifluoride dihydrate	8	UN2851	II	8	IB2, T7, TP2	157	CORROSIVE
	Boron trifluoride dimethyl etherate	4.3	UN2965	I	4.3, 8, 3	A19, T10, TP2, TP7	139	DANGEROUS WHEN WET*
	Boron trifluoride propionic acid complex, liquid	8	UN1743	II	8	B2, IB2, T8, TP2, TP12	157	CORROSIVE
	Boron trifluoride propionic acid complex, solid	8	UN3420	II	8	B2, IB8, IP2, IP4, T3, TP33	157	CORROSIVE
	Box toe gum, see **Nitrocellulose** *etc.*							
	Bromates, inorganic, aqueous solution, n.o.s.	5.1	UN3213	II	5.1	IB2, T4, TP1	140	OXIDIZER
				III	5.1	IB2, T4, TP1	140	
	Bromates, inorganic, n.o.s.	5.1	UN1450	II	5.1	IB8, IP2, IP4, T3, TP33	141	OXIDIZER
+	**Bromine**	8	UN1744	I	8, 6.1	1, B9, B64, B85, N34, N43, T22, TP2, TP10, TP12, TP13	154	CORROSIVE, POISON INHALATION HAZARD*
	Bromine azide	Forbidden						
	Bromine chloride	2.3	UN2901		2.3, 8, 5.1	2, B9, B14	124	POISON GAS*
+	**Bromine pentafluoride**	5.1	UN1745	I	5.1, 6.1 , 8	1, B9, B14, B30, B72, T22, TP2, TP12, TP13, TP38, TP44	144	OXIDIZER, POISON INHALATION HAZARD*

Symbols	Hazardous materials descriptions and proper shipping names	Hazard class or Division	Identification Numbers	PG	Label Codes	Special provisions (§172.102)	ERG Guide No.	Placard Advisory Consult §172.504 & §172.505 *Placard any quantity
(1)	(2)	(3)	(4)	(5)	(6)	(7)		
+	**Bromine solutions**	8	UN1744	I	8, 6.1	1, B9, B64, B85, N34, N43, T22, TP2, TP10, TP12, TP13	154	CORROSIVE, POISON INHALATION HAZARD*
+	**Bromine solutions**	8	UN1744	I	8, 6.1	2, B9, B64, B85, N34, N43, T22, TP2, TP10, TP12, TP13	154	CORROSIVE, POISON INHALATION HAZARD*
+	**Bromine trifluoride**	5.1	UN1746	I	5.1, 6.1 , 8	2, B9, B14, B32, B74, T22, TP2, TP12, TP13, TP38, TP45	144	OXIDIZER, POISON INHALATION HAZARD*
	4-Bromo-1,2-dinitrobenzene	Forbidden						
	4-Bromo-1,2-dinitrobenzene (unstable at 59 degrees C.)	Forbidden						
	1-Bromo-3-chloropropane	6.1	UN2688	III	6.1	IB3, T4, TP1	159	POISON
	1-Bromo-3-methylbutane	3	UN2341	III	3	B1, IB3, T2, TP1	130	FLAMMABLE
	1-Bromo-3-nitrobenzene (unstable at 56 degrees C)	Forbidden						
	2-Bromo-2-nitropropane-1,3-diol	4.1	UN3241	III	4.1	46, IB8, IP3	133	FLAMMABLE SOLID
	Bromoacetic acid solid	8	UN3425	II	8	A7, IB8, IP2, IP4, N34, T3, TP33	156	CORROSIVE
	Bromoacetic acid solution	8	UN1938	II	8	A7, B2, IB2, T7, TP2	156	CORROSIVE

Symbols	Hazardous materials descriptions and proper shipping names	Hazard class or Division	Identification Numbers	PG	Label Codes	Special provisions (§172.102)	ERG Guide No.	Placard Advisory Consult §172.504 & §172.505 *Placard any quantity
(1)	(2)	(3)	(4)	(5)	(6)	(7)		
				III	8	B2, IB3, T7, TP2	156	CORROSIVE
+	**Bromoacetone**	6.1	UN1569	II	6.1, 3	2, T20, TP2, TP13	131	POISON INHALATION HAZARD*
	Bromoacetyl bromide	8	UN2513	II	8	B2, IB2, T8, TP2, TP12	156	CORROSIVE
	Bromobenzene	3	UN2514	III	3	B1, IB3, T2, TP1	130	FLAMMABLE
	Bromobenzyl cyanides, liquid	6.1	UN1694	I	6.1	T14, TP2, TP13	159	POISON
	Bromobenzyl cyanides, solid	6.1	UN3449	I	6.1	T6, TP33	159	POISON
	1-Bromobutane	3	UN1126	II	3	IB2, T4, TP1	130	FLAMMABLE
	2-Bromobutane	3	UN2339	II	3	B1, IB2, T4, TP1	130	FLAMMABLE
	Bromochloromethane	6.1	UN1887	III	6.1	IB3, T4, TP1	160	POISON
	2-Bromoethyl ethyl ether	3	UN2340	II	3	IB2, T4, TP1	130	FLAMMABLE
	Bromoform	6.1	UN2515	III	6.1	IB3, T4, TP1	159	POISON
	Bromomethylpropanes	3	UN2342	II	3	IB2, T4, TP1	130	FLAMMABLE
	2-Bromopentane	3	UN2343	II	3	IB2, T4, TP1	130	FLAMMABLE
	Bromopropanes	3	UN2344	II	3	IB2, T4, TP1	129	FLAMMABLE
				III	3	IB3, T2, TP1	129	FLAMMABLE
	3-Bromopropyne	3	UN2345	II	3	IB2, T4, TP1	130	FLAMMABLE
	Bromosilane	Forbidden						
	Bromotoluene-alpha, see **Benzyl bromide**							

Symbols	Hazardous materials descriptions and proper shipping names	Hazard class or Division	Identification Numbers	PG	Label Codes	Special provisions (§172.102)	ERG Guide No.	Placard Advisory Consult §172.504 & §172.505 *Placard any quantity
(1)	(2)	(3)	(4)	(5)	(6)	(7)		
	Bromotrifluoroethylene	2.1	UN2419		2.1		116	FLAMMABLE GAS
	Bromotrifluoromethane *or* **Refrigerant gas, R 13B1**	2.2	UN1009		2.2	T50	126	NONFLAMMABLE GAS
	Brucine	6.1	UN1570	I	6.1	IB7, IP1, T6, TP33	152	POISON
	Bursters, *explosive*	1.1D	UN0043	II	1.1D		112	EXPLOSIVES 1.1*
	Butadienes, stabilized *or* **Butadienes and Hydrocarbon mixture, stabilized** *containing more than 40% Butadienes*	2.1	UN1010		2.1	T50	116P	FLAMMABLE GAS
	Butane *see also* **Petroleum gases, liquefied**	2.1	UN1011		2.1	19, T50	115	FLAMMABLE GAS
	Butane, butane mixtures and mixtures having similar properties in cartridges each not exceeding 500 grams, see **Receptacles,** *etc.*							
	Butanedione	3	UN2346	II	3	IB2, T4, TP1	127	FLAMMABLE
	1,2,4-Butanetriol trinitrate	Forbidden						
	Butanols	3	UN1120	II	3	IB2, T4, TP1, TP29	129	FLAMMABLE
				III	3	B1, IB3, T2, TP1	129	FLAMMABLE
	tert-Butoxycarbonyl azide	Forbidden						
	Butyl acetates	3	UN1123	II	3	IB2, T4, TP1	129	FLAMMABLE
				III	3	B1, IB3, T2, TP1	129	FLAMMABLE

Sym-bols	Hazardous materials descriptions and proper shipping names	Hazard class or Division	Identifica-tion Numbers	PG	Label Codes	Special provisions (§172.102)	ERG Guide No.	Placard Advisory Consult §172.504 & §172.505 *Placard any quantity
(1)	(2)	(3)	(4)	(5)	(6)	(7)		
	Butyl acid phosphate	8	UN1718	III	8	IB3, T4, TP1	153	CORROSIVE
	Butyl acrylates, stabilized	3	UN2348	III	3	B1, IB3, T2, TP1	130P	FLAMMABLE
	Butyl alcohols, see **Butanols**							
	Butyl benzenes	3	UN2709	III	3	B1, IB3, T2, TP1	128	FLAMMABLE
	n-Butyl bromide, see **1-Bromobutane**							
	n-Butyl chloride, see **Chlorobutanes**							
D	**sec-Butyl chloroformate**	6.1	NA2742	I	6.1, 3, 8	2, B9, B14, B32, B74, T20, TP4, TP12, TP13, TP38, TP45	155	POISON INHALATION HAZARD*
	n-Butyl chloroformate	6.1	UN2743	I	6.1, 8, 3	2, B9, B14, B32, B74, T20, TP2, TP13, TP38, TP45	155	POISON INHALATION HAZARD*
	Butyl ethers, see **Dibutyl ethers**							
	Butyl ethyl ether, see **Ethyl butyl ether**							
	n-Butyl formate	3	UN1128	II	3	IB2, T4, TP1	129	FLAMMABLE
	tert-Butyl hydroperoxide, with more than 90 percent with water	Forbidden						
	tert-Butyl hypochlorite	4.2	UN3255	I	4.2, 8		135	SPONTANEOUSLY COMBUSTIBLE
	N-n-Butyl imidazole	6.1	UN2690	II	6.1	IB2, T7, TP2	152	POISON

Symbols	Hazardous materials descriptions and proper shipping names	Hazard class or Division	Identification Numbers	PG	Label Codes	Special provisions (§172.102)	ERG Guide No.	Placard Advisory Consult §172.504 & §172.505 *Placard any quantity
(1)	(2)	(3)	(4)	(5)	(6)	(7)		
	tert-Butyl isocyanate	6.1	UN2484	I	6.1, 3	1, B9, B14, B30, B72, T22, TP2, TP13, TP38, TP44	155	POISON INHALATION HAZARD*
	n-Butyl isocyanate	6.1	UN2485	I	6.1, 3	2, B9, B14, B32, B74, B77, T20, TP2, TP13, TP38, TP45	155	POISON INHALATION HAZARD*
	Butyl mercaptans	3	UN2347	II	3	A3, A6, IB2, T4, TP1	130	FLAMMABLE
	n-Butyl methacrylate, stabilized	3	UN2227	III	3	B1, IB3, T2, TP1	130P	FLAMMABLE
	Butyl methyl ether	3	UN2350	II	3	IB2, T4, TP1	127	FLAMMABLE
	Butyl nitrites	3	UN2351	I	3	T11, TP1, TP8, TP27	129	FLAMMABLE
				II	3	IB2, T4, TP1	129	FLAMMABLE
				III	3	B1, IB3, T2, TP1	129	FLAMMABLE
	tert-Butyl peroxyacetate, with more than 76 percent in solution	Forbidden						
	n-Butyl peroxydicarbonate, with more than 52 percent in solution	Forbidden						
	tert-Butyl peroxyisobutyrate, with more than 77 percent in solution	Forbidden						
	Butyl phosphoric acid, see **Butyl acid phosphate**							

Symbols	Hazardous materials descriptions and proper shipping names	Hazard class or Division	Identification Numbers	PG	Label Codes	Special provisions (§172.102)	ERG Guide No.	Placard Advisory Consult §172.504 & §172.505 *Placard any quantity
(1)	(2)	(3)	(4)	(5)	(6)	(7)		
	Butyl propionates	3	UN1914	III	3	B1, IB3, T2, TP1	130	FLAMMABLE
	5-tert-Butyl-2,4,6-trinitro-m-xylene *or* **Musk xylene**	4.1	UN2956	III	4.1	159	149	FLAMMABLE SOLID
	Butyl vinyl ether, stabilized	3	UN2352	II	3	IB2, T4, TP1	127P	FLAMMABLE
	n-Butylamine	3	UN1125	II	3, 8	IB2, T7, TP1	132	FLAMMABLE
	N-Butylaniline	6.1	UN2738	II	6.1	IB2, T7, TP2	153	POISON
	tert-Butylcyclohexylchloroformate	6.1	UN2747	III	6.1	IB3, T4, TP1	156	POISON
	Butylene *see also* **Petroleum gases, liquefied**	2.1	UN1012		2.1	19, T50	115	FLAMMABLE GAS
	1,2-Butylene oxide, stabilized	3	UN3022	II	3	IB2, T4, TP1	127P	FLAMMABLE
	Butyltoluenes	6.1	UN2667	III	6.1	IB3, T4, TP1	152	POISON
	Butyltrichlorosilane	8	UN1747	II	8, 3	A7, B2, B6, IB2, N34, T7, TP2, TP13	155	CORROSIVE
	1,4-Butynediol	6.1	UN2716	III	6.1	A1, IB8, IP3, T1, TP33	153	POISON
	Butyraldehyde	3	UN1129	II	3	IB2, T4, TP1	129	FLAMMABLE
	Butyraldoxime	3	UN2840	III	3	B1, IB3, T2, TP1	129	FLAMMABLE
	Butyric acid	8	UN2820	III	8	IB3, T4, TP1	153	CORROSIVE
	Butyric anhydride	8	UN2739	III	8	IB3, T4, TP1	156	CORROSIVE
	Butyronitrile	3	UN2411	II	3, 6.1	IB2, T7, TP1, TP13	131	FLAMMABLE

Symbols	Hazardous materials descriptions and proper shipping names	Hazard class or Division	Identification Numbers	PG	Label Codes	Special provisions (§172.102)	ERG Guide No.	Placard Advisory Consult §172.504 & §172.505 *Placard any quantity
(1)	(2)	(3)	(4)	(5)	(6)	(7)		
	Butyryl chloride	3	UN2353	II	3, 8	IB2, T8, TP2, TP12, TP13	132	FLAMMABLE
	Cacodylic acid	6.1	UN1572	II	6.1	IB8, IP2, IP4, T3, TP33	151	POISON
	Cadmium compounds	6.1	UN2570	I	6.1	IB7, IP1, T6, TP33	154	POISON
				II	6.1	IB8, IP2, IP4, T3, TP33	154	POISON
				III	6.1	IB8, IP3, T1, TP33	154	POISON
	Caesium hydroxide	8	UN2682	II	8	IB8, IP2, IP4, T3, TP33	157	CORROSIVE
	Caesium hydroxide solution	8	UN2681	II	8	B2, IB2, T7, TP2	154	CORROSIVE
				III	8	IB3, T4, TP1	154	CORROSIVE
	Calcium	4.3	UN1401	II	4.3	IB7, IP2, T3, TP33	138	DANGEROUS WHEN WET*
	Calcium arsenate	6.1	UN1573	II	6.1	IB8, IP2, IP4, T3, TP33	151	POISON
	Calcium arsenate and calcium arsenite, mixtures, solid	6.1	UN1574	II	6.1	IB8, IP2, IP4, T3, TP33	151	POISON
	Calcium bisulfite solution, see **Bisulfites, aqueous solutions, n.o.s.**							

Symbols	Hazardous materials descriptions and proper shipping names	Hazard class or Division	Identification Numbers	PG	Label Codes	Special provisions (§172.102)	ERG Guide No.	Placard Advisory Consult §172.504 & §172.505 *Placard any quantity
(1)	(2)	(3)	(4)	(5)	(6)	(7)		
	Calcium carbide	4.3	UN1402	I	4.3	A1, A8, B55, B59, IB4, IP1, N34, T9, TP7, TP33	138	DANGEROUS WHEN WET*
				II	4.3	A1, A8, B55, B59, IB7, IP2, N34, T3, TP33	138	DANGEROUS WHEN WET*
	Calcium chlorate	5.1	UN1452	II	5.1	A9, IB8, IP2, IP4, N34, T3, TP33	140	OXIDIZER
	Calcium chlorate aqueous solution	5.1	UN2429	II	5.1	A2, IB2, N41, T4, TP1	140	OXIDIZER
				III	5.1	A2, IB2, N41, T4, TP1	140	OXIDIZER
	Calcium chlorite	5.1	UN1453	II	5.1	A9, IB8, IP2, IP4, N34, T3, TP33	140	OXIDIZER
	Calcium cyanamide *with more than 0.1 percent of calcium carbide*	4.3	UN1403	III	4.3	A1, A19, IB8, IP4, T1, TP33	138	DANGEROUS WHEN WET*
	Calcium cyanide	6.1	UN1575	I	6.1	IB7, IP1, N79, N80, T6, TP33	157	POISON
	Calcium dithionite *or* **Calcium hydrosulfite**	4.2	UN1923	II	4.2	A19, A20, IB6, IP2, T3, TP33	135	SPONTANEOUSLY COMBUSTIBLE
	Calcium hydride	4.3	UN1404	I	4.3	A19, N40	138	DANGEROUS WHEN WET*
	Calcium hydrosulfite, *see* **Calcium dithionite**							

Symbols	Hazardous materials descriptions and proper shipping names	Hazard class or Division	Identification Numbers	PG	Label Codes	Special provisions (§172.102)	ERG Guide No.	Placard Advisory Consult §172.504 & §172.505 *Placard any quantity
(1)	(2)	(3)	(4)	(5)	(6)	(7)		
	Calcium hypochlorite, dry *or* **Calcium hypochlorite mixtures dry** *with more than 39 percent available chlorine (8.8 percent available oxygen)*	5.1	UN1748	II	5.1	165, 166, A7, A9, IB8, IP2, IP4, IP13, N34, W9	140	OXIDIZER
				III	5.1	165, 171, A7, A9, IB8, IP4, IP13, N34, W9	140	OXIDIZER
	Calcium hypochlorite, hydrated *or* **Calcium hypochlorite, hydrated mixtures,** *with not less than 5.5 percent but not more than 16 percent water*	5.1	UN2880	II	5.1	165, 166, IB8, IP2, IP4, IP13, W9	140	OXIDIZER
				III	5.1	165, 171, IB8, IP4, IP13, W9	140	OXIDIZER
	Calcium hypochlorite mixtures, dry, *with more than 10 percent but not more than 39 percent available chlorine*	5.1	UN2208	III	5.1	165, A1, A29, IB8, IP3, IP13, N34, W9	140	OZIDIZER
	Calcium manganese silicon	4.3	UN2844	III	4.3	A1, A19, IB8, IP2, IP4, T1, TP33	138	DANGEROUS WHEN WET*
	Calcium nitrate	5.1	UN1454	III	5.1	34, IB8, IP3, T1, TP33	140	OXIDIZER
A	**Calcium oxide**	8	UN1910	III	8	IB8, IP3, T1, TP33	157	CORROSIVE
	Calcium perchlorate	5.1	UN1455	II	5.1	IB6, IP2, T3, TP33	140	OXIDIZER
	Calcium permanganate	5.1	UN1456	II	5.1	IB6, IP2, T3, TP33	140	OXIDIZER

Sym-bols	Hazardous materials descriptions and proper shipping names	Hazard class or Division	Identifica-tion Numbers	PG	Label Codes	Special provisions (§172.102)	ERG Guide No.	Placard Advisory Consult §172.504 & §172.505 *Placard any quantity
(1)	(2)	(3)	(4)	(5)	(6)	(7)		
	Calcium peroxide	5.1	UN1457	II	5.1	IB6, IP2, T3, TP33	140	OXIDIZER
	Calcium phosphide	4.3	UN1360	I	4.3, 6.1	A8, A19, N40	139	DANGEROUS WHEN WET*
	Calcium, pyrophoric *or* **Calcium alloys, pyrophoric**	4.2	UN1855	I	4.2		135	SPONTANEOUSLY COMBUSTIBLE
	Calcium resinate	4.1	UN1313	III	4.1	A1, A19, IB6, T1, TP33	133	FLAMMABLE SOLID
	Calcium resinate, fused	4.1	UN1314	III	4.1	A1, A19, IB4, T1, TP33	133	FLAMMABLE SOLID
	Calcium selenate, see **Selenates** *or* **Selenites**							
	Calcium silicide	4.3	UN1405	II	4.3	A19, IB7, IP2, T3, TP33	138	DANGEROUS WHEN WET*
				III	4.3	A1, A19, IB8, IP4, T1, TP33	138	DANGEROUS WHEN WET*
	Camphor oil	3	UN1130	III	3	B1, IB3, T2, TP1	128	FLAMMABLE
	Camphor, *synthetic*	4.1	UN2717	III	4.1	A1, IB8, IP3, T1, TP33	133	FLAMMABLE SOLID
	Cannon primers, see **Primers, tubular**							
	Caproic acid	8	UN2829	III	8	IB3, T4, TP1	153	CORROSIVE
	Caps, blasting, see **Detonators,** *etc.*							

Sym-bols	Hazardous materials descriptions and proper shipping names	Hazard class or Division	Identifica-tion Numbers	PG	Label Codes	Special provisions (§172.102)	ERG Guide No.	Placard Advisory Consult §172.504 & §172.505 *Placard any quantity
(1)	(2)	(3)	(4)	(5)	(6)	(7)		
	Carbamate pesticides, liquid, flammable, toxic, *flash point less than 23 degrees C*	3	UN2758	I	3, 6.1	T14, TP2, TP13, TP27	131	FLAMMABLE
				II	3, 6.1	IB2, T11, TP2, TP13, TP27	131	FLAMMABLE
	Carbamate pesticides, liquid, toxic	6.1	UN2992	I	6.1	T14, TP2, TP13, TP27	151	POISON
				II	6.1	IB2, T11, TP2, TP13, TP27	151	POISON
				III	6.1	IB3, T7, TP2, TP28	151	POISON
	Carbamate pesticides, liquid, toxic, flammable, *flash point not less than 23 degrees C*	6.1	UN2991	I	6.1, 3	T14, TP2, TP13, TP27	131	POISON
				II	6.1, 3	IB2, T11, TP2, TP13, TP27	131	POISON
				III	6.1, 3	B1, IB3, T7, TP2, TP28	131	POISON
	Carbamate pesticides, solid, toxic	6.1	UN2757	I	6.1	IB7, IP1, T6, TP33	151	POISON
				II	6.1	IB8, IP2, IP4, T3, TP33	151	POISON
				III	6.1	IB8, IP3, T1, TP33	151	POISON
	Carbolic acid, see **Phenol, solid** *or* **Phenol, molten**							

Symbols	Hazardous materials descriptions and proper shipping names	Hazard class or Division	Identification Numbers	PG	Label Codes	Special provisions (§172.102)	ERG Guide No.	Placard Advisory Consult §172.504 & §172.505 *Placard any quantity
(1)	(2)	(3)	(4)	(5)	(6)	(7)		
	Carbolic acid solutions, see **Phenol solutions**							
I	**Carbon, activated**	4.2	UN1362	III	4.2	IB8, IP3, T1, TP33	133	SPONTANEOUSLY COMBUSTIBLE
I	**Carbon,** ***animal or vegetable origin***	4.2	UN1361	II	4.2	IB6, T3, TP33	133	SPONTANEOUSLY COMBUSTIBLE
				III	4.2	IB8, IP3, T1, TP33	133	SPONTANEOUSLY COMBUSTIBLE
	Carbon bisulfide, see **Carbon disulfide**							
	Carbon dioxide	2.2	UN1013		2.2		120	NONFLAMMABLE GAS
	Carbon dioxide and nitrous oxide mixtures	2.2	UN1015		2.2		126	NONFLAMMABLE GAS
	Carbon dioxide and oxygen mixtures, compressed	2.2	UN1014		2.2, 5.1	77, A14	122	NONFLAMMABLE GAS
	Carbon dioxide, refrigerated liquid	2.2	UN2187		2.2	T75, TP5	120	NONFLAMMABLE GAS
A W	**Carbon dioxide, solid** *or* **Dry ice**	9	UN1845	III	None		120	CLASS 9
	Carbon disulfide	3	UN1131	I	3, 6.1	B16, T14, TP2, TP7, TP13	131	FLAMMABLE
	Carbon monoxide, compressed	2.3	UN1016		2.3, 2.1	4	119	POISON GAS*

Symbols	Hazardous materials descriptions and proper shipping names	Hazard class or Division	Identification Numbers	PG	Label Codes	Special provisions (§172.102)	ERG Guide No.	Placard Advisory Consult §172.504 & §172.505 *Placard any quantity
(1)	(2)	(3)	(4)	(5)	(6)	(7)		
	Carbon monoxide and hydrogen mixture, compressed	2.3	UN2600		2.3, 2.1	6	119	POISON GAS*
D	**Carbon monoxide, refrigerated liquid** *(cryogenic liquid)*	2.3	NA9202		2.3, 2.1	4, T75, TP5	168	POISON GAS*
	Carbon tetrabromide	6.1	UN2516	III	6.1	IB8, IP3, T1, TP33	151	POISON
	Carbon tetrachloride	6.1	UN1846	II	6.1	IB2, N36, T7, TP2	151	POISON
	Carbonyl chloride, see **Phosgene**							
	Carbonyl fluoride	2.3	UN2417		2.3, 8	2	125	POISON GAS*
	Carbonyl sulfide	2.3	UN2204		2.3, 2.1	3, B14	119	POISON GAS*
	Cartridge cases, empty primed, see **Cases, cartridge, empty, with primer**							
	Cartridges, actuating, for aircraft ejector seat catapult, fire extinguisher, canopy removal or apparatus, see **Cartridges, power device**							
	Cartridges, explosive, see **Charges, demolition**							
	Cartridges, flash	1.1G	UN0049	II	1.1G		112	EXPLOSIVES 1.1*
	Cartridges, flash	1.3G	UN0050	II	1.3G		112	EXPLOSIVES 1.3*
	Cartridges for weapons, blank	1.1C	UN0326	II	1.1C		112	EXPLOSIVES 1.1*
	Cartridges for weapons, blank	1.2C	UN0413	II	1.2C		112	EXPLOSIVES 1.2*

Symbols	Hazardous materials descriptions and proper shipping names	Hazard class or Division	Identification Numbers	PG	Label Codes	Special provisions (§172.102)	ERG Guide No.	Placard Advisory Consult §172.504 & §172.505 *Placard any quantity
(1)	(2)	(3)	(4)	(5)	(6)	(7)		
	Cartridges for weapons, blank *or* **Cartridges, small arms, blank**	1.4S	UN0014	II	None		114	EXPLOSIVES 1.4
	Cartridges for weapons, blank *or* **Cartridges, small arms, blank**	1.3C	UN0327	II	1.3C		112	EXPLOSIVES 1.3*
	Cartridges for weapons, blank *or* **Cartridges, small arms, blank**	1.4C	UN0338	II	1.4C		114	EXPLOSIVES 1.4
	Cartridges for weapons, inert projectile	1.2C	UN0328	II	1.2C		112	EXPLOSIVES 1.2*
	Cartridges for weapons, inert projectile *or* **Cartridges, small arms**	1.4S	UN0012	II	None		114	EXPLOSIVES 1.4
	Cartridges for weapons, inert projectile *or* **Cartridges, small arms**	1.4C	UN0339	II	1.4C		114	EXPLOSIVES 1.4
	Cartridges for weapons, inert projectile *or* **Cartridges, small arms**	1.3C	UN0417	II	1.3C		112	EXPLOSIVES 1.3*
	Cartridges for weapons, *with bursting charge*	1.1F	UN0005	II	1.1F		112	EXPLOSIVES 1.1*
	Cartridges for weapons, *with bursting charge*	1.1E	UN0006	II	1.1E		112	EXPLOSIVES 1.1*
	Cartridges for weapons, *with bursting charge*	1.2F	UN0007	II	1.2F		112	EXPLOSIVES 1.2*
	Cartridges for weapons, *with bursting charge*	1.2E	UN0321	II	1.2E		112	EXPLOSIVES 1.2*
	Cartridges for weapons, *with bursting charge*	1.4F	UN0348	II	1.4F		114	EXPLOSIVES 1.4

Symbols	Hazardous materials descriptions and proper shipping names	Hazard class or Division	Identification Numbers	PG	Label Codes	Special provisions (§172.102)	ERG Guide No.	Placard Advisory Consult §172.504 & §172.505 *Placard any quantity
(1)	(2)	(3)	(4)	(5)	(6)	(7)		
	Cartridges for weapons, *with bursting charge*	1.4E	UN0412	II	1.4E		114	EXPLOSIVES 1.4
	Cartridges, oil well	1.3C	UN0277	II	1.3C		112	EXPLOSIVES 1.3*
	Cartridges, oil well	1.4C	UN0278	II	1.4C		114	EXPLOSIVES 1.4
	Cartridges, power device	1.3C	UN0275	II	1.3C		112	EXPLOSIVES 1.3*
	Cartridges, power device	1.4C	UN0276	II	1.4C	110	114	EXPLOSIVES 1.4
	Cartridges, power device	1.4S	UN0323	II	1.4S	110	114	EXPLOSIVES 1.4
	Cartridges, power device	1.2C	UN0381	II	1.2C		112	EXPLOSIVES 1.2*
D	**Cartridges power device** *(used to project fastening devices)*	ORM-D			None		—	NONE
	Cartridges, safety, blank, see **Cartridges for weapons, blank** *(UN 0014)*							
	Cartridges, safety, see **Cartridges for weapons,** *other than blank or* **Cartridges, power device** *(UN 0323)*							
	Cartridges, signal	1.3G	UN0054	II	1.3G		112	EXPLOSIVES 1.3*
	Cartridges, signal	1.4G	UN0312	II	1.4G		114	EXPLOSIVES 1.4
	Cartridges, signal	1.4S	UN0405	II	1.4S		114	EXPLOSIVES 1.4
D	**Cartridges, small arms**	ORM-D			None		—	NONE
	Cartridges, sporting, see **Cartridges for weapons,** *other than blank*							

Symbols	Hazardous materials descriptions and proper shipping names	Hazard class or Division	Identification Numbers	PG	Label Codes	Special provisions (§172.102)	ERG Guide No.	Placard Advisory Consult §172.504 & §172.505 *Placard any quantity
(1)	(2)	(3)	(4)	(5)	(6)	(7)		
	Cartridges, starter, jet engine, see **Cartridges, power device**							
	Cases, cartridge, empty with primer	1.4S	UN0055	II	1.4S	50	114	EXPLOSIVES 1.4
	Cases, cartridges, empty with primer	1.4C	UN0379	II	1.4C	50	114	EXPLOSIVES 1.4
	Cases, combustible, empty, without primer	1.4C	UN0446	II	1.4C		114	EXPLOSIVES 1.4
	Cases, combustible, empty, without primer	1.3C	UN0447	II	1.3C		112	EXPLOSIVES 1.3*
	Casinghead gasoline see **Gasoline**							
A W	**Castor beans** *or* **Castor meal** *or* **Castor pomace** *or* **Castor flake**	9	UN2969	II	None	IB8, IP2, IP4, T3, TP33	171	CLASS 9
G	**Caustic alkali liquids, n.o.s.**	8	UN1719	II	8	B2, IB2, T11, TP2, TP27	154	CORROSIVE
				III	8	IB3, T7, TP1, TP28	154	CORROSIVE
	Caustic potash, see **Potassium hydroxide** *etc.*							
	Caustic soda, (etc.) see **Sodium hydroxide** *etc.*							
	Cells, containing sodium	4.3	UN3292	II	4.3		138	DANGEROUS WHEN WET*
	Celluloid, *in block, rods, rolls, sheets, tubes, etc., except scrap*	4.1	UN2000	III	4.1		133	FLAMMABLE SOLID

Sym-bols	Hazardous materials descriptions and proper shipping names	Hazard class or Division	Identification Numbers	PG	Label Codes	Special provisions (§172.102)	ERG Guide No.	Placard Advisory Consult §172.504 & §172.505 *Placard any quantity
(1)	(2)	(3)	(4)	(5)	(6)	(7)		
	Celluloid, scrap	4.2	UN2002	III	4.2	IB8, IP3	135	SPONTANEOUSLY COMBUSTIBLE
	Cement, see **Adhesives** *containing flammable liquid*							
	Cerium, *slabs, ingots, or rods*	4.1	UN1333	II	4.1	IB8, IP2, IP4, N34	170	FLAMMABLE SOLID
	Cerium, *turnings or gritty powder*	4.3	UN3078	II	4.3	A1, IB7, IP2, T3, TP33	138	DANGEROUS WHEN WET*
	Cesium *or* **Caesium**	4.3	UN1407	I	4.3	A7, A19, IB4, IP1, N34, N40	138	DANGEROUS WHEN WET*
	Cesium nitrate *or* **Caesium nitrate**	5.1	UN1451	III	5.1	A1, A29, IB8, IP3, T1, TP33	140	OXIDIZER
D	**Charcoal** *briquettes, shell, screenings, wood, etc.*	4.2	NA1361	III	4.2	IB8, T1, TP33	133	SPONTANEOUSLY COMBUSTIBLE
	Charges, bursting, plastics bonded	1.1D	UN0457	II	1.1D		112	EXPLOSIVES 1.1*
	Charges, bursting, plastics bonded	1.2D	UN0458	II	1.2D		112	EXPLOSIVES 1.2*
	Charges, bursting, plastics bonded	1.4D	UN0459	II	1.4D		114	EXPLOSIVES 1.4
	Charges, bursting, plastics bonded	1.4S	UN0460	II	1.4S		114	EXPLOSIVES 1.4
	Charges, demolition	1.1D	UN0048	II	1.1D		112	EXPLOSIVES 1.1*
	Charges, depth	1.1D	UN0056	II	1.1D		112	EXPLOSIVES 1.1*
	Charges, expelling, explosive, for fire extinguishers, see **Cartridges, power device**							

Symbols	Hazardous materials descriptions and proper shipping names	Hazard class or Division	Identification Numbers	PG	Label Codes	Special provisions (§172.102)	ERG Guide No.	Placard Advisory Consult §172.504 & §172.505 *Placard any quantity
(1)	(2)	(3)	(4)	(5)	(6)	(7)		
	Charges, explosive, commercial *without detonator*	1.1D	UN0442	II	1.1D		112	EXPLOSIVES 1.1*
	Charges, explosive, commercial *without detonator*	1.2D	UN0443	II	1.2D		112	EXPLOSIVES 1.2*
	Charges, explosive, commercial *without detonator*	1.4D	UN0444	II	1.4D		114	EXPLOSIVES 1.4
	Charges, explosive, commercial *without detonator*	1.4S	UN0445	II	1.4S		114	EXPLOSIVES 1.4
	Charges, propelling	1.1C	UN0271	II	1.1C		112	EXPLOSIVES 1.1*
	Charges, propelling	1.3C	UN0272	II	1.3C		112	EXPLOSIVES 1.3*
	Charges, propelling	1.2C	UN0415	II	1.2C		112	EXPLOSIVES 1.2*
	Charges, propelling	1.4C	UN0491	II	1.4C		114	EXPLOSIVES 1.4
	Charges, propelling, for cannon	1.3C	UN0242	II	1.3C		112	EXPLOSIVES 1.3*
	Charges, propelling, for cannon	1.1C	UN0279	II	1.1C		112	EXPLOSIVES 1.1*
	Charges, propelling, for cannon	1.2C	UN0414	II	1.2C		112	EXPLOSIVES 1.2*
	Charges, shaped, flexible, linear	1.4D	UN0237	II	1.4D		114	EXPLOSIVES 1.4
	Charges, shaped, flexible, linear	1.1D	UN0288	II	1.1D	101	112	EXPLOSIVES 1.1*
	Charges, shaped, *without detonator*	1.1D	UN0059	II	1.1D		112	EXPLOSIVES 1.1*
	Charges, shaped, *without detonator*	1.2D	UN0439	II	1.2D		112	EXPLOSIVES 1.2*
	Charges, shaped, *without detonator*	1.4D	UN0440	II	1.4D		114	EXPLOSIVES 1.4
	Charges, shaped, *without detonator*	1.4S	UN0441	II	1.4S		114	EXPLOSIVES 1.4

Symbols	Hazardous materials descriptions and proper shipping names	Hazard class or Division	Identification Numbers	PG	Label Codes	Special provisions (§172.102)	ERG Guide No.	Placard Advisory Consult §172.504 & §172.505 *Placard any quantity
(1)	(2)	(3)	(4)	(5)	(6)	(7)		
	Charges, supplementary explosive	1.1D	UN0060	II	1.1D		112	EXPLOSIVES 1.1*
D	**Chemical kit**	8	NA1760	II	8		154	CORROSIVE
	Chemical kits	9	UN3316		9	15	171	CLASS 9
	Chloral, anhydrous, stabilized	6.1	UN2075	II	6.1	IB2, T7, TP2	153	POISON
	Chlorate and borate mixtures	5.1	UN1458	II	5.1	A9, IB8, IP2, IP4, N34, T3, TP33	140	OXIDIZER
				III	5.1	A9, IB8, IP3, N34, T1, TP33	140	OXIDIZER
	Chlorate and magnesium chloride mixture solid	5.1	UN1459	II	5.1	A9, IB8, IP2, IP4, N34, T3, TP33	140	OXIDIZER
				III	5.1	A9, IB8, IP3, N34, T1, TP33	140	OXIDIZER
	Chlorate and magnesium chloride mixture solution	5.1	UN3407	II	5.1	A9, IB2, N34, T4, TP1	140	OXIDIZER
				III	5.1	A9, IB2, N34, T4, TP1	140	OXIDIZER
	Chlorate of potash, see **Potassium chlorate**							
	Chlorate of soda, see **Sodium chlorate**							
	Chlorates, inorganic, aqueous solution, n.o.s.	5.1	UN3210	II	5.1	IB2, T4, TP1	140	OXIDIZER
				III	5.1	IB2, T4, TP1	140	OXIDIZER

Sym-bols	Hazardous materials descriptions and proper shipping names	Hazard class or Division	Identifica-tion Numbers	PG	Label Codes	Special provisions (§172.102)	ERG Guide No.	Placard Advisory Consult §172.504 & §172.505 *Placard any quantity
(1)	(2)	(3)	(4)	(5)	(6)	(7)		
	Chlorates, inorganic, n.o.s.	5.1	UN1461	II	5.1	A9, IB6, IP2, N34, T3, TP33	140	OXIDIZER
	Chloric acid aqueous solution, *with not more than 10 percent chloric acid*	5.1	UN2626	II	5.1	IB2, T4, TP1	140	OXIDIZER
	Chloride of phosphorus, see **Phosphorus trichloride**							
	Chloride of sulfur, see **Sulfur chloride**							
	Chlorinated lime, see **Calcium hypochlorite mixtures,** *etc.*							
	Chlorine	2.3	UN1017		2.3, 8	2, B9, B14, T50, TP19	124	POISON GAS*
	Chlorine azide	Forbidden						
D	**Chlorine dioxide, hydrate, frozen**	5.1	NA9191	II	5.1, 6.1		143	OXIDIZER
	Chlorine dioxide (not hydrate)	Forbidden						
	Chlorine pentafluoride	2.3	UN2548		2.3, 5.1 , 8	1, B7, B9, B14	124	POISON GAS*
	Chlorine trifluoride	2.3	UN1749		2.3, 5.1 , 8	2, B7, B9, B14	124	POISON GAS*
	Chlorite solution	8	UN1908	II	8	A3, A6, A7, B2, IB2, N34, T7, TP2, TP24	154	CORROSIVE

Symbols	Hazardous materials descriptions and proper shipping names	Hazard class or Division	Identification Numbers	PG	Label Codes	Special provisions (§172.102)	ERG Guide No.	Placard Advisory Consult §172.504 & §172.505 *Placard any quantity
(1)	(2)	(3)	(4)	(5)	(6)	(7)		
				III	8	A3, A6, A7, B2, IB3, N34, T4, TP2, TP24	154	CORROSIVE
	Chlorites, inorganic, n.o.s.	5.1	UN1462	II	5.1	A7, IB6, IP2, N34, T3, TP33	143	OXIDIZER
	1-Chloro-1,1-difluoroethane *or* **Refrigerant gas R 142b**	2.1	UN2517		2.1	T50	115	FLAMMABLE GAS
	3-Chloro-4-methylphenyl isocyanate, liquid	6.1	UN2236	II	6.1	IB2	156	POISON
	3-Chloro-4-methylphenyl isocyanate, solid	6.1	UN3428	II	6.1	IB8, IP2, IP4, T3, TP33	156	POISON
	1-Chloro-1,2,2,2-tetrafluoroethane *or* **Refrigerant gas R 124**	2.2	UN1021		2.2	T50	126	NONFLAMMABLE GAS
	4-Chloro-o-toluidine hydrochloride, solid	6.1	UN1579	III	6.1	IB8, IP3, T1, TP33	153	POISON
	4-Chloro-o-toluidine hydrochloride, solution	6.1	UN3410	III	6.1	IB3, T4, T1	153	POISON
	1-Chloro-2,2,2-trifluoroethane *or* **Refrigerant gas R 133a**	2.2	UN1983		2.2	T50	126	NONFLAMMABLE GAS
	Chloroacetic acid, molten	6.1	UN3250	II	6.1, 8	IB1, T7, TP3, TP28	153	POISON
	Chloroacetic acid, solid	6.1	UN1751	II	6.1, 8	A3, A7, IB8, IP4, N34, T3, TP33	153	POISON
	Chloroacetic acid, solution	6.1	UN1750	II	6.1, 8	A7, IB2, N34, T7, TP2	153	POISON

Symbols	Hazardous materials descriptions and proper shipping names	Hazard class or Division	Identification Numbers	PG	Label Codes	Special provisions (§172.102)	ERG Guide No.	Placard Advisory Consult §172.504 & §172.505 *Placard any quantity
(1)	(2)	(3)	(4)	(5)	(6)	(7)		
	Chloroacetone, stabilized	6.1	UN1695	I	6.1, 3, 8	2, B9, B14, B32, B74, N12, N32, N34, T20, TP2, TP13, TP38, TP45	131	POISON INHALATION HAZARD*
	Chloroacetone (unstabilized)	Forbidden						
+	**Chloroacetonitrile**	6.1	UN2668	II	6.1, 3	2, B9, B14, B32, B74, IB9, T20, TP2, TP38, TP45	131	POISON INHALATION HAZARD*
	Chloroacetophenone, CN, liquid	6.1	UN3416	II	6.1	A3, IB2, N12, N32, N33, N34, T3, TP2, TP13	153	POISON
	Chloroacetophenone, CN, solid	6.1	UN1697	II	6.1	A3, IB8, IP2, IP4, N12, N32, N33, N34, T3, TP13, TP33	153	POISON
	Chloroacetyl chloride	6.1	UN1752	I	6.1, 8	2, B3, B8, B9, B14, B32, B74, B77, N34, N43, T20, TP2, TP13, TP38, TP45	156	POISON INHALATION HAZARD*
	Chloroanilines, liquid	6.1	UN2019	II	6.1	IB2, T7, TP2	152	POISON
	Chloroanilines, solid	6.1	UN2018	II	6.1	IB8, IP2, IP4, T3, TP33	152	POISON
	Chloroanisidines	6.1	UN2233	III	6.1	IB8, IP3, T1, TP33	152	POISON
	Chlorobenzene	3	UN1134	III	3	B1, IB3, T2, TP1	130	FLAMMABLE

Symbols (1)	Hazardous materials descriptions and proper shipping names (2)	Hazard class or Division (3)	Identification Numbers (4)	PG (5)	Label Codes (6)	Special provisions (§172.102) (7)	ERG Guide No.	Placard Advisory Consult §172.504 & §172.505 *Placard any quantity
	Chlorobenzol, see **Chlorobenzene**							
	Chlorobenzotrifluorides	3	UN2234	III	3	B1, IB3, T2, TP1	130	FLAMMABLE
	Chlorobenzyl chlorides, liquid	6.1	UN2235	III	6.1	IB3, T4, TP1	153	POISON
	Chlorobenzyl chlorides, solid	6.1	UN3427	III	6.1	IB8, IP3, T1, TP33	153	POISON
	Chlorobutanes	3	UN1127	II	3	IB2, T4, TP1	130	FLAMMABLE
	Chlorocresols solution	6.1	UN2669	II	6.1	IB2, T7, TP2	152	POISON
				III	6.1	IB3, T7, TP2	152	POISON
	Chlorocresols, solid	6.1	UN3437	II	6.1	IB8, IP2, IP4, T3, TP33	152	POISON
	Chlorodifluorobromomethane *or* **Refrigerant gas R 12B1**	2.2	UN1974		2.2	T50	126	NONFLAMMABLE GAS
	Chlorodifluoromethane and chloropentafluoroethane mixture *or* **Refrigerant gas R 502** *with fixed boiling point, with approximately 49 percent chlorodifluoromethane*	2.2	UN1973		2.2	T50	126	NONFLAMMABLE GAS
	Chlorodifluoromethane *or* **Refrigerant gas R 22**	2.2	UN1018		2.2	T50	126	NONFLAMMABLE GAS
+	**Chlorodinitrobenzenes, liquid**	6.1	UN1577	II	6.1	IB2, T7, TP2	153	POISON
+	**Chlorodinitrobenzenes, solid**	6.1	UN3441	II	6.1	IB8, IP2, IP4, T3, TP33	153	POISON

Symbols	Hazardous materials descriptions and proper shipping names	Hazard class or Division	Identification Numbers	PG	Label Codes	Special provisions (§172.102)	ERG Guide No.	Placard Advisory Consult §172.504 & §172.505 *Placard any quantity
(1)	(2)	(3)	(4)	(5)	(6)	(7)		
	2-Chloroethanal	6.1	UN2232	I	6.1	2, B9, B14, B32, B74, T20, TP2, TP13, TP38, TP45	153	POISON INHALATION HAZARD*
	Chloroform	6.1	UN1888	III	6.1	IB3, N36, T7, TP2	151	POISON
G	**Chloroformates, toxic, corrosive, flammable, n.o.s.**	6.1	UN2742	II	6.1, 8, 3	5, IB1, T7, TP2	155	POISON INHALATION HAZARD*
G	**Chloroformates, toxic, corrosive, n.o.s.**	6.1	UN3277	II	6.1, 8	IB2, T8, TP2, TP13, TP28	154	POISON
	Chloromethyl chloroformate	6.1	UN2745	II	6.1, 8	IB2, T7, TP2, TP13	157	POISON
	Chloromethyl ethyl ether	3	UN2354	II	3, 6.1	IB2, T7, TP1, TP13	131	FLAMMABLE
	Chloronitroanilines	6.1	UN2237	III	6.1	IB8, IP3, T1, TP33	153	POISON
+	**Chloronitrobenzene, liquid** *ortho*	6.1	UN3409	II	6.1	IB2, T7, TP2	152	POISON
+	**Chloronitrobenzenes, solid** *meta or para*	6.1	UN1578	II	6.1	IB8, IP2, IP4, T3, TP33	152	POISON
	Chloronitrotoluenes, liquid	6.1	UN2433	III	6.1	IB3, T4, TP1	152	POISON
	Chloronitrotoluenes, solid	6.1	UN3457	III	6.1	IB8, IP3, T1, TP33	152	POISON
	Chloropentafluoroethane *or* **Refrigerant gas R 115**	2.2	UN1020		2.2	T50	126	NONFLAMMABLE GAS
	Chlorophenolates, liquid *or* **Phenolates, liquid**	8	UN2904	III	8	IB3	154	CORROSIVE
	Chlorophenolates, solid *or* **Phenolates, solid**	8	UN2905	III	8	IB8, IP3, T1, TP33	154	CORROSIVE

Sym-bols	Hazardous materials descriptions and proper shipping names	Hazard class or Division	Identification Numbers	PG	Label Codes	Special provisions (§172.102)	ERG Guide No.	Placard Advisory Consult §172.504 & §172.505 *Placard any quantity
(1)	(2)	(3)	(4)	(5)	(6)	(7)		
	Chlorophenols, liquid	6.1	UN2021	III	6.1	IB3, T4, TP1	153	POISON
	Chlorophenols, solid	6.1	UN2020	III	6.1	IB8, IP3, T1, TP1, TP33	153	POISON
	Chlorophenyltrichlorosilane	8	UN1753	II	8	A7, B2, B6, IB2, N34, T7, TP2	156	CORROSIVE
+	**Chloropicrin**	6.1	UN1580	I	6.1	2, B7, B9, B14, B32, B46, B74, T20, TP2, TP13, TP38, TP45	154	POISON INHALATION HAZARD*
	Chloropicrin and methyl bromide mixtures	2.3	UN1581		2.3	2, B9, B14, T50	123	POISON GAS*
	Chloropicrin and methyl chloride mixtures	2.3	UN1582		2.3	2, T50	119	POISON GAS*
	Chloropicrin mixture, flammable (pressure not exceeding 14.7 psia at 115 degrees F flash point below 100 degrees F) see **Toxic liquids, flammable,** *etc.*							
	Chloropicrin mixtures, n.o.s.	6.1	UN1583	I	6.1	5	154	POISON INHALATION HAZARD*
				II	6.1	IB2	154	POISON
				III	6.1	IB3	154	POISON

Sym-bols	Hazardous materials descriptions and proper shipping names	Hazard class or Division	Identifica-tion Numbers	PG	Label Codes	Special provisions (§172.102)	ERG Guide No.	Placard Advisory Consult §172.504 & §172.505 *Placard any quantity
(1)	(2)	(3)	(4)	(5)	(6)	(7)		
D	**Chloropivaloyl chloride**	6.1	NA9263	I	6.1, 8	2, B9, B14, B32, B74, T20, TP4, TP12, TP13, TP38, TP45	156	POISON INHALATION HAZARD*
	Chloroplatinic acid, solid	8	UN2507	III	8	IB8, IP3, T1, TP33	154	CORROSIVE
	Chloroprene, stabilized	3	UN1991	I	3, 6.1	B57, T14, TP2, TP13	131P	FLAMMABLE
	Chloroprene, uninhibited	Forbidden						
	1-Chloropropane	3	UN1278	II	3	IB2, IP8, N34, T7, TP2	129	FLAMMABLE
	2-Chloropropane	3	UN2356	I	3	N36, T11, TP2, TP13	129	FLAMMABLE
	3-Chloropropanol-1	6.1	UN2849	III	6.1	IB3, T4, TP1	153	POISON
	2-Chloropropene	3	UN2456	I	3	A3, N36, T11, TP2	130P	FLAMMABLE
	2-Chloropropionic acid	8	UN2511	III	8	IB3, T4, TP2	153	CORROSIVE
	2-Chloropyridine	6.1	UN2822	II	6.1	IB2, T7, TP2	153	POISON
	Chlorosilanes, corrosive, flammable, n.o.s.	8	UN2986	II	8, 3	IB2, T11, TP2, TP27	155	CORROSIVE
	Chlorosilanes, corrosive, n.o.s.	8	UN2987	II	8	B2, IB2, T14, TP2, TP27	156	CORROSIVE
	Chlorosilanes, flammable, corrosive, n.o.s.	3	UN2985	II	3, 8	IB1, T11, TP2, TP13, TP27	155	FLAMMABLE

Symbols	Hazardous materials descriptions and proper shipping names	Hazard class or Division	Identification Numbers	PG	Label Codes	Special provisions (§172.102)	ERG Guide No.	Placard Advisory Consult §172.504 & §172.505 *Placard any quantity
(1)	(2)	(3)	(4)	(5)	(6)	(7)		
	Chlorosilanes, toxic, corrosive, n.o.s.	6.1	UN3361	II	6.1, 8	IB1, T11, TP2, TP13	156	POISON
	Chlorosilanes toxic, corrisive, flammable, n.o.s.	6.1	UN3362	II	6.1, 3, 8	IB1, T11, TP2, TP13	155	POISON
	Chlorosilanes, water-reactive, flammable, corrosive, n.o.s.	4.3	UN2988	I	4.3, 3, 8	A2, T10,TP2, TP7, TP13	139	DANGEROUS WHEN WET*
+	**Chlorosulfonic acid** *(with or without sulfur trioxide)*	8	UN1754	I	8, 6.1	2, B9, B10, B14, B32, B74, T20, TP2, TP12, TP38, TP45	137	CORROSIVE, POISON INHALATION HAZARD*
	Chlorotoluenes	3	UN2238	III	3	B1, IB3, T2, TP1	129	FLAMMABLE
	Chlorotoluidines, liquid	6.1	UN3429	III	6.1	IB3, T4, TP1	153	POISON
	Chlorotoluidines, solid	6.1	UN2239	III	6.1	IB8, IP3, T1, TP33	153	POISON
	Chlorotrifluoromethane and trifluoromethane azeotropic mixture *or* **Refrigerant gas R 503** *with approximately 60 percent chlorotrifluoromethane*	2.2	UN2599		2.2		126	NONFLAMMABLE GAS
	Chlorotrifluoromethane *or* **Refrigerant gas R 13**	2.2	UN1022		2.2		126	NONFLAMMABLE GAS
	Chromic acid solution	8	UN1755	II	8	B2, IB2, T8, TP2, TP12	154	CORROSIVE
				III	8	IB3, T4, TP1, TP12	154	CORROSIVE

Symbols	Hazardous materials descriptions and proper shipping names	Hazard class or Division	Identification Numbers	PG	Label Codes	Special provisions (§172.102)	ERG Guide No.	Placard Advisory Consult §172.504 & §172.505 *Placard any quantity
(1)	(2)	(3)	(4)	(5)	(6)	(7)		
	Chromic anhydride, see **Chromium trioxide, anhydrous**							
	Chromic fluoride, solid	8	UN1756	II	8	IB8, IP2, IP4, T3, TP33	154	CORROSIVE
	Chromic fluoride, solution	8	UN1757	II	8	B2, IB2, T7, TP2	154	CORROSIVE
				III	8	IB3, T4, TP1	154	CORROSIVE
	Chromium nitrate	5.1	UN2720	III	5.1	A1, A29, IB8, IP3, T1, TP33	141	OXIDIZER
	Chromium oxychloride	8	UN1758	I	8	A3, A6, A7, B10, N34, T10, TP2, TP12	137	CORROSIVE
	Chromium trioxide, anhydrous	5.1	UN1463	II	5.1, 8	IB8, IP4, T3, TP33	141	OXIDIZER
	Chromosulfuric acid	8	UN2240	I	8	A3, A6, A7, B4, B6, N34, T10, TP2, TP12, TP13	154	CORROSIVE
	Chromyl chloride, see **Chromium oxychloride**							
	Cigar and cigarette lighters, charged with fuel, see **Lighters** *or* **Lighter refills** *containing flammable gas*							
	Coal briquettes, hot	Forbidden						
	Coal gas, compressed	2.3	UN1023		2.3, 2.1	3	119	POISON GAS*

Sym-bols	Hazardous materials descriptions and proper shipping names	Hazard class or Division	Identification Numbers	PG	Label Codes	Special provisions (§172.102)	ERG Guide No.	Placard Advisory Consult §172.504 & §172.505 *Placard any quantity
(1)	(2)	(3)	(4)	(5)	(6)	(7)		
	Coal tar distillates, flammable	3	UN1136	II	3	IB2, T4, TP1	128	FLAMMABLE
				III	3	B1, IB3, T4, TP1, TP29	128	FLAMMABLE
	Coal tar dye, corrosive, liquid, n.o.s, see **Dyes, liquid** *or* **solid, n.o.s.** *or* **Dye intermediates, liquid** *or* **solid, n.o.s.,** *corrosive*							
	Coating solution *(includes surface treatments or coatings used for industrial or other purposes such as vehicle undercoating, drum or barrel lining)*	3	UN1139	I	3	T11, TP1, TP8, TP27	127	FLAMMABLE
				II	3	149, IB2, T4, TP1, TP8	127	FLAMMABLE
				III	3	B1, IB3, T2, TP1	127	FLAMMABLE
	Cobalt naphthenates, powder	4.1	UN2001	III	4.1	A19, IB8, IP3, T1, TP33	133	FLAMMABLE SOLID
	Cobalt resinate, precipitated	4.1	UN1318	III	4.1	A1, A19, IB6, T1, TP33	133	FLAMMABLE SOLID
	Coke, hot	Forbidden						
	Collodion, see **Nitrocellulose** *etc.*							
D G	**Combustible liquid, n.o.s.**	Comb liq	NA1993	III	None	IB3, T1, T4, TP1	128	COMBUSTIBLE (BULK)
G	**Components, explosive train, n.o.s.**	1.2B	UN0382	II	1.2B	101	112	EXPLOSIVES 1.2*

Sym-bols	Hazardous materials descriptions and proper shipping names	Hazard class or Division	Identifica-tion Numbers	PG	Label Codes	Special provisions (§172.102)	ERG Guide No.	Placard Advisory Consult §172.504 & §172.505 *Placard any quantity
(1)	(2)	(3)	(4)	(5)	(6)	(7)		
G	**Components, explosive train, n.o.s.**	1.4B	UN0383	II	1.4B	101	114	EXPLOSIVES 1.4
G	**Components, explosive train, n.o.s.**	1.4S	UN0384	II	1.4S	101	114	EXPLOSIVES 1.4
G	**Components, explosive train, n.o.s.**	1.1B	UN0461	II	1.1B	101	112	EXPLOSIVES 1.1*
	Composition B, see **Hexolite**, *etc.*							
D G	**Compounds, cleaning liquid**	8	NA1760	I	8	A7, B10, T14, TP2, TP27	154	CORROSIVE
				II	8	B2, IB2, N37, T11, TP2, TP27	154	CORROSIVE
				III	8	IB3, N37, T7, TP1, TP28	154	CORROSIVE
D G	**Compounds, cleaning liquid**	3	NA1993	I	3	T11, TP1	128	FLAMMABLE
				II	3	IB2, T7, TP1, TP8, TP28	128	FLAMMABLE
				III	3	B1, B52, IB3, T4, TP1, TP29	128	FLAMMABLE
D G	**Compounds, tree killing, liquid** *or* **Compounds, weed killing, liquid**	8	NA1760	I	8	A7, B10, T14, TP2, TP27	154	CORROSIVE
				II	8	B2, IB2, N37, T11, TP2, TP27	154	CORROSIVE
				III	8	IB3, N37, T7, TP1, TP28	154	CORROSIVE
D G	**Compounds, tree killing, liquid** *or* **Compounds, weed killing, liquid**	3	NA1993	I	3	T11, TP1	128	FLAMMABLE

Symbols	Hazardous materials descriptions and proper shipping names	Hazard class or Division	Identification Numbers	PG	Label Codes	Special provisions (§172.102)	ERG Guide No.	Placard Advisory Consult §172.504 & §172.505 *Placard any quantity
(1)	(2)	(3)	(4)	(5)	(6)	(7)		
				II	3	IB2, T7, TP1, TP8, TP28	128	FLAMMABLE
				III	3	B1, B52, IB3, T4, TP1, TP29	128	FLAMMABLE
D G	**Compounds, tree killing, liquid** *or* **Compounds, weed killing, liquid**	6.1	NA2810	I	6.1	T14, TP2, TP13, TP27	153	POISON
				II	6.1	IB2, T11, TP2, TP27	153	POISON
				III	6.1	IB3, T7, TP1, TP28	153	POISON
G	**Compressed gas, flammable, n.o.s.**	2.1	UN1954		2.1		115	FLAMMABLE GAS
G	**Compressed gas, n.o.s.**	2.2	UN1956		2.2		126	NONFLAMMABLE GAS
G	**Compressed gas, oxidizing, n.o.s.**	2.2	UN3156		2.2, 5.1	A14	122	NONFLAMMABLE GAS
G I	**Compressed gas, toxic, corrosive, n.o.s.** *Inhalation Hazard Zone A*	2.3	UN3304		2.3, 8	1	123	POISON GAS*
G I	**Compressed gas, toxic, corrosive, n.o.s.** *Inhalation Hazard Zone B*	2.3	UN3304		2.3, 8	2, B9, B14	123	POISON GAS*
G I	**Compressed gas, toxic, corrosive, n.o.s.** *Inhalation Hazard Zone C*	2.3	UN3304		2.3, 8	3, B14	123	POISON GAS*
G I	**Compressed gas, toxic, corrosive, n.o.s.** *Inhalation Hazard Zone D*	2.3	UN3304		2.3, 8	4	123	POISON GAS*

Sym-bols	Hazardous materials descriptions and proper shipping names	Hazard class or Division	Identifica-tion Numbers	PG	Label Codes	Special provisions (§172.102)	ERG Guide No.	Placard Advisory Consult §172.504 & §172.505 *Placard any quantity
(1)	(2)	(3)	(4)	(5)	(6)	(7)		
G I	**Compressed gas, toxic, flammable, corrosive, n.o.s.** *Inhalation Hazard Zone A*	2.3	UN3305		2.3, 2.1 , 8	1	119	POISON GAS*
G I	**Compressed gas, toxic, flammable, corrosive, n.o.s.** *Inhalation Hazard Zone B*	2.3	UN3305		2.3, 2.1 , 8	2, B9, B14	119	POISON GAS*
G I	**Compressed gas, toxic, flammable, corrosive, n.o.s.** *Inhalation Hazard Zone C*	2.3	UN3305		2.3, 2.1 , 8	3, B14	119	POISON GAS*
G I	**Compressed gas, toxic, flammable, corrosive, n.o.s.** *Inhalation Hazard Zone D*	2.3	UN3305		2.3, 2.1 , 8	4	119	POISON GAS*
G	**Compressed gas, toxic, flammable, n.o.s.** *Inhalation hazard Zone A*	2.3	UN1953		2.3, 2.1	1	119	POISON GAS*
G	**Compressed gas, toxic, flammable, n.o.s.** *Inhalation Hazard Zone B*	2.3	UN1953		2.3, 2.1	2, B9, B14	119	POISON GAS*
G	**Compressed gas, toxic, flammable, n.o.s.** *Inhalation Hazard Zone C*	2.3	UN1953		2.3, 2.1	3, B14	119	POISON GAS*
G	**Compressed gas, toxic, flammable, n.o.s.** *Inhalation Hazard Zone D*	2.3	UN1953		2.3, 2.1	4	119	POISON GAS*
G	**Compressed gas, toxic, n.o.s.** *Inhalation Hazard Zone A*	2.3	UN1955		2.3	1	123	POISON GAS*
G	**Compressed gas, toxic, n.o.s.** *Inhalation Hazard Zone B*	2.3	UN1955		2.3	2, B9, B14	123	POISON GAS*

Sym-bols	Hazardous materials descriptions and proper shipping names	Hazard class or Division	Identifica-tion Numbers	PG	Label Codes	Special provisions (§172.102)	ERG Guide No.	Placard Advisory Consult §172.504 & §172.505 *Placard any quantity
(1)	(2)	(3)	(4)	(5)	(6)	(7)		
G	**Compressed gas, toxic, n.o.s.** *Inhalation Hazard Zone C*	2.3	UN1955		2.3	3, B14	123	POISON GAS*
G	**Compressed gas, toxic, n.o.s.** *Inhalation Hazard Zone D*	2.3	UN1955		2.3	4	123	POISON GAS*
G I	**Compressed gas, toxic, oxidizing, corrosive, n.o.s.** *Inhalation Hazard Zone A*	2.3	UN3306		2.3, 5.1 , 8	1	124	POISON GAS*
G I	**Compressed gas, toxic, oxidizing, corrosive, n.o.s.** *Inhalation Hazard Zone B*	2.3	UN3306		2.3, 5.1 , 8	2, B9, B14	124	POISON GAS*
G I	**Compressed gas, toxic, oxidizing, corrosive, n.o.s.** *Inhalation Hazard Zone C*	2.3	UN3306		2.3, 5.1 , 8	3, B14	124	POISON GAS*
G I	**Compressed gas, toxic, oxidizing, corrosive, n.o.s.** *Inhalation Hazard Zone D*	2.3	UN3306		2.3, 5.1 , 8	4	124	POISON GAS*
G	**Compressed gas, toxic, oxidizing, n.o.s.** *Inhalation Hazard Zone A*	2.3	UN3303		2.3, 5.1	1	124	POISON GAS*
G	**Compressed gas, toxic, oxidizing, n.o.s.** *Inhalation Hazard Zone B*	2.3	UN3303		2.3, 5.1	2, B9, B14	124	POISON GAS*
G	**Compressed gas, toxic, oxidizing, n.o.s.** *Inhalation Hazard Zone C*	2.3	UN3303		2.3, 5.1	3, B14	124	POISON GAS*
G	**Compressed gas, toxic, oxidizing, n.o.s.** *Inhalation Hazard Zone D*	2.3	UN3303		2.3, 5.1	4	124	POISON GAS*

Sym-bols	Hazardous materials descriptions and proper shipping names	Hazard class or Division	Identification Numbers	PG	Label Codes	Special provisions (§172.102)	ERG Guide No.	Placard Advisory Consult §172.504 & §172.505 *Placard any quantity
(1)	(2)	(3)	(4)	(5)	(6)	(7)		
D	**Consumer commodity**	ORM-D			None		—	NONE
	Contrivances, water-activated, *with burster, expelling charge or propelling charge*	1.2L	UN0248	II	1.2L	101	112	EXPLOSIVES 1.2*
	Contrivances, water-activated, *with burster, expelling charge or propelling charge*	1.3L	UN0249	II	1.3L	101	112	EXPLOSIVES 1.3*
	Copper acetoarsenite	6.1	UN1585	II	6.1	IB8, IP2, IP4, T3, TP33	151	POISON
	Copper acetylide	Forbidden						
	Copper amine azide	Forbidden						
	Copper arsenite	6.1	UN1586	II	6.1	IB8, IP2, IP4, T3, TP33	151	POISON
	Copper based pesticides, liquid, flammable, toxic, *flash point less than 23 degrees C*	3	UN2776	I	3, 6.1	T14, TP2, TP13, TP27	131	FLAMMABLE
				II	3, 6.1	IB2, T11, TP2, TP13, TP27	131	FLAMMABLE
	Copper based pesticides, liquid, toxic	6.1	UN3010	I	6.1	T14, TP2, TP13, TP27	151	POISON
				II	6.1	IB2, T11, TP2, TP13, TP27	151	POISON
				III	6.1	IB3, T7, TP2, TP28	151	POISON

Symbols	Hazardous materials descriptions and proper shipping names	Hazard class or Division	Identification Numbers	PG	Label Codes	Special provisions (§172.102)	ERG Guide No.	Placard Advisory Consult §172.504 & §172.505 *Placard any quantity
(1)	(2)	(3)	(4)	(5)	(6)	(7)		
	Copper based pesticides, liquid, toxic, flammable *flashpoint not less than 23 degrees C*	6.1	UN3009	I	6.1, 3	T14, TP2, TP13, TP27	131	POISON
				II	6.1, 3	IB2, T11, TP2, TP13, TP27	131	POISON
				III	6.1, 3	B1, IB3, T7, TP2, TP28	131	POISON
	Copper based pesticides, solid, toxic	6.1	UN2775	I	6.1	IB7, IP1, T6, TP33	151	POISON
				II	6.1	IB8, IP2, IP4, T3, TP33	151	POISON
				III	6.1	IB8, IP3, T1, TP33	151	POISON
	Copper chlorate	5.1	UN2721	II	5.1	A1, IB8, IP2, IP4, T3, TP33	141	OXIDIZER
	Copper chloride	8	UN2802	III	8	IB8, IP3, T1, TP33	154	CORROSIVE
	Copper cyanide	6.1	UN1587	II	6.1	IB8, IP2, IP4, T3, TP33	151	POISON
	Copper selenate, see **Selenates** *or* **Selenites**							
	Copper selenite, see **Selenates** *or* **Selenites**							
	Copper tetramine nitrate	Forbidden						
A W	**Copra**	4.2	UN1363	III	4.2	IB8, IP3, IP7	135	SPONTANEOUSLY COMBUSTIBLE

Symbols	Hazardous materials descriptions and proper shipping names	Hazard class or Division	Identification Numbers	PG	Label Codes	Special provisions (§172.102)	ERG Guide No.	Placard Advisory Consult §172.504 & §172.505 *Placard any quantity
(1)	(2)	(3)	(4)	(5)	(6)	(7)		
	Cord, detonating, *flexible*	1.1D	UN0065	II	1.1D	102	112	EXPLOSIVES 1.1*
	Cord, detonating, *flexible*	1.4D	UN0289	II	1.4D		114	EXPLOSIVES 1.4
	Cord detonating *or* **Fuse detonating** *metal clad*	1.2D	UN0102	II	1.2D		112	EXPLOSIVES 1.2*
	Cord, detonating *or* **Fuse, detonating** *metal clad*	1.1D	UN0290	II	1.1D		112	EXPLOSIVES 1.1*
	Cord, detonating, mild effect *or* **Fuse, detonating, mild effect** *metal clad*	1.4D	UN0104	II	1.4D		114	EXPLOSIVES 1.4
	Cord, igniter	1.4G	UN0066	II	1.4G		114	EXPLOSIVES 1.4
	Cordeau detonant fuse, see **Cord, detonating,** *etc;* **Cord, detonating,** *flexible*							
	Cordite, see **Powder, smokeless**							
G	**Corrosive liquid, acidic, inorganic, n.o.s.**	8	UN3264	I	8	A6, B10, T14, TP2, TP27	154	CORROSIVE
				II	8	A6, B2, IB2, T11, TP2, TP27	154	CORROSIVE
				III	8	IB3, T7, TP1, TP28	154	CORROSIVE
G	**Corrosive liquid, acidic, organic, n.o.s.**	8	UN3265	I	8	A6, B10, T14, TP2, TP27	153	CORROSIVE
				II	8	B2, IB2, T11, TP2, TP27	153	CORROSIVE
				III	8	IB3, T7, TP1, TP28	153	CORROSIVE

Symbols	Hazardous materials descriptions and proper shipping names	Hazard class or Division	Identification Numbers	PG	Label Codes	Special provisions (§172.102)	ERG Guide No.	Placard Advisory Consult §172.504 & §172.505 *Placard any quantity
(1)	(2)	(3)	(4)	(5)	(6)	(7)		
G	**Corrosive liquid, basic, inorganic, n.o.s.**	8	UN3266	I	8	A6, T14, TP2, TP27	154	CORROSIVE
				II	8	B2, IB2, T11, TP2, TP27	154	CORROSIVE
				III	8	IB3, T7, TP1, TP28	154	CORROSIVE
G	**Corrosive liquid, basic, organic, n.o.s.**	8	UN3267	I	8	A6, B10, T14, TP2, TP27	153	CORROSIVE
				II	8	B2, IB2, T11, TP2, TP27	153	CORROSIVE
				III	8	IB3, T7, TP1, TP28	153	CORROSIVE
G	**Corrosive liquid, self-heating, n.o.s.**	8	UN3301	I	8, 4.2	A6, B10	136	CORROSIVE
				II	8, 4.2	B2, IB1	136	CORROSIVE
G	**Corrosive liquids, flammable, n.o.s.**	8	UN2920	I	8, 3	A6, B10, T14, TP2, TP27	132	CORROSIVE
				II	8, 3	B2, IB2, T11, TP2, TP27	132	CORROSIVE
G	**Corrosive liquids, n.o.s.**	8	UN1760	I	8	A6, A7, B10, T14, TP2, TP27	154	CORROSIVE
				II	8	B2, IB2, T11, TP2, TP27	154	CORROSIVE
				III	8	IB3, T7, TP1, TP28	154	CORROSIVE
G	**Corrosive liquids, oxidizing, n.o.s.**	8	UN3093	I	8, 5.1	A6, A7	140	CORROSIVE

Symbols	Hazardous materials descriptions and proper shipping names	Hazard class or Division	Identification Numbers	PG	Label Codes	Special provisions (§172.102)	ERG Guide No.	Placard Advisory Consult §172.504 & §172.505 *Placard any quantity
(1)	(2)	(3)	(4)	(5)	(6)	(7)		
				II	8, 5.1	A6, A7, IB2	140	CORROSIVE
G	**Corrosive liquids, toxic, n.o.s.**	8	UN2922	I	8, 6.1	A6, A7, B10, T14, TP2, TP13, TP27	154	CORROSIVE
				II	8, 6.1	B3, IB2, T7, TP2	154	CORROSIVE
				III	8, 6.1	IB3, T7, TP1, TP28	154	CORROSIVE
G	**Corrosive liquids, water-reactive, n.o.s.**	8	UN3094	I	8, 4.3	A6, A7	138	CORROSIVE, DANGEROUS WHEN WET*
				II	8, 4.3	A6, A7	138	CORROSIVE, DANGEROUS WHEN WET*
G	**Corrosive solid, acidic, inorganic, n.o.s.**	8	UN3260	I	8	IB7, IP1, T6, TP33	154	CORROSIVE
				II	8	IB8, IP2, IP4, T3, TP33	154	CORROSIVE
				III	8	IB8, IP3, T1, TP33	154	CORROSIVE
G	**Corrosive solid, acidic, organic, n.o.s.**	8	UN3261	I	8	IB7, IP1, T6, TP33	154	CORROSIVE
				II	8	IB8, IP2, IP4, T3, TP33	154	CORROSIVE
				III	8	IB8, IP3, T1, TP33	154	CORROSIVE
G	**Corrosive solid, basic, inorganic, n.o.s.**	8	UN3262	I	8	IB7, IP1, T6, TP33	154	CORROSIVE

Sym-bols	Hazardous materials descriptions and proper shipping names	Hazard class or Division	Identifica-tion Numbers	PG	Label Codes	Special provisions (§172.102)	ERG Guide No.	Placard Advisory Consult §172.504 & §172.505 *Placard any quantity
(1)	(2)	(3)	(4)	(5)	(6)	(7)		
				II	8	IB8, IP2, IP4, T3, TP33	154	CORROSIVE
				III	8	IB8, IP3, T1, TP33	154	CORROSIVE
G	**Corrosive solid, basic, organic, n.o.s.**	8	UN3263	I	8	IB7, IP1, T6, TP33	154	CORROSIVE
				II	8	IB8, IP2, IP4, T3, TP33	154	CORROSIVE
				III	8	IB8, IP3, T1, TP33	154	CORROSIVE
G	**Corrosive solids, flammable, n.o.s.**	8	UN2921	I	8, 4.1	IB6, T6, TP33	134	CORROSIVE
				II	8, 4.1	IB8, IP2, IP4, T3, TP33	134	CORROSIVE
G	**Corrosive solids, n.o.s.**	8	UN1759	I	8	IB7, IP1, T6, TP33	154	CORROSIVE
				II	8	128, IB8, IP2, IP4, T3, TP33	154	CORROSIVE
				III	8	128, IB8, IP3, T1, TP33	154	CORROSIVE
G	**Corrosive solids, oxidizing, n.o.s.**	8	UN3084	I	8, 5.1	T6, TP33	140	CORROSIVE
				II	8, 5.1	IB6, IP2, T3, TP33	140	CORROSIVE
G	**Corrosive solids, self-heating, n.o.s.**	8	UN3095	I	8, 4.2	T6, TP33	136	CORROSIVE
				II	8, 4.2	IB6, IP2, T3, TP33	136	CORROSIVE
G	**Corrosive solids, toxic, n.o.s.**	8	UN2923	I	8, 6.1	IB7, T6, TP33	154	CORROSIVE
				II	8, 6.1	IB8, IP2, IP4, T3, TP33	154	CORROSIVE

Symbols	Hazardous materials descriptions and proper shipping names	Hazard class or Division	Identification Numbers	PG	Label Codes	Special provisions (§172.102)	ERG Guide No.	Placard Advisory Consult §172.504 & §172.505
(1)	(2)	(3)	(4)	(5)	(6)	(7)		*Placard any quantity
				III	8, 6.1	IB8, IP3, T1, TP33	154	CORROSIVE
G	**Corrosive solids, water-reactive, n.o.s.**	8	UN3096	I	8, 4.3	IB4, IP1, T6, TP33	138	CORROSIVE, DANGEROUS WHEN WET*
				II	8, 4.3	IB6, IP2, T3, TP33	138	CORROSIVE, DANGEROUS WHEN WET*
D W	**Cotton**	9	NA1365		9	137, IB8, IP2, IP4, W41	133	CLASS 9
A W	**Cotton waste, oily**	4.2	UN1364	III	4.2	IB8, IP3, IP7	133	SPONTANEOUSLY COMBUSTIBLE
A I W	**Cotton, wet**	4.2	UN1365	III	4.2	IB8, IP3, IP7	133	SPONTANEOUSLY COMBUSTIBLE
	Coumarin derivative pesticides, liquid, flammable, toxic, *flashpoint less than 23 degrees C*	3	UN3024	I	3, 6.1	T14, TP2, TP13, TP27	131	FLAMMABLE
				II	3, 6.1	IB2, T11, TP2, TP13, TP27	131	FLAMMABLE
	Coumarin derivative pesticides, liquid, toxic	6.1	UN3026	I	6.1	T14, TP2, TP13, TP27	151	POISON
				II	6.1	IB2, T11, TP2, TP27	151	POISON
				III	6.1	IB3, T7, TP1, TP28	151	POISON

Sym-bols	Hazardous materials descriptions and proper shipping names	Hazard class or Division	Identification Numbers	PG	Label Codes	Special provisions (§172.102)	ERG Guide No.	Placard Advisory Consult §172.504 & §172.505 *Placard any quantity
(1)	(2)	(3)	(4)	(5)	(6)	(7)		
	Coumarin derivative pesticides, liquid, toxic, flammable, *flash point not less than 23 degrees C*	6.1	UN3025	I	6.1, 3	T14, TP2, TP13, TP27	131	POISON
				II	6.1, 3	IB2, T11, TP2, TP13, TP27	131	POISON
				III	6.1, 3	B1, IB3, T7, TP1, TP28	131	POISON
	Coumarin derivative pesticides, solid, toxic	6.1	UN3027	I	6.1	IB7, IP1, T6, TP33	151	POISON
				II	6.1	IB8, IP2, IP4, T3, TP33	151	POISON
				III	6.1	IB8, IP3, T1, TP33	151	POISON
	Cresols, liquid	6.1	UN2076	II	6.1, 8	IB8, IP2, IP4, T7, TP2	153	POISON
	Cresols, solid	6.1	UN3455	ii	6.1, 8	IB8, IP2, IP4, T3, TP33	153	POISON
	Cresylic acid	6.1	UN2022	II	6.1, 8	IB2, T7, TP2, TP13	153	POISON
	Crotonaldehyde, stabilized	6.1	UN1143	I	6.1, 3	2, B9, B14, B32, B74, B77, T20, TP2, TP13, TP38, TP45	131P	POISON INHALATION HAZARD*
	Crotonic acid *liquid*	8	UN2823	III	8	IB8, T1	153	CORROSIVE
	Crotonic acid, *solid*	8	UN2823	III	8	IB8, IP3, T1, TP33	153	CORROSIVE

Sym-bols	Hazardous materials descriptions and proper shipping names	Hazard class or Division	Identification Numbers	PG	Label Codes	Special provisions (§172.102)	ERG Guide No.	Placard Advisory Consult §172.504 & §172.505 *Placard any quantity
(1)	(2)	(3)	(4)	(5)	(6)	(7)		
	Crotonylene	3	UN1144	I	3	T11, TP2	128	FLAMMABLE
	Cupriethylenediamine solution	8	UN1761	II	8, 6.1	IB2, T7, TP2	154	CORROSIVE
				III	8, 6.1	IB3, T7, TP1, TP28	154	CORROSIVE
	Cutters, cable, explosive	1.4S	UN0070	II	1.4S		112	EXPLOSIVES 1.4
	Cyanide or cyanide mixtures, dry, see **Cyanides, inorganic, solid, n.o.s.**							
	Cyanide solutions, n.o.s.	6.1	UN1935	I	6.1	B37, T14, TP2, TP13, TP27	157	POISON
				II	6.1	IB2, T11, TP2, TP13, TP27	157	POISON
				III	6.1	IB3, T7, TP2, TP13, TP28	157	POISON
	Cyanides, inorganic, solid, n.o.s.	6.1	UN1588	I	6.1	IB7, IP1, N74, N75, T6, TP33	157	POISON
				II	6.1	IB8, IP2, IP4, N74, N75, T3, TP33	157	POISON
				III	6.1	IB8, IP3, N74, N75, T1, TP33	157	POISON
	Cyanogen	2.3	UN1026		2.3, 2.1	2	119	POISON GAS*
	Cyanogen bromide	6.1	UN1889	I	6.1, 8	A6, A8, T6, TP33	157	POISON
	Cyanogen chloride, stabilized	2.3	UN1589		2.3, 8	1	125	POISON GAS*

Sym-bols	Hazardous materials descriptions and proper shipping names	Hazard class or Division	Identifica-tion Numbers	PG	Label Codes	Special provisions (§172.102)	ERG Guide No.	Placard Advisory Consult §172.504 & §172.505 *Placard any quantity
(1)	(2)	(3)	(4)	(5)	(6)	(7)		
	Cyanuric chloride	8	UN2670	II	8	IB8, IP2, IP4, T3, TP33	157	CORROSIVE
	Cyanuric triazide	Forbidden						
	Cyclobutane	2.1	UN2601		2.1		115	FLAMMABLE GAS
	Cyclobutyl chloroformate	6.1	UN2744	II	6.1, 8, 3	IB1, T7, TP2, TP13	155	POISON
	1,5,9-Cyclododecatriene	6.1	UN2518	III	6.1	IB3, T4, TP1	153	POISON
	Cycloheptane	3	UN2241	II	3	IB2, T4, TP1	128	FLAMMABLE
	Cycloheptatriene	3	UN2603	II	3, 6.1	IB2, T7, TP1, TP13	131	FLAMMABLE
	Cycloheptene	3	UN2242	II	3	B1, IB2, T4, TP1	128	FLAMMABLE
	Cyclohexane	3	UN1145	II	3	IB2, T4, TP1	128	FLAMMABLE
	Cyclohexanone	3	UN1915	III	3	B1, IB3, T2, TP1	127	FLAMMABLE
	Cyclohexene	3	UN2256	II	3	IB2, T4, TP1	130	FLAMMABLE
	Cyclohexenyltrichlorosilane	8	UN1762	II	8	A7, B2, IB2, N34, T7, TP2, TP13	156	CORROSIVE
	Cyclohexyl acetate	3	UN2243	III	3	B1, IB3, T2, TP1	130	FLAMMABLE
	Cyclohexyl isocyanate	6.1	UN2488	I	6.1, 3	2, B9, B14, B32, B74, B77, T20, TP2, TP13, TP38, TP45	155	POISON INHALATION HAZARD*
	Cyclohexyl mercaptan	3	UN3054	III	3	B1, IB3, T2, TP1	129	FLAMMABLE
	Cyclohexylamine	8	UN2357	II	8, 3	IB2, T7, TP2	132	CORROSIVE

Sym-bols	Hazardous materials descriptions and proper shipping names	Hazard class or Division	Identifica-tion Numbers	PG	Label Codes	Special provisions (§172.102)	ERG Guide No.	Placard Advisory Consult §172.504 & §172.505 *Placard any quantity
(1)	(2)	(3)	(4)	(5)	(6)	(7)		
	Cyclohexyltrichlorosilane	8	UN1763	II	8	A7, B2, IB2, N34, T7, TP2, TP13	156	CORROSIVE
	Cyclonite and cyclotetramethylene-tetranitramine mixtures, wetted *or* **desensitized** *see* **RDX and HMX mixtures, wetted** *or* **desensitized** *etc.*							
	Cyclonite and HMX mixtures, wetted *or* **desensitized** *see* **RDX and HMX mixtures, wetted** *or* **desensitized** *etc.*							
	Cyclonite and octogen mixtures, wetted *or* **desensitized** *see* **RDX and HMX mixtures, wetted** *or* **desensi-tized** *etc.*							
	Cyclonite, *see* **Cyclotrimethylenetrin-itramine,** *etc.*							
	Cyclooctadiene phosphines, *see* **9-Phosphabicyclononanes**							
	Cyclooctadienes	3	UN2520	III	3	B1, IB3, T2, TP1	130P	FLAMMABLE
	Cyclooctatetraene	3	UN2358	II	3	IB2, T4, TP1	128P	FLAMMABLE
	Cyclopentane	3	UN1146	II	3	IB2, T7, TP1	128	FLAMMABLE
	Cyclopentane, methyl, see **Methylcyclopentane**							
	Cyclopentanol	3	UN2244	III	3	B1, IB3, T2, TP1	129	FLAMMABLE

Symbols	Hazardous materials descriptions and proper shipping names	Hazard class or Division	Identification Numbers	PG	Label Codes	Special provisions (§172.102)	ERG Guide No.	Placard Advisory Consult §172.504 & §172.505 *Placard any quantity
(1)	(2)	(3)	(4)	(5)	(6)	(7)		
	Cyclopentanone	3	UN2245	III	3	B1, IB3, T2, TP1	128	FLAMMABLE
	Cyclopentene	3	UN2246	II	3	IB2, IP8, T7, TP2	128	FLAMMABLE
	Cyclopropane	2.1	UN1027		2.1	T50	115	FLAMMABLE GAS
	Cyclotetramethylene tetranitramine (dry or unphlegmatized) (HMX)	Forbidden						
	Cyclotetramethylenetetranitramine, desensitized *or* **Octogen, desensitized** *or* **HMX, desensitized**	1.1D	UN0484	II	1.1D		112	EXPLOSIVES 1.1*
	Cyclotetramethylenetetranitramine, wetted *or* **HMX, wetted** *or* **Octogen, wetted** *with not less than 15 percent water, by mass*	1.1D	UN0226	II	1.1D		112	EXPLOSIVES 1.1*
	Cyclotrimethylenenitramine and oxygen, mixtures, wetted *or* **desensitized** *see* **RDX and HMX mixtures, wetted** *or* **desensitized** *etc.*							
	Cyclotrimethylenetrinitramine and cyclotetramethylenetetranitramine mixtures, wetted *or* **desensitized** *see* **RDX and HMX mixtures, wetted** *or* **desensitized** *etc.*							
	Cyclotrimethylenetrinitramine and HMX mixtures, wetted *or* **desensitized** *see* **RDX and HMX mixtures, wetted** *or* **desensitized** *etc.*							

Symbols	Hazardous materials descriptions and proper shipping names	Hazard class or Division	Identification Numbers	PG	Label Codes	Special provisions (§172.102)	ERG Guide No.	Placard Advisory Consult §172.504 & §172.505 *Placard any quantity
(1)	(2)	(3)	(4)	(5)	(6)	(7)		
	Cyclotrimethylenetrinitramine, desensitized *or* **Cyclonite, desensitized** *or* **Hexogen, desensitized** *or* **RDX, desensitized**	1.1D	UN0483	II	1.1D		112	EXPLOSIVES 1.1*
	Cyclotrimethylenetrinitramine, wetted *or* **Cyclonite, wetted** *or* **Hexogen, wetted** *or* **RDX, wetted** *with not less than 15 percent water by mass*	1.1D	UN0072	II	1.1D		112	EXPLOSIVES 1.1*
	Cymenes	3	UN2046	III	3	B1, IB3, T2, TP1	130	FLAMMABLE
	Dangerous Goods in Machinery *or* **Dangerous Goods in Apparatus**	9	UN3363			136	171	CLASS 9
	Decaborane	4.1	UN1868	II	4.1, 6.1	A19, A20, IB6, IP2, T3, TP33	134	FLAMMABLE SOLID
	Decahydronaphthalene	3	UN1147	III	3	B1, IB3, T2, TP1	130	FLAMMABLE
	n-Decane	3	UN2247	III	3	B1, IB3, T2, TP1	128	FLAMMABLE
	Deflagrating metal salts of aromatic nitroderivatives, n.o.s	1.3C	UN0132	II	1.3C		112	EXPLOSIVES 1.3*
	Delay electric igniter, see **Igniters**							
D	**Denatured alcohol**	3	NA1987	II	3	172, T8, T31	127	FLAMMABLE
				III	3	172, B1, T7, T30	127	FLAMMABLE
	Depth charges, see **Charges, depth**							
G	**Desensitized explosive, liquid, n.o.s.**	3	UN3379	I	3	164	128	FLAMMABLE

Symbols	Hazardous materials descriptions and proper shipping names	Hazard class or Division	Identification Numbers	PG	Label Codes	Special provisions (§172.102)	ERG Guide No.	Placard Advisory Consult §172.504 & §172.505 *Placard any quantity
(1)	(2)	(3)	(4)	(5)	(6)	(7)		
G	**Desensitized explosive, solid, n.o.s.**	4.1	UN3380	I	4.1	164	133	FLAMMABLE SOLID
	Detonating relays, see **Detonators,** *etc.*							
	Detonator assemblies, non-electric *for blasting*	1.1B	UN0360	II	1.1B		112	EXPLOSIVES 1.1*
	Detonator assemblies, non-electric, *for blasting*	1.4B	UN0361	II	1.4B	103	114	EXPLOSIVES 1.4
	Detonator assemblies, non-electric *for blasting*	1.4S	UN0500	II	1.4S		114	EXPLOSIVES 1.4
	Detonators, electric, *for blasting*	1.1B	UN0030	II	1.1B		112	EXPLOSIVES 1.1*
	Detonators, electric, *for blasting*	1.4B	UN0255	II	1.4B	103	114	EXPLOSIVES 1.4
	Detonators, electric *for blasting*	1.4S	UN0456	II	1.4S		114	EXPLOSIVES 1.4
	Detonators for ammunition	1.1B	UN0073	II	1.1B		112	EXPLOSIVES 1.1*
	Detonators for ammunition	1.2B	UN0364	II	1.2B		112	EXPLOSIVES 1.2*
	Detonators for ammunition	1.4B	UN0365	II	1.4B	103	114	EXPLOSIVES 1.4
	Detonators for ammunition	1.4S	UN0366	II	1.4S		114	EXPLOSIVES 1.4
	Detonators, non-electric, *for blasting*	1.1B	UN0029	II	1.1B		112	EXPLOSIVES 1.1*
	Detonators, non-electric, *for blasting*	1.4B	UN0267	II	1.4B	103	114	EXPLOSIVES 1.4
	Detonators, non-electric, *for blasting*	1.4S	UN0455	II	1.4S		114	EXPLOSIVES 1.4
	Deuterium, compressed	2.1	UN1957		2.1		115	FLAMMABLE GAS

Symbols	Hazardous materials descriptions and proper shipping names	Hazard class or Division	Identification Numbers	PG	Label Codes	Special provisions (§172.102)	ERG Guide No.	Placard Advisory Consult §172.504 & §172.505 *Placard any quantity
(1)	(2)	(3)	(4)	(5)	(6)	(7)		
	Devices, small, hydrocarbon gas powered *or* **Hydrocarbon gas refills for small devices** *with release device*	2.1	UN3150		2.1		115	FLAMMABLE GAS
	Di-n-amylamine	3	UN2841	III	3, 6.1	B1, IB3, T4, TP1	131	FLAMMABLE
	Di-n-butyl peroxydicarbonate, with more than 52 percent in solution	Forbidden						
	Di-n-butylamine	8	UN2248	II	8, 3	IB2, T7, TP2	132	CORROSIVE
	2,2-Di-(tert-butylperoxy) butane, with more than 55 percent in solution	Forbidden						
	Di-(tert-butylperoxy) phthalate, with more than 55 percent in solution	Forbidden						
	2,2-Di-(4,4-di-tert-butylperoxycyclohexyl) propane, with more than 42 percent with inert solid	Forbidden						
	Di-2,4-dichlorobenzoyl peroxide, with more than 75 percent with water	Forbidden						
	1,2-Di-(dimethylamino)ethane	3	UN2372	II	3	IB2, T4, TP1	129	FLAMMABLE
	Di-2-ethylhexyl phosphoric acid, see **Diisooctyl acid phosphate**							
	Di-(1-hydroxytetrazole) (dry)	Forbidden						
	Di-(1-naphthoyl) peroxide	Forbidden						
	a,ai-Di-(nitroxy) methylether	Forbidden						
	Di-(beta-nitroxyethyl) ammonium nitrate	Forbidden						

Sym-bols	Hazardous materials descriptions and proper shipping names	Hazard class or Division	Identification Numbers	PG	Label Codes	Special provisions (§172.102)	ERG Guide No.	Placard Advisory Consult §172.504 & §172.505 *Placard any quantity
(1)	(2)	(3)	(4)	(5)	(6)	(7)		
	Diacetone alcohol	3	UN1148	II	3	IB2, T4, TP1	129	FLAMMABLE
				III	3	B1, IB3, T2, TP1	129	FLAMMABLE
	Diacetone alcohol peroxides, with more than 57 percent in solution with more than 9 percent hydrogen peroxide, less than 26 percent diacetone alcohol and less than 9 percent water; total active oxygen content more than 9 percent by mass	Forbidden						
	Diacetyl, see **Butanedione**							
	Diacetyl peroxide, solid, or with more than 25 percent in solution	Forbidden						
	Diagnostic specimen	6.2				A82	158	NONE
	Diallylamine	3	UN2359	II	3, 6.1, 8	IB2, T7, TP1	132	FLAMMABLE
	Diallylether	3	UN2360	II	3, 6.1	IB2, N12, T7, TP1, TP13	131P	FLAMMABLE
	4,4´-Diaminodiphenyl methane	6.1	UN2651	III	6.1	IB8, IP3, T1, TP33	153	POISON
	p-Diazidobenzene	Forbidden						
	1,2-Diazidoethane	Forbidden						
	1,1i-Diazoaminonaphthalene	Forbidden						
	Diazoaminotetrazole (dry)	Forbidden						
	Diazodinitrophenol (dry)	Forbidden						

Symbols	Hazardous materials descriptions and proper shipping names	Hazard class or Division	Identification Numbers	PG	Label Codes	Special provisions (§172.102)	ERG Guide No.	Placard Advisory Consult §172.504 & §172.505 *Placard any quantity
(1)	(2)	(3)	(4)	(5)	(6)	(7)		
	Diazodinitrophenol, wetted *with not less than 40 percent water or mixture of alcohol and water, by mass*	1.1A	UN0074	II	1.1A	111, 117	112	EXPLOSIVES 1.1*
	Diazodiphenylmethane	Forbidden						
	Diazonium nitrates (dry)	Forbidden						
	Diazonium perchlorates (dry)	Forbidden						
	1,3-Diazopropane	Forbidden						
	Dibenzyl peroxydicarbonate, with more than 87 percent with water	Forbidden						
	Dibenzyldichlorosilane	8	UN2434	II	8	B2, IB2, T7, TP2, TP13	156	CORROSIVE
	Diborane	2.3	UN1911		2.3, 2.1	1	119	POISON GAS*
D	**Diborane mixtures**	2.1	NA1911		2.1	5	119	FLAMMABLE GAS
	Dibromoacetylene	Forbidden						
	1,2-Dibromobutan-3-one	6.1	UN2648	II	6.1	IB2	154	POISON
	Dibromochloropropane	6.1	UN2872	II	6.1	IB2, T7, TP2	159	POISON
				III	6.1	IB3, T4, TP1	159	POISON
A	**Dibromodifluoromethane,** *R12B2*	9	UN1941	III	None	T11, TP2	171	CLASS 9
	1,2-Dibromoethane, see **Ethylene dibromide**							
	Dibromomethane	6.1	UN2664	III	6.1	IB3, T4, TP1	160	POISON

Symbols	Hazardous materials descriptions and proper shipping names	Hazard class or Division	Identification Numbers	PG	Label Codes	Special provisions (§172.102)	ERG Guide No.	Placard Advisory Consult §172.504 & §172.505 *Placard any quantity
(1)	(2)	(3)	(4)	(5)	(6)	(7)		
	Dibutyl ethers	3	UN1149	III	3	B1, IB3, T2, TP1	128	FLAMMABLE
	Dibutylaminoethanol	6.1	UN2873	III	6.1	IB3, T4, TP1	153	POISON
	N,Ni-Dichlorazodicarbonamidine (salts of) (dry)	Forbidden						
	1,1-Dichloro-1-nitroethane	6.1	UN2650	II	6.1	IB2, T7, TP2	153	POISON
D	**3,5-Dichloro-2,4,6-trifluoropyridine**	6.1	NA9264	I	6.1	2, B9, B14, B32, B74, T20, TP4, TP12, TP13, TP38, TP45	151	POISON INHALATION HAZARD*
	Dichloroacetic acid	8	UN1764	II	8	A3, A6, A7, B2, IB2, N34, T8, TP2, TP12	153	CORROSIVE
	1,3-Dichloroacetone	6.1	UN2649	II	6.1	IB8, IP2, IP4, T3, TP33	153	POISON
	Dichloroacetyl chloride	8	UN1765	II	8	A3, A6, A7, B2, B6, IB2, N34, T7, TP2	156	CORROSIVE
	Dichloroacetylene	Forbidden						
+	**Dichloroanilines, liquid**	6.1	UN1590	II	6.1	IB2, T7, TP2	153	POISON
	Dichloroanilines, solid	6.1	UN3442	II	6.1	IB8, IP2, IP4, T3, TP33	153	POISON
+	**o-Dichlorobenzene**	6.1	UN1591	III	6.1	IB3, T4, TP1	152	POISON
	2,2'-Dichlorodiethyl ether	6.1	UN1916	II	6.1, 3	IB2, N33, N34, T7, TP2	152	POISON

Symbols	Hazardous materials descriptions and proper shipping names	Hazard class or Division	Identification Numbers	PG	Label Codes	Special provisions (§172.102)	ERG Guide No.	Placard Advisory Consult §172.504 & §172.505 *Placard any quantity
(1)	(2)	(3)	(4)	(5)	(6)	(7)		
	Dichlorodifluoromethane and difluoroethane azeotropic mixture *or* **Refrigerant gas R 500** *with approximately 74 percent dichlorodifluoromethane*	2.2	UN2602		2.2	T50	126	NONFLAMMABLE GAS
	Dichlorodifluoromethane *or* **Refrigerant gas R 12**	2.2	UN1028		2.2	T50	126	NONFLAMMABLE GAS
	Dichlorodimethyl ether, symmetrical	6.1	UN2249	I	6.1, 3		131	POISON
	1,1-Dichloroethane	3	UN2362	II	3	IB2, T4, TP1	130	FLAMMABLE
	1,2-Dichloroethane, see **Ethylene dichloride**							
	Dichloroethyl sulfide	Forbidden						
	1,2-Dichloroethylene	3	UN1150	II	3	IB2, T7, TP2	130P	FLAMMABLE
	Dichlorofluoromethane *or* **Refrigerant gas R 21**	2.2	UN1029		2.2	T50	126	NONFLAMMABLE GAS
	Dichloroisocyanuric acid, dry *or* **Dichloroisocyanuric acid salts**	5.1	UN2465	II	5.1	28, IB8, IP4, T3, TP33	140	OXIDIZER
	Dichloroisopropyl ether	6.1	UN2490	II	6.1	IB2, T7, TP2	153	POISON
	Dichloromethane	6.1	UN1593	III	6.1	IB3, IP8, N36, T7, TP2	160	POISON
	Dichloropentanes	3	UN1152	III	3	B1, IB3, T2, TP1	130	FLAMMABLE
	Dichlorophenyl isocyanates	6.1	UN2250	II	6.1	IB8, IP2, IP4, T3, TP33	156	POISON

Sym-bols	Hazardous materials descriptions and proper shipping names	Hazard class or Division	Identification Numbers	PG	Label Codes	Special provisions (§172.102)	ERG Guide No.	Placard Advisory Consult §172.504 & §172.505 *Placard any quantity
(1)	(2)	(3)	(4)	(5)	(6)	(7)		
	Dichlorophenyltrichlorosilane	8	UN1766	II	8	A7, B2, B6, IB2, N34, T7, TP2, TP13	156	CORROSIVE
	1,2-Dichloropropane	3	UN1279	II	3	IB2, N36, T4, TP1	130	FLAMMABLE
	1,3-Dichloropropanol-2	6.1	UN2750	II	6.1	IB2, T7, TP2	153	POISON
	Dichloropropene and propylene dichloride mixture, see **1,2-Dichloropropane**							
	Dichloropropenes	3	UN2047	II	3	IB2, T4, TP1	129	FLAMMABLE
				III	3	B1, IB3, T2, TP1	129	FLAMMABLE
	Dichlorosilane	2.3	UN2189		2.3, 2.1 , 8	2, B9, B14	119	POISON GAS*
	1,2-Dichloro-1,1,2,2-tetrafluoroethane *or* **Refrigerant gas R 114**	2.2	UN1958		2.2	T50	126	NONFLAMMABLE GAS
	Dichlorovinylchloroarsine	Forbidden						
	Dicycloheptadiene, see **Bicyclo [2,2,1] hepta-2,5-diene, stabilized**							
	Dicyclohexylamine	8	UN2565	III	8	IB3, T4, TP1	153	CORROSIVE
	Dicyclohexylammonium nitrite	4.1	UN2687	III	4.1	IB8, IP3, T1, TP33	133	FLAMMABLE SOLID
	Dicyclopentadiene	3	UN2048	III	3	B1, IB3, T2, TP1	130	FLAMMABLE
	Didymium nitrate	5.1	UN1465	III	5.1	A1, IB8, IP3, T1, TP33	140	OXIDIZER

Symbols	Hazardous materials descriptions and proper shipping names	Hazard class or Division	Identification Numbers	PG	Label Codes	Special provisions (§172.102)	ERG Guide No.	Placard Advisory Consult §172.504 & §172.505 *Placard any quantity
(1)	(2)	(3)	(4)	(5)	(6)	(7)		
D	**Diesel fuel**	3	NA1993	III	None	144, B1, IB3, T4, TP1, TP29	128	COMBUSTIBLE (BULK ONLY)
I	**Diesel fuel**	3	UN1202	III	3	144, B1, IB3, T2, TP1	128	FLAMMABLE
	Diethanol nitrosamine dinitrate (dry)	Forbidden						
	Diethoxymethane	3	UN2373	II	3	IB2, T4, TP1	127	FLAMMABLE
	3,3-Diethoxypropene	3	UN2374	II	3	IB2, T4, TP1	127	FLAMMABLE
	Diethyl carbonate	3	UN2366	III	3	B1, IB3, T2, TP1	128	FLAMMABLE
	Diethyl cellosolve, see **Ethylene glycol diethyl ether**							
	Diethyl ether *or* **Ethyl ether**	3	UN1155	I	3	T11, TP2	127	FLAMMABLE
	Diethyl ketone	3	UN1156	II	3	IB2, T4, TP1	127	FLAMMABLE
	Diethyl peroxydicarbonate, with more than 27 percent in solution	Forbidden						
	Diethyl sulfate	6.1	UN1594	II	6.1	IB2, T7, TP2	152	POISON
	Diethyl sulfide	3	UN2375	II	3	IB2, T7, TP1, TP13	129	FLAMMABLE
	Diethylamine	3	UN1154	II	3, 8	A3, IB2, N34, T7, TP1	132	FLAMMABLE
	2-Diethylaminoethanol	8	UN2686	II	8, 3	B2, IB2, T7, TP2	132	CORROSIVE
	3-Diethylamino-propylamine	3	UN2684	III	3, 8	B1, IB3, T4, TP1	132	FLAMMABLE
+	**N,N-Diethylaniline**	6.1	UN2432	III	6.1	IB3, T4, TP1	153	POISON

Symbols	Hazardous materials descriptions and proper shipping names	Hazard class or Division	Identification Numbers	PG	Label Codes	Special provisions (§172.102)	ERG Guide No.	Placard Advisory Consult §172.504 & §172.505 *Placard any quantity
(1)	(2)	(3)	(4)	(5)	(6)	(7)		
	Diethylbenzene	3	UN2049	III	3	B1, IB3, T2, TP1	130	FLAMMABLE
	Diethyldichlorosilane	8	UN1767	II	8, 3	A7, B6, IB2, N34, T7, TP2, TP13	155	CORROSIVE
	Diethylene glycol dinitrate	Forbidden						
	Diethyleneglycol dinitrate, desensitized *with not less than 25 percent non-volatile water-insoluble phlegmatizer, by mass*	1.1D	UN0075	II	1.1D		112	EXPLOSIVES 1.1*
	Diethylenetriamine	8	UN2079	II	8	B2, IB2, T7, TP2	154	CORROSIVE
	N,N-Diethylethylenediamine	8	UN2685	II	8, 3	IB2, T7, TP2	132	CORROSIVE
	Diethylgold bromide	Forbidden						
	Diethylthiophosphoryl chloride	8	UN2751	II	8	B2, IB2, T7, TP2	155	CORROSIVE
	Diethylzinc	4.2	UN1366	I	4.2, 4.3	173, B11, T21, TP2, TP7	135	SPONTANEOUSLY COMBUSTIBLE, DANGEROUS WHEN WET*
	Difluorochloroethanes, see **1-Chloro-1, 1-difluoroethanes**							
	1,1-Difluoroethane *or* **Refrigerant gas R 152a**	2.1	UN1030		2.1	T50	115	FLAMMABLE GAS
	1,1-Difluoroethylene *or* **Refrigerant gas R 1132a**	2.1	UN1959		2.1		116P	FLAMMABLE GAS

Symbols	Hazardous materials descriptions and proper shipping names	Hazard class or Division	Identification Numbers	PG	Label Codes	Special provisions (§172.102)	ERG Guide No.	Placard Advisory Consult §172.504 & §172.505 *Placard any quantity
(1)	(2)	(3)	(4)	(5)	(6)	(7)		
	Difluoromethane *or* **Refrigerant gas R 32**	2.1	UN3252		2.1	T50	115	FLAMMABLE GAS
	Difluorophosphoric acid, anhydrous	8	UN1768	II	8	A6, A7, B2, IB2, N5, N34, T8, TP2, TP12	154	CORROSIVE
	2,3-Dihydropyran	3	UN2376	II	3	IB2, T4, TP1	127	FLAMMABLE
	1,8-Dihydroxy-2,4,5,7-tetranitroanthraquinone (chrysamminic acid)	Forbidden						
	Diiodoacetylene	Forbidden						
	Diisobutyl ketone	3	UN1157	III	3	B1, IB3, T2, TP1	128	FLAMMABLE
	Diisobutylamine	3	UN2361	III	3, 8	B1, IB3, T4, TP1	132	FLAMMABLE
	Diisobutylene, isomeric compounds	3	UN2050	II	3	IB2, T4, TP1	128	FLAMMABLE
	Diisooctyl acid phosphate	8	UN1902	III	8	IB3, T4, TP1	153	CORROSIVE
	Diisopropyl ether	3	UN1159	II	3	IB2, T4, TP1	127	FLAMMABLE
	Diisopropylamine	3	UN1158	II	3, 8	IB2, T7, TP1	132	FLAMMABLE
	Diisopropylbenzene hydroperoxide, with more than 72 percent in solution	Forbidden						
	Diketene, stabilized	6.1	UN2521	I	6.1, 3	2, B9, B14, B32, B74, T20, TP2, TP13, TP38, TP45	131P	POISON INHALATION HAZARD*
	1,2-Dimethoxyethane	3	UN2252	II	3	IB2, T4, TP1	127	FLAMMABLE
	1,1-Dimethoxyethane	3	UN2377	II	3	IB2, T7, TP1	127	FLAMMABLE

Symbols	Hazardous materials descriptions and proper shipping names	Hazard class or Division	Identification Numbers	PG	Label Codes	Special provisions (§172.102)	ERG Guide No.	Placard Advisory Consult §172.504 & §172.505 *Placard any quantity
(1)	(2)	(3)	(4)	(5)	(6)	(7)		
	Dimethyl carbonate	3	UN1161	II	3	IB2, T4, TP1	129	FLAMMABLE
	Dimethyl chlorothiophosphate, see **Dimethyl thiophosphoryl chloride**							
	2,5-Dimethyl-2,5-dihydroperoxy hexane, with more than 82 percent with water	Forbidden						
	Dimethyl disulfide	3	UN2381	II	3	IB2, T4, TP1	130	FLAMMABLE
	Dimethyl ether	2.1	UN1033		2.1	T50	115	FLAMMABLE GAS
	Dimethyl-N-propylamine	3	UN2266	II	3, 8	IB2, T7, TP2, TP13	130	FLAMMABLE
	Dimethyl sulfate	6.1	UN1595	I	6.1, 8	2, B9, B14, B32, B74, B77, T20, TP2, TP13, TP38, TP45	156	POISON INHALATION HAZARD*
	Dimethyl sulfide	3	UN1164	II	3	IB2, IP8, T7, TP2	130	FLAMMABLE
	Dimethyl thiophosphoryl chloride	6.1	UN2267	II	6.1, 8	IB2, T7, TP2	156	POISON
	Dimethylamine, anhydrous	2.1	UN1032		2.1	T50	118	FLAMMABLE GAS
	Dimethylamine solution	3	UN1160	II	3, 8	IB2, T7, TP1	132	FLAMMABLE
	2-Dimethylaminoacetonitrile	3	UN2378	II	3, 6.1	IB2, T7, TP1	131	FLAMMABLE
	2-Dimethylaminoethanol	8	UN2051	II	8, 3	B2, IB2, T7, TP2	132	CORROSIVE
	2-Dimethylaminoethyl acrylate	6.1	UN3302	II	6.1	IB2,T7, TP2	152	POISON
	2-Dimethylaminoethyl methacrylate	6.1	UN2522	II	6.1	IB2, T7, TP2	153P	POISON
	N,N-Dimethylaniline	6.1	UN2253	II	6.1	IB1, T7, TP2	153	POISON

Symbols	Hazardous materials descriptions and proper shipping names	Hazard class or Division	Identification Numbers	PG	Label Codes	Special provisions (§172.102)	ERG Guide No.	Placard Advisory Consult §172.504 & §172.505 *Placard any quantity
(1)	(2)	(3)	(4)	(5)	(6)	(7)		
	2,3-Dimethylbutane	3	UN2457	II	3	IB2, T7, TP1	128	FLAMMABLE
	1,3-Dimethylbutylamine	3	UN2379	II	3, 8	IB2, T7, TP1	132	FLAMMABLE
	Dimethylcarbamoyl chloride	8	UN2262	II	8	B2, IB2,T7, TP2	156	CORROSIVE
	Dimethylcyclohexanes	3	UN2263	II	3	IB2, T4, TP1	128	FLAMMABLE
	N,N-Dimethylcyclohexylamine	8	UN2264	II	8, 3	B2, IB2, T7, TP2	132	CORROSIVE
	Dimethyldichlorosilane	3	UN1162	II	3, 8	B77, IB2, T7, TP2, TP13	155	FLAMMABLE
	Dimethyldiethoxysilane	3	UN2380	II	3	IB2, T4, TP1	127	FLAMMABLE
	Dimethyldioxanes	3	UN2707	II	3	IB2, T4, TP1	127	FLAMMABLE
				III	3	B1, IB3, T2, TP1	127	FLAMMABLE
	N,N-Dimethylformamide	3	UN2265	III	3	B1, IB3, T2, TP2	129	FLAMMABLE
	Dimethylhexane dihydroperoxide (dry)	Forbidden						
	Dimethylhydrazine, symmetrical	6.1	UN2382	I	6.1, 3	2, B9, B14, B32, B74, B77, T20, TP2, TP13, TP38, TP45	131	POISON INHALATION HAZARD*
	Dimethylhydrazine, unsymmetrical	6.1	UN1163	I	6.1, 3, 8	2, B7, B9, B14, B32, B74, T20, TP2, TP13, TP38, TP45	131	POISON INHALATION HAZARD*
	2,2-Dimethylpropane	2.1	UN2044		2.1		115	FLAMMABLE GAS

Sym-bols	Hazardous materials descriptions and proper shipping names	Hazard class or Division	Identification Numbers	PG	Label Codes	Special provisions (§172.102)	ERG Guide No.	Placard Advisory Consult §172.504 & §172.505 *Placard any quantity
(1)	(2)	(3)	(4)	(5)	(6)	(7)		
	Dimethylzinc	4.2	UN1370	I	4.2, 4.3	173, B11, B16, T21, TP2, TP7	135	SPONTANEOUSLY COMBUSTIBLE, DANGEROUS WHEN WET*
	Dinitro-o-cresol	6.1	UN1598	II	6.1	IB8, IP2, IP4, T3, TP33	153	POISON
	1,3-Dinitro-5,5-dimethyl hydantoin	Forbidden						
	Dinitro-7,8-dimethylglycoluril (dry)	Forbidden						
	1,3-Dinitro-4,5-dinitrosobenzene	Forbidden						
	1,4-Dinitro-1,1,4,4-tetramethylolbutane-tetranitrate (dry)	Forbidden						
	2,4-Dinitro-1,3,5-trimethylbenzene	Forbidden						
	Dinitroanilines	6.1	UN1596	II	6.1	IB8, IP2, IP4, T3, TP33	153	POISON
	Dinitrobenzenes, liquid	6.1	UN1597	II	6.1	11, IB2, T7, TP2	152	POISON
				III	6.1	11, IB3, T7, TP2	152	POISON
	Dinitrobenzenes, solid	6.1	UN3443	II	6.1	IB8, IP2, IP4, T3, TP33	152	POISON
	Dinitrochlorobenzene, see **Chlorodinitrobenzene**							
	1,2-Dinitroethane	Forbidden						
	1,1-Dinitroethane (dry)	Forbidden						

Symbols	Hazardous materials descriptions and proper shipping names	Hazard class or Division	Identification Numbers	PG	Label Codes	Special provisions (§172.102)	ERG Guide No.	Placard Advisory Consult §172.504 & §172.505 *Placard any quantity
(1)	(2)	(3)	(4)	(5)	(6)	(7)		
	Dinitrogen tetroxide	2.3	UN1067		2.3, 5.1 , 8	1, B7, B14, B45, B46, B61, B66, B67, B77, T50, TP21	124	POISON GAS*
	Dinitroglycoluril *or* **Dingu**	1.1D	UN0489	II	1.1D		112	EXPLOSIVES 1.1*
	Dinitromethane	Forbidden						
	Dinitrophenol, *dry or wetted with less than 15 percent water, by mass*	1.1D	UN0076	II	1.1D, 6.1		112	EXPLOSIVES 1.1*
	Dinitrophenol solutions	6.1	UN1599	II	6.1	IB2, T7, TP2	153	POISON
				III	6.1	IB3, T4, TP1	153	POISON
	Dinitrophenol, wetted *with not less than 15 percent water, by mass*	4.1	UN1320	I	4.1, 6.1	23, A8, A19, A20, N41	113	FLAMMABLE SOLID
	Dinitrophenolates *alkali metals, dry or wetted with less than 15 percent water, by mass*	1.3C	UN0077	II	1.3C, 6.1		112	EXPLOSIVES 1.3*
	Dinitrophenolates, wetted *with not less than 15 percent water, by mass*	4.1	UN1321	I	4.1, 6.1	23, A8, A19, A20, N41	113	FLAMMABLE SOLID
	Dinitropropylene glycol	Forbidden						
	Dinitroresorcinol, *dry or wetted with less than 15 percent water, by mass*	1.1D	UN0078	II	1.1D		112	EXPLOSIVES 1.1*
	2,4-Dinitroresorcinol (heavy metal salts of) (dry)	Forbidden						

Symbols	Hazardous materials descriptions and proper shipping names	Hazard class or Division	Identification Numbers	PG	Label Codes	Special provisions (§172.102)	ERG Guide No.	Placard Advisory Consult §172.504 & §172.505 *Placard any quantity
(1)	(2)	(3)	(4)	(5)	(6)	(7)		
	4,6-Dinitroresorcinol (heavy metal salts of) (dry)	Forbidden						
	Dinitroresorcinol, wetted *with not less than 15 percent water, by mass*	4.1	UN1322	I	4.1	23, A8, A19, A20, N41	113	FLAMMABLE SOLID
	3,5-Dinitrosalicylic acid (lead salt) (dry)	Forbidden						
	Dinitrosobenzene	1.3C	UN0406	II	1.3C		112	EXPLOSIVES 1.3*
	Dinitrosobenzylamidine and salts of (dry)	Forbidden						
	2,2-Dinitrostilbene	Forbidden						
	Dinitrotoluenes, *liquid*	6.1	UN2038	II	6.1	IB2, T7, TP2	152	POISON
	Dinitrotoluenes, molten	6.1	UN1600	II	6.1	T7, TP3	152	POISON
	Dinitrotoluenes, solid	6.1	UN3454	II	6.1	IB8, IP2, IP4, T3, TP33	152	POISON
	1,9-Dinitroxy pentamethylene-2,4, 6, 8-tetramine (dry)	Forbidden						
	Dioxane	3	UN1165	II	3	IB2, T4, TP1	127	FLAMMABLE
	Dioxolane	3	UN1166	II	3	IB2, T4, TP1	127	FLAMMABLE
	Dipentene	3	UN2052	III	3	B1, IB3, T2, TP1	128	FLAMMABLE
	Diphenylamine chloroarsine	6.1	UN1698	I	6.1	T6, TP33	154	POISON
	Diphenylchloroarsine, liquid	6.1	UN1699	I	6.1	A8, B14, B32, N33, N34, T14, TP2, TP13, TP27	151	POISON

Symbols	Hazardous materials descriptions and proper shipping names	Hazard class or Division	Identification Numbers	PG	Label Codes	Special provisions (§172.102)	ERG Guide No.	Placard Advisory Consult §172.504 & §172.505 *Placard any quantity
(1)	(2)	(3)	(4)	(5)	(6)	(7)		
	Diphenylchloroarsine, solid	6.1	UN3450	I	6.1	IB7, IP1, T6, TP33	151	POISON
	Diphenyldichlorosilane	8	UN1769	II	8	A7, B2, IB2, N34, T7, TP2, TP13	156	CORROSIVE
	Diphenylmethyl bromide	8	UN1770	II	8	IB8, IP2, IP4, T3, TP33	153	CORROSIVE
	Dipicryl sulfide, *dry or wetted with less than 10 percent water, by mass*	1.1D	UN0401	II	1.1D		112	EXPLOSIVES 1.1*
	Dipicryl sulfide, wetted *with not less than 10 percent water, by mass*	4.1	UN2852	I	4.1	162, A2, N41, N84	113	FLAMMABLE SOLID
	Dipicrylamine, *see* **Hexanitrodiphenylamine**							
	Dipropionyl peroxide, with more than 28 percent in solution	Forbidden						
	Di-n-propyl ether	3	UN2384	II	3	IB2, T4, TP1	127	FLAMMABLE
	Dipropyl ketone	3	UN2710	III	3	B1, IB3, T2, TP1	128	FLAMMABLE
	Dipropylamine	3	UN2383	II	3, 8	IB2, T7, TP1	132	FLAMMABLE
G	**Disinfectant, liquid, corrosive, n.o.s.**	8	UN1903	I	8	A6, A7, B10, T14, TP2, TP27	153	CORROSIVE
G	**Disinfectants, liquid, corrosive n.o.s.**	8	UN1903	II	8	B2, IB2, T7, TP2	153	CORROSIVE
				III	8	IB3, T4, TP1	153	CORROSIVE
G	**Disinfectants, liquid, toxic, n.o.s**	6.1	UN3142	I	6.1	A4, T14, TP2, TP27	151	POISON

Symbols	Hazardous materials descriptions and proper shipping names	Hazard class or Division	Identification Numbers	PG	Label Codes	Special provisions (§172.102)	ERG Guide No.	Placard Advisory Consult §172.504 & §172.505 *Placard any quantity
(1)	(2)	(3)	(4)	(5)	(6)	(7)		
				II	6.1	IB2, T11, TP2, TP27	151	POISON
				III	6.1	IB3, T7, TP1, TP28	151	POISON
G	**Disinfectants, solid, toxic, n.o.s.**	6.1	UN1601	I	6.1	IB7, IP1, T6, TP33	151	POISON
				II	6.1	IB8, IP2, IP4, T3, TP33	151	POISON
				III	6.1	IB8, IP3, T1, TP33	151	POISON
	Disodium trioxosilicate	8	UN3253	III	8	IB8, IP3, T1, TP33	154	CORROSIVE
G	**Dispersant gases, n.o.s.** *see* **Refrigerant gases, n.o.s.**							
	Divinyl ether, stabilized	3	UN1167	I	3	A3, T11, TP2	128P	FLAMMABLE
	Dodecyltrichlorosilane	8	UN1771	II	8	A7, B2, B6, IB2, N34, T7, TP2, TP13	156	CORROSIVE
	Dry ice, *see* **Carbon dioxide, solid**							
G	**Dyes, liquid, corrosive n.o.s.** *or* **Dye intermediates, liquid, corrosive, n.o.s.**	8	UN2801	I	8	11, A6, B10, T14, TP2, TP27	154	CORROSIVE
				II	8	11, B2, IB2, T11, TP2, TP27	154	CORROSIVE
				III	8	11, IB3, T7, TP1, TP28	154	CORROSIVE

Sym-bols	Hazardous materials descriptions and proper shipping names	Hazard class or Division	Identifica-tion Numbers	PG	Label Codes	Special provisions (§172.102)	ERG Guide No.	Placard Advisory Consult §172.504 & §172.505 *Placard any quantity
(1)	(2)	(3)	(4)	(5)	(6)	(7)		
G	**Dyes, liquid, toxic, n.o.s** *or* **Dye intermediates, liquid, toxic, n.o.s.**	6.1	UN1602	I	6.1		151	POISON
				II	6.1	IB2	151	POISON
				III	6.1	IB3	151	POISON
G	**Dyes, solid, corrosive, n.o.s.** *or* **Dye intermediates, solid, corrosive, n.o.s.**	8	UN3147	I	8	IB7, IP1, T6, TP33	154	CORROSIVE
				II	8	IB8, IP2, IP4, T3, TP33	154	CORROSIVE
				III	8	IB8, IP3, T1, TP33	154	CORROSIVE
G	**Dyes, solid, toxic, n.o.s.** *or* **Dye intermediates, solid, toxic, n.o.s.**	6.1	UN3143	I	6.1	A5, IB7, IP1, T6, TP33	151	POISON
				II	6.1	IB8, IP2, IP4, T3, TP33	151	POISON
				III	6.1	IB8, IP3, T1, TP33	151	POISON
	Dynamite, see **Explosive, blasting, type A**							
	Electrolyte (acid or alkali) for batteries, see **Battery fluid, acid** *or* **Battery fluid, alkali**							
	Elevated temperature liquid, flammable, n.o.s., *with flash point above 37.8 C, at or above its flash point*	3	UN3256	III	3	IB1, T3, TP3, TP29	128	FLAMMABLE

Symbols	Hazardous materials descriptions and proper shipping names	Hazard class or Division	Identification Numbers	PG	Label Codes	Special provisions (§172.102)	ERG Guide No.	Placard Advisory Consult §172.504 & §172.505 *Placard any quantity
(1)	(2)	(3)	(4)	(5)	(6)	(7)		
	Elevated temperature liquid, n.o.s., *at or above 100 C and below its flash point (including molten metals, molten salts, etc.)*	9	UN3257	III	9	IB1, T3, TP3, TP29	128	CLASS 9
	Elevated temperature solid, n.o.s., *at or above 240 C, see §173.247(h)(4)*	9	UN3258	III	9		171	CLASS 9
	Engines, internal combustion, *flammable gas powered*	9	UN3166		9	135	128	CLASS 9
	Engines, internal combustion, *flammable liquid powered*	9	UN3166		9	135	128	CLASS 9
G	**Environmentally hazardous substances, liquid, n.o.s.**	9	UN3082	III	9	8, 146, IB3, T4, TP1, TP29	171	CLASS 9
G	**Environmentally hazardous substances, solid, n.o.s.**	9	UN3077	III	9	8, 146, B54, IB8, IP3, N20, T1, TP33	171	CLASS 9
	Epibromohydrin	6.1	UN2558	I	6.1, 3	T14, TP2, TP13	131	POISON
+	**Epichlorohydrin**	6.1	UN2023	II	6.1, 3	IB2, T7, TP2, TP13	131P	POISON
	1,2-Epoxy-3-ethoxypropane	3	UN2752	III	3	B1, IB3, T2, TP1	127	FLAMMABLE
	Esters, n.o.s.	3	UN3272	II	3	IB2, T7, TP1, TP8, TP28	127	FLAMMABLE
				III	3	B1, IB3, T4, TP1, TP29	127	FLAMMABLE
	Etching acid, liquid, n.o.s., see **Hydrofluoric acid, solution** *etc.*							

Symbols	Hazardous materials descriptions and proper shipping names	Hazard class or Division	Identification Numbers	PG	Label Codes	Special provisions (§172.102)	ERG Guide No.	Placard Advisory Consult §172.504 & §172.505 *Placard any quantity
(1)	(2)	(3)	(4)	(5)	(6)	(7)		
	Ethane	2.1	UN1035		2.1		115	FLAMMABLE GAS
D	**Ethane-Propane mixture, refrigerated liquid**	2.1	NA1961		2.1	T75, TP5	115	FLAMMABLE GAS
	Ethane, refrigerated liquid	2.1	UN1961		2.1	T75, TP5	115	FLAMMABLE GAS
	Ethanol amine dinitrate	Forbidden						
	Ethanol *or* **Ethyl alcohol** *or* **Ethanol solutions** *or* **Ethyl alcohol solutions**	3	UN1170	II	3	24, IB2, T4, TP1	127	FLAMMABLE
				III	3	24, B1, IB3, T2, TP1	127	FLAMMABLE
	Ethanolamine *or* **Ethanolamine solutions**	8	UN2491	III	8	IB3, T4, TP1	153	CORROSIVE
	Ether, see **Diethyl ether**							
	Ethers, n.o.s.	3	UN3271	II	3	IB2, T7, TP1, TP8, TP28	127	FLAMMABLE
				III	3	B1, IB3, T4, TP1, TP29	127	FLAMMABLE
	Ethyl acetate	3	UN1173	II	3	IB2, T4, TP1	129	FLAMMABLE
	Ethyl acrylate, stabilized	3	UN1917	II	3	IB2, T4, TP1, TP13	129P	FLAMMABLE
	Ethyl alcohol, *see* **Ethanol**							
	Ethyl aldehyde, see **Acetaldehyde**							
	Ethyl amyl ketone	3	UN2271	III	3	B1, IB3, T2, TP1	128	FLAMMABLE
	N-Ethyl-N-benzylaniline	6.1	UN2274	III	6.1	IB3, T4, TP1	153	POISON

Sym-bols	Hazardous materials descriptions and proper shipping names	Hazard class or Division	Identification Numbers	PG	Label Codes	Special provisions (§172.102)	ERG Guide No.	Placard Advisory Consult §172.504 & §172.505 *Placard any quantity
(1)	(2)	(3)	(4)	(5)	(6)	(7)		
	Ethyl borate	3	UN1176	II	3	IB2, T4, TP1	129	FLAMMABLE
	Ethyl bromide	6.1	UN1891	II	6.1	IB2, IP8, T7, TP2, TP13	131	POISON
	Ethyl bromoacetate	6.1	UN1603	II	6.1, 3	IB2, T7, TP2	155	POISON
	Ethyl butyl ether	3	UN1179	II	3	B1, IB2, T4, TP1	127	FLAMMABLE
	Ethyl butyrate	3	UN1180	III	3	B1, IB3, T2, TP1	130	FLAMMABLE
	Ethyl chloride	2.1	UN1037		2.1	B77, T50	115	FLAMMABLE GAS
	Ethyl chloroacetate	6.1	UN1181	II	6.1, 3	IB2, T7, TP2	155	POISON
	Ethyl chloroformate	6.1	UN1182	I	6.1, 3, 8	2, B9, B14, B32, B74, N34, T20, TP2, TP13, TP38, TP45	155	POISON INHALATION HAZARD*
	Ethyl 2-chloropropionate	3	UN2935	III	3	B1, IB3, T2, TP1	129	FLAMMABLE
+	**Ethyl chlorothioformate**	8	UN2826	II	8, 6.1, 3	2, B9, B14, B32, B74, T20, TP2, TP38, TP45	155	CORROSIVE, POISON INHALATION HAZARD*
	Ethyl crotonate	3	UN1862	II	3	IB2, T4, TP2	130	FLAMMABLE
	Ethyl ether, *see* **Diethyl ether**							
	Ethyl fluoride *or* **Refrigerant gas R161**	2.1	UN2453		2.1		115	FLAMMABLE GAS
	Ethyl formate	3	UN1190	II	3	IB2, T4, TP1	129	FLAMMABLE
	Ethyl hydroperoxide	Forbidden						

Sym-bols	Hazardous materials descriptions and proper shipping names	Hazard class or Division	Identification Numbers	PG	Label Codes	Special provisions (§172.102)	ERG Guide No.	Placard Advisory Consult §172.504 & §172.505 *Placard any quantity
(1)	(2)	(3)	(4)	(5)	(6)	(7)		
	Ethyl isobutyrate	3	UN2385	II	3	IB2, T4, TP1	129	FLAMMABLE
+	**Ethyl isocyanate**	3	UN2481	I	3, 6.1	1, B9, B14, B30, B72, T22, TP2, TP13, TP38, TP44	155	FLAMMABLE, POISON INHALATION HAZARD*
	Ethyl lactate	3	UN1192	III	3	B1, IB3, T2, TP1	129	FLAMMABLE
	Ethyl mercaptan	3	UN2363	I	3	A6, T11, TP2, TP13	129	FLAMMABLE
	Ethyl methacrylate, stabilized	3	UN2277	II	3	IB2, T4, TP1	130P	FLAMMABLE
	Ethyl methyl ether	2.1	UN1039		2.1		115	FLAMMABLE GAS
	Ethyl methyl ketone *or* **Methyl ethyl ketone**	3	UN1193	II	3	IB2, T4, TP1	127	FLAMMABLE
	Ethyl nitrite solutions	3	UN1194	I	3, 6.1		131	FLAMMABLE
	Ethyl orthoformate	3	UN2524	III	3	B1, IB3, T2, TP1	129	FLAMMABLE
	Ethyl oxalate	6.1	UN2525	III	6.1	IB3, T4, TP1	156	POISON
	Ethyl perchlorate	Forbidden						
D	**Ethyl phosphonothioic dichloride, anhydrous**	6.1	NA2927	I	6.1, 8	2, B9, B14, B32, B74, T20, TP4, TP12, TP13, TP38, TP45	154	POISON INHALATION HAZARD*

Symbols	Hazardous materials descriptions and proper shipping names	Hazard class or Division	Identification Numbers	PG	Label Codes	Special provisions (§172.102)	ERG Guide No.	Placard Advisory Consult §172.504 & §172.505 *Placard any quantity
(1)	(2)	(3)	(4)	(5)	(6)	(7)		
D	**Ethyl phosphonous dichloride, anhydrous** *pyrophoric liquid*	6.1	NA2845	I	6.1, 4.2	2, B9, B14, B32, B74, T20, TP4, TP12, TP13, TP38, TP45	135	POISON INHALATION HAZARD*
D	**Ethyl phosphorodichloridate**	6.1	NA2927	I	6.1, 8	2, B9, B14, B32, B74, T20, TP4, TP12, TP13, TP38, TP45	154	POISON INHALATION HAZARD*
	Ethyl propionate	3	UN1195	II	3	IB2, T4, TP1	129	FLAMMABLE
	Ethyl propyl ether	3	UN2615	II	3	IB2, T4, TP1	127	FLAMMABLE
	Ethyl silicate, see **Tetraethyl silicate**							
	Ethylacetylene, stabilized	2.1	UN2452		2.1		116P	FLAMMABLE GAS
	Ethylamine	2.1	UN1036		2.1	B77, T50	118	FLAMMABLE GAS
	Ethylamine, aqueous solution *with not less than 50 percent but not more than 70 percent ethylamine*	3	UN2270	II	3, 8	IB2, T7, TP1	132	FLAMMABLE
	N-Ethylaniline	6.1	UN2272	III	6.1	IB3, T4, TP1	153	POISON
	2-Ethylaniline	6.1	UN2273	III	6.1	IB3, T4, TP1	153	POISON
	Ethylbenzene	3	UN1175	II	3	IB2, T4, TP1	130	FLAMMABLE
	N-Ethylbenzyltoluidines liquid	6.1	UN2753	III	6.1	IB3, T7, TP1	153	POISON
	N-Ethylbenzyltoluidines, solid	6.1	UN3460	III	6.1	IB8, IP3, T1, TP33	153	POISON
	2-Ethylbutanol	3	UN2275	III	3	B1, IB3, T2, TP1	129	FLAMMABLE

Symbols	Hazardous materials descriptions and proper shipping names	Hazard class or Division	Identification Numbers	PG	Label Codes	Special provisions (§172.102)	ERG Guide No.	Placard Advisory Consult §172.504 & §172.505 *Placard any quantity
(1)	(2)	(3)	(4)	(5)	(6)	(7)		
	2-Ethylbutyl acetate	3	UN1177	III	3	B1, IB3, T2, TP1	130	FLAMMABLE
	2-Ethylbutyraldehyde	3	UN1178	II	3	B1, IB2, T4, TP1	130	FLAMMABLE
	Ethyldichloroarsine	6.1	UN1892	I	6.1	2, B9, B14, B32, B74, T20, TP2, TP13, TP38, TP45	151	POISON INHALATION HAZARD*
	Ethyldichlorosilane	4.3	UN1183	I	4.3, 8, 3	A2, A3, A7, N34, T10, TP2, TP7, TP13	139	DANGEROUS WHEN WET*
	Ethylene, acetylene and propylene in mixture, refrigerated liquid *with at least 71.5 percent ethylene with not more than 22.5 percent acetylene and not more than 6 percent propylene*	2.1	UN3138		2.1	T75, TP5	115	FLAMMABLE GAS
	Ethylene chlorohydrin	6.1	UN1135	I	6.1, 3	2, B9, B14, B32, B74, T20, TP2, TP13, TP38, TP45	131	POISON INHALATION HAZARD*
	Ethylene	2.1	UN1962		2.1		116P	FLAMMABLE GAS
	Ethylene diamine diperchlorate	Forbidden						
	Ethylene dibromide	6.1	UN1605	I	6.1	2, B9, B14, B32, B74, B77, T20, TP2, TP13, TP38, TP45	154	POISON INHALATION HAZARD*

Symbols	Hazardous materials descriptions and proper shipping names	Hazard class or Division	Identification Numbers	PG	Label Codes	Special provisions (§172.102)	ERG Guide No.	Placard Advisory Consult §172.504 & §172.505 *Placard any quantity
(1)	(2)	(3)	(4)	(5)	(6)	(7)		
	Ethylene dibromide and methyl bromide liquid mixtures, see **Methyl bromide and ethylene dibromide, liquid mixtures**							
	Ethylene dichloride	3	UN1184	II	3, 6.1	IB2, N36, T7, TP1	131	FLAMMABLE
	Ethylene glycol diethyl ether	3	UN1153	II	3	IB2, T4, TP1	127	FLAMMABLE
				III	3	B1, IB3, T2, TP1	127	FLAMMABLE
	Ethylene glycol dinitrate	Forbidden						
	Ethylene glycol monoethyl ether	3	UN1171	III	3	B1, IB3, T2, TP1	127	FLAMMABLE
	Ethylene glycol monoethyl ether acetate	3	UN1172	III	3	B1, IB3, T2, TP1	129	FLAMMABLE
	Ethylene glycol monomethyl ether	3	UN1188	III	3	B1, IB3, T2, TP1	127	FLAMMABLE
	Ethylene glycol monomethyl ether acetate	3	UN1189	III	3	B1, IB3, T2, TP1	129	FLAMMABLE
	Ethylene oxide and carbon dioxide mixture *with more than 87 percent ethylene oxide*	2.3	UN3300		2.3, 2.1	4	119P	POISON GAS*
	Ethylene oxide and carbon dioxide mixtures *with more than 9 percent but not more than 87 percent ethylene oxide*	2.1	UN1041		2.1	T50	115	FLAMMABLE GAS
	Ethylene oxide and carbon dioxide mixtures *with not more than 9 percent ethylene oxide*	2.2	UN1952		2.2		126	NONFLAMMABLE GAS

Symbols	Hazardous materials descriptions and proper shipping names	Hazard class or Division	Identification Numbers	PG	Label Codes	Special provisions (§172.102)	ERG Guide No.	Placard Advisory Consult §172.504 & §172.505 *Placard any quantity
(1)	(2)	(3)	(4)	(5)	(6)	(7)		
	Ethylene oxide and chlorotetrafluoroethane mixture *with not more than 8.8 percent ethylene oxide*	2.2	UN3297		2.2	T50	126	NONFLAMMABLE GAS
	Ethylene oxide and dichlorodifluoromethane mixture, *with not more than 12.5 percent ethylene oxide*	2.2	UN3070		2.2	T50	126	NONFLAMMABLE GAS
	Ethylene oxide and pentafluoroethane mixture *with not more than 7.9 percent ethylene oxide*	2.2	UN3298		2.2	T50	126	NONFLAMMABLE GAS
	Ethylene oxide and propylene oxide mixtures, *with not more than 30 percent ethylene oxide*	3	UN2983	I	3, 6.1	5, A11, N4, N34, T14, TP2, TP7, TP13	129P	FLAMMABLE
	Ethylene oxide and tetrafluoroethane mixture *with not more than 5.6 percent ethylene oxide*	2.2	UN3299		2.2	T50	126	NONFLAMMABLE GAS
	Ethylene oxide *or* **Ethylene oxide with nitrogen** *up to a total pressure of 1MPa (10 bar) at 50 degrees C*	2.3	UN1040		2.3, 2.1	4, T50, TP20	119P	POISON GAS*
	Ethylene, refrigerated liquid *(cryogenic liquid)*	2.1	UN1038		2.1	T75, TP5	115	FLAMMABLE GAS
	Ethylenediamine	8	UN1604	II	8, 3	IB2, T7, TP2	132	CORROSIVE
	Ethyleneimine, stabilized	6.1	UN1185	I	6.1, 3	1, B9, B14, B30, B72, B77, N25, N32, T22, TP2, TP13, TP38, TP44	131P	POISON INHALATION HAZARD*

Sym-bols	Hazardous materials descriptions and proper shipping names	Hazard class or Division	Identification Numbers	PG	Label Codes	Special provisions (§172.102)	ERG Guide No.	Placard Advisory Consult §172.504 & §172.505 *Placard any quantity
(1)	(2)	(3)	(4)	(5)	(6)	(7)		
	Ethylhexaldehyde, see **Octyl aldehydes** *etc.*							
	2-Ethylhexyl chloroformate	6.1	UN2748	II	6.1, 8	IB2, T7, TP2, TP13	156	POISON
	2-Ethylhexylamine	3	UN2276	III	3, 8	B1, IB3, T4, TP1	132	FLAMMABLE
	Ethylphenyldichlorosilane	8	UN2435	II	8	A7, B2, IB2, N34, T7, TP2, TP13	156	CORROSIVE
	1-Ethylpiperidine	3	UN2386	II	3, 8	IB2, T7, TP1	132	FLAMMABLE
	N-Ethyltoluidines	6.1	UN2754	II	6.1	IB2, T7, TP2	153	POISON
	Ethyltrichlorosilane	3	UN1196	II	3, 8	A7, IB1, N34, T7, TP2, TP13	155	FLAMMABLE
	Etiologic agent, see **Infectious substances,** *etc.*							
	Explosive articles, see **Articles, explosive, n.o.s.** *etc.*							
	Explosive, blasting, type A	1.1D	UN0081	II	1.1D		112	EXPLOSIVES 1.1*
	Explosive, blasting, type B	1.1D	UN0082	II	1.1D		112	EXPLOSIVES 1.1*
	Explosive, blasting, type B *or* **Agent blasting, Type B**	1.5D	UN0331	II	1.5D	105, 106	112	EXPLOSIVES 1.5
	Explosive, blasting, type C	1.1D	UN0083	II	1.1D	123	112	EXPLOSIVES 1.1*
	Explosive, blasting, type D	1.1D	UN0084	II	1.1D		112	EXPLOSIVES 1.1*
	Explosive, blasting, type E	1.1D	UN0241	II	1.1D		112	EXPLOSIVES 1.1*

Sym-bols	Hazardous materials descriptions and proper shipping names	Hazard class or Division	Identifica-tion Numbers	PG	Label Codes	Special provisions (§172.102)	ERG Guide No.	Placard Advisory Consult §172.504 & §172.505 *Placard any quantity
(1)	(2)	(3)	(4)	(5)	(6)	(7)		
	Explosive, blasting, type E *or* **Agent blasting, Type E**	1.5D	UN0332	II	1.5D	105, 106	112	EXPLOSIVES 1.5
	Explosive, forbidden. See §173.54	Forbidden						
	Explosive substances, see **Substances, explosive, n.o.s.** *etc.*							
	Explosives, slurry, see **Explosive, blasting, type E**							
	Explosives, water gels, see **Explosive, blasting, type E**							
	Extracts, aromatic, liquid	3	UN1169	II	3	149, IB2, T4, TP1, TP8	127	FLAMMABLE
				III	3	B1, IB3, T2, TP1	127	FLAMMABLE
	Extracts, flavoring, liquid	3	UN1197	II	3	149, IB2, T4, TP1, TP8	127	FLAMMABLE
				III	3	B1, IB3, T2, TP1	127	FLAMMABLE
	Fabric with animal or vegetable oil, see **Fibers** *or* **fabrics,** *etc.*							
	Ferric arsenate	6.1	UN1606	II	6.1	IB8, IP2, IP4, T3, TP33	151	POISON
	Ferric arsenite	6.1	UN1607	II	6.1	IB8, IP2, IP4, T3, TP33	151	POISON
	Ferric chloride, anhydrous	8	UN1773	III	8	IB8, IP3, T1, TP33	157	CORROSIVE
	Ferric chloride, solution	8	UN2582	III	8	B15, IB3, T4, TP1	154	CORROSIVE

Sym-bols	Hazardous materials descriptions and proper shipping names	Hazard class or Division	Identification Numbers	PG	Label Codes	Special provisions (§172.102)	ERG Guide No.	Placard Advisory Consult §172.504 & §172.505 *Placard any quantity
(1)	(2)	(3)	(4)	(5)	(6)	(7)		
	Ferric nitrate	5.1	UN1466	III	5.1	A1, A29, IB8, IP3, T1, TP33	140	OXIDIZER
	Ferrocerium	4.1	UN1323	II	4.1	59, A19, IB8, IP2, IP4, T3, TP33	170	FLAMMABLE SOLID
	Ferrosilicon, *with 30 percent or more but less than 90 percent silicon*	4.3	UN1408	III	4.3, 6.1	A1, A19, B6, IB8, IP4, IP7, T1, TP33	139	DANGEROUS WHEN WET*
	Ferrous arsenate	6.1	UN1608	II	6.1	IB8, IP2, IP4, T3, TP33	151	POISON
D	**Ferrous chloride, solid**	8	NA1759	II	8	IB8, IP2, IP4, T3, TP33	154	CORROSIVE
D	**Ferrous chloride, solution**	8	NA1760	II	8	B3, IB2, T11, TP2, TP27	154	CORROSIVE
	Ferrous metal borings *or* **Ferrous metal shavings** *or* **Ferrous metal turnings** *or* **Ferrous metal cuttings** *in a form liable to self-heating*	4.2	UN2793	III	4.2	A1, A19, IB8, IP3, IP7	170	SPONTANEOUSLY COMBUSTIBLE
	Fertilizer ammoniating solution *with free ammonia*	2.2	UN1043		2.2		125	NONFLAMMABLE GAS
A I W	**Fibers, animal** *or* **Fibers, vegetable** *burnt, wet or damp*	4.2	UN1372	III	4.2		133	SPONTANEOUSLY COMBUSTIBLE
I W	**Fibers, vegetable, dry**	4.1	UN3360	III	4.1	137	133	FLAMMABLE SOLID

Symbols	Hazardous materials descriptions and proper shipping names	Hazard class or Division	Identification Numbers	PG	Label Codes	Special provisions (§172.102)	ERG Guide No.	Placard Advisory Consult §172.504 & §172.505 *Placard any quantity
(1)	(2)	(3)	(4)	(5)	(6)	(7)		
A W	**Fibers** *or* **Fabrics, animal** *or* **vegetable** *or* **Synthentic, n.o.s.** *with animal or vegetable oil*	4.2	UN1373	III	4.2	137, IB8, IP3, T1, TP33	133	SPONTANEOUSLY COMBUSTIBLE
	Fibers *or* **Fabrics impregnated with weakly nitrated nitrocellulose, n.o.s.**	4.1	UN1353	III	4.1	A1, IB8, IP3	133	FLAMMABLE SOLID
	Films, nitrocellulose base, from which gelatine has been removed; film scrap, see **Celluloid scrap**							
	Films, nitrocellulose base, *gelatine coated (except scrap)*	4.1	UN1324	III	4.1		133	FLAMMABLE SOLID
	Fire extinguisher charges, *corrosive liquid*	8	UN1774	II	8	N41	154	CORROSIVE
	Fire extinguisher charges, expelling, explosive, see **Cartridges, power device**							
	Fire extinguishers *containing compressed or liquefied gas*	2.2	UN1044		2.2	18, 110	126	NONFLAMMABLE GAS
	Firelighters, solid *with flammable liquid*	4.1	UN2623	III	4.1	A1, A19	133	FLAMMABLE SOLID
	Fireworks	1.1G	UN0333	II	1.1G	108	112	EXPLOSIVES 1.1*
	Fireworks	1.2G	UN0334	II	1.2G	108	112	EXPLOSIVES 1,2*
	Fireworks	1.3G	UN0335	II	1.3G	108	112	EXPLOSIVES 1.3*
	Fireworks	1.4G	UN0336	II	1.4G	108	114	EXPLOSIVES 1.4

Symbols	Hazardous materials descriptions and proper shipping names	Hazard class or Division	Identification Numbers	PG	Label Codes	Special provisions (§172.102)	ERG Guide No.	Placard Advisory Consult §172.504 & §172.505 *Placard any quantity
(1)	(2)	(3)	(4)	(5)	(6)	(7)		
	Fireworks	1.4S	UN0337	II	1.4S	108	114	EXPLOSIVES 1.4
	First aid kits	9	UN3316		9	15	171	CLASS 9
W	**Fish meal, stabilized** *or* **Fish scrap, stabilized**	9	UN2216	III	None	155, IB8, IP3, T1, TP33	171	CLASS 9
	Fish meal, unstablized *or* **Fish scrap, unstabilized**	4.2	UN1374	II	4.2	155, A1, A19, IB8, IP2, IP4, T3, TP33	133	SPONTANEOUSLY COMBUSTIBLE
	Fissile radioactive materials, see **Radioactive material, fissile, n.o.s.**							
	Flammable compressed gas, see **Compressed** *or* **Liquefied gas, flammable,** *etc.*							
	Flammable compressed gas (small receptacles not fitted with a dispersion device, not refillable), see **Receptacles,** *etc.*							
	Flammable gas in lighters, see **Lighters** *or* **lighter refills,** *cigarettes, containing flammable gas*							
G	**Flammable liquid, toxic, corrosive, n.o.s.**	3	UN3286	I	3, 6.1, 8	T14, TP2, TP13, TP27	131	FLAMMABLE
				II	3, 6.1, 8	IB2, T11, TP2, TP13, TP27	131	FLAMMABLE
G	**Flammable liquids, corrosive, n.o.s.**	3	UN2924	I	3, 8	T14, TP2	132	FLAMMABLE

Symbols	Hazardous materials descriptions and proper shipping names	Hazard class or Division	Identification Numbers	PG	Label Codes	Special provisions (§172.102)	ERG Guide No.	Placard Advisory Consult §172.504 & §172.505 *Placard any quantity
(1)	(2)	(3)	(4)	(5)	(6)	(7)		
				II	3, 8	IB2, T11, TP2, TP27	132	FLAMMABLE
				III	3, 8	B1, IB3, T7, TP1, TP28	132	FLAMMABLE
G	**Flammable liquids, n.o.s.**	3	UN1993	I	3	T11, TP1, TP27	128	FLAMMABLE
				II	3	IB2, T7, TP1, TP8, TP28	128	FLAMMABLE
				III	3	B1, B52, IB3, T4, TP1, TP29	128	FLAMMABLE
G	**Flammable liquids, toxic, n.o.s.**	3	UN1992	I	3, 6.1	T14, TP2, TP13, TP27	131	FLAMMABLE
				II	3, 6.1	IB2, T7, TP2, TP13	131	FLAMMABLE
				III	3, 6.1	B1, IB3, T7, TP1, TP28	131	FLAMMABLE
G	**Flammable solid, corrosive, inorganic, n.o.s.**	4.1	UN3180	II	4.1, 8	A1, IB6, IP2, T3, TP33	134	FLAMMABLE SOLID
				III	4.1, 8	A1, IB6, T1, TP33	134	FLAMMABLE SOLID
G	**Flammable solid, inorganic, n.o.s.**	4.1	UN3178	II	4.1	A1, IB8, IP2, IP4, T3, TP33	133	FLAMMABLE SOLID
				III	4.1	A1, IB8, IP3, T1, TP33	133	FLAMMABLE SOLID

Symbols	Hazardous materials descriptions and proper shipping names	Hazard class or Division	Identification Numbers	PG	Label Codes	Special provisions (§172.102)	ERG Guide No.	Placard Advisory Consult §172.504 & §172.505 *Placard any quantity
(1)	(2)	(3)	(4)	(5)	(6)	(7)		
G	**Flammable solid, organic, molten, n.o.s.**	4.1	UN3176	II	4.1	IB1, T3, TP3, TP26	133	FLAMMABLE SOLID
				III	4.1	IB1, T1, TP3, TP26	133	FLAMMABLE SOLID
G	**Flammable solid, oxidizing, n.o.s.**	4.1	UN3097	II	4.1, 5.1	131	140	FLAMMABLE SOLID
				III	4.1, 5.1	131, T1, TP33	140	FLAMMABLE SOLID
G	**Flammable solid, toxic, inorganic, n.o.s.**	4.1	UN3179	II	4.1, 6.1	A1, IB6, IP2, T3, TP33	134	FLAMMABLE SOLID
				III	4.1, 6.1	A1, IB6, T1, TP33	134	FLAMMABLE SOLID
G	**Flammable solids, corrosive, organic, n.o.s.**	4.1	UN2925	II	4.1, 8	A1, IB6, IP2, T3, TP33	134	FLAMMABLE SOLID
				III	4.1, 8	A1, IB6, T1, TP33	134	FLAMMABLE SOLID
G	**Flammable solids, organic, n.o.s.**	4.1	UN1325	II	4.1	A1, IB8, IP2, IP4, T3, TP33	133	FLAMMABLE SOLID
				III	4.1	A1, IB8, IP3, T1, TP33	133	FLAMMABLE SOLID
G	**Flammable solids, toxic, organic, n.o.s.**	4.1	UN2926	II	4.1, 6.1	A1, IB6, IP2, T3, TP33	134	FLAMMABLE SOLID
				III	4.1, 6.1	A1, IB6, T1, TP33	134	FLAMMABLE SOLID

Symbols	Hazardous materials descriptions and proper shipping names	Hazard class or Division	Identification Numbers	PG	Label Codes	Special provisions (§172.102)	ERG Guide No.	Placard Advisory Consult §172.504 & §172.505 *Placard any quantity
(1)	(2)	(3)	(4)	(5)	(6)	(7)		
	Flares, aerial	1.3G	UN0093	II	1.3G		112	EXPLOSIVES 1.3*
	Flares, aerial	1.4G	UN0403	II	1.4G		114	EXPLOSIVES 1.4
	Flares, aerial	1.4S	UN0404	II	1.4S		114	EXPLOSIVES 1.4
	Flares, aerial	1.1G	UN0420	II	1.1G		112	EXPLOSIVES 1.1*
	Flares, aerial	1.2G	UN0421	II	1.2G		112	EXPLOSIVES 1.2*
	Flares, airplane, see **Flares, aerial**							
	Flares, signal, see **Cartridges, signal**							
	Flares, surface	1.3G	UN0092	II	1.3G		112	EXPLOSIVES 1.3*
	Flares, surface	1.1G	UN0418	II	1.1G		112	EXPLOSIVES 1.1*
	Flares, surface	1.2G	UN0419	II	1.2G		112	EXPLOSIVES 1.2*
	Flares, water-activated, see **Contrivances, water-activated,** *etc.*							
	Flash powder	1.1G	UN0094	II	1.1G		112	EXPLOSIVES 1.1*
	Flash powder	1.3G	UN0305	II	1.3G		112	EXPLOSIVES 1.3*
	Flue dusts, poisonous, see **Arsenical dust**							
	Fluoric acid, see **Hydrofluoric acid,** *etc.*							
	Fluorine, compressed	2.3	UN1045		2.3, 5.1 , 8	1	124	POISON GAS*
	Fluoroacetic acid	6.1	UN2642	I	6.1	IB7, IP1, T6, TP33	154	POISON

Sym-bols	Hazardous materials descriptions and proper shipping names	Hazard class or Division	Identification Numbers	PG	Label Codes	Special provisions (§172.102)	ERG Guide No.	Placard Advisory Consult §172.504 & §172.505 *Placard any quantity
(1)	(2)	(3)	(4)	(5)	(6)	(7)		
	Fluoroanilines	6.1	UN2941	III	6.1	IB3, T4, TP1	153	POISON
	Fluorobenzene	3	UN2387	II	3	IB2, T4, TP1	130	FLAMMABLE
	Fluoroboric acid	8	UN1775	II	8	A6, A7, B2, B15, IB2, N3, N34, T7, TP2	154	CORROSIVE
	Fluorophosphoric acid anhydrous	8	UN1776	II	8	A6, A7, B2, IB2, N3, N34, T8, TP2, TP12	154	CORROSIVE
	Fluorosilicates, n.o.s.	6.1	UN2856	III	6.1	IB8, IP3, T1, TP33	151	POISON
	Fluorosilicic acid	8	UN1778	II	8	A6, A7, B2, B15, IB2, N3, N34, T8, TP2, TP12	154	CORROSIVE
	Fluorosulfonic acid	8	UN1777	I	8	A3, A6, A7, A10, B6, B10, N3, N36, T10, TP2, TP12	137	CORROSIVE
	Fluorotoluenes	3	UN2388	II	3	IB2, T4, TP1	130	FLAMMABLE
	Forbidden materials. See §173.21	Forbidden						
	Formaldehyde, solutions, flammable	3	UN1198	III	3, 8	B1, IB3, T4, TP1	132	FLAMMABLE
	Formaldehyde, solutions, *with not less than 25 percent formaldehyde*	8	UN2209	III	8	IB3, T4, TP1	132	CORROSIVE
	Formalin, see **Formaldehyde, solutions**							

Symbols	Hazardous materials descriptions and proper shipping names	Hazard class or Division	Identification Numbers	PG	Label Codes	Special provisions (§172.102)	ERG Guide No.	Placard Advisory Consult §172.504 & §172.505 *Placard any quantity
(1)	(2)	(3)	(4)	(5)	(6)	(7)		
	Formic acid	8	UN1779	II	8	B2, B28, IB2, T7, TP2	153	CORROSIVE
	Fracturing devices, explosive, *without detonators for oil wells*	1.1D	UN0099	II	1.1D		112	EXPLOSIVES 1.1*
	Fuel, aviation, turbine engine	3	UN1863	I	3	144, T11, TP1, TP8, TP28	128	FLAMMABLE
				II	3	144, IB2, T4, TP1, TP8	128	FLAMMABLE
				III	3	144, B1, IB3, T2, TP1	128	FLAMMABLE
D	**Fuel oil** *(No. 1, 2, 4, 5, or 6)*	3	NA1993	III	3	144, B1, IB3, T4, TP1, TP29	128	FLAMMABLE
	Fuel system components (including fuel control units (FCU), carburetors, fuel lines, fuel pumps) see **Dangerous Goods in Apparatus** *or* **Dangerous Goods in Machinery**							
	Fulminate of mercury (dry)	Forbidden						
	Fulminate of mercury, wet, see **Mercury fulminate,** *etc.*							
	Fulminating gold	Forbidden						
	Fulminating mercury	Forbidden						
	Fulminating platinum	Forbidden						

Sym-bols	Hazardous materials descriptions and proper shipping names	Hazard class or Division	Identification Numbers	PG	Label Codes	Special provisions (§172.102)	ERG Guide No.	Placard Advisory Consult §172.504 & §172.505 *Placard any quantity
(1)	(2)	(3)	(4)	(5)	(6)	(7)		
	Fulminating silver	Forbidden						
	Fulminic acid	Forbidden						
	Fumaryl chloride	8	UN1780	II	8	B2, IB2, T7, TP2	156	CORROSIVE
	Fumigated lading, see §§172.302(g), 173.9 and 176.76(h)							
	Fumigated transport vehicle or freight container see §173.9							
	Furaldehydes	6.1	UN1199	II	6.1, 3	IB2, T7, TP2	132P	POISON
	Furan	3	UN2389	I	3	T12, TP2, TP13	128	FLAMMABLE
	Furfuryl alcohol	6.1	UN2874	III	6.1	IB3, T4, TP1	153	POISON
	Furfurylamine	3	UN2526	III	3, 8	B1, IB3, T4, TP1	132	FLAMMABLE
	Fuse, detonating, *metal clad, see* **Cord, detonating,** *metal clad*							
	Fuse, detonating, mild effect, *metal clad, see* **Cord, detonating, mild effect,** *metal clad*							
	Fuse, igniter *tubular metal clad*	1.4G	UN0103	II	1.4G		114	EXPLOSIVES 1.4
	Fuse, non-detonating *instantaneous or quickmatch*	1.3G	UN0101	II	1.3G		112	EXPLOSIVES 1.3*
	Fuse, safety	1.4S	UN0105	II	1.4S		114	EXPLOSIVES 1.4
D	**Fusee** *(railway or highway)*	4.1	NA1325	II	4.1		133	FLAMMABLE SOLID

Symbols	Hazardous materials descriptions and proper shipping names	Hazard class or Division	Identification Numbers	PG	Label Codes	Special provisions (§172.102)	ERG Guide No.	Placard Advisory Consult §172.504 & §172.505 *Placard any quantity
(1)	(2)	(3)	(4)	(5)	(6)	(7)		
	Fusel oil	3	UN1201	II	3	IB2, T4, TP1	127	FLAMMABLE
				III	3	B1, IB3, T2, TP1	127	FLAMMABLE
	Fuses, tracer, see **Tracers for ammunition**							
	Fuzes, combination, percussion and time, see **Fuzes, detonating** *(UN 0257, UN 0367);* **Fuzes, igniting** *(UN 0317, UN 0368)*							
	Fuzes, detonating	1.1B	UN0106	II	1.1B		112	EXPLOSIVES 1.1*
	Fuzes, detonating	1.2B	UN0107	II	1.2B		112	EXPLOSIVES 1.2*
	Fuzes, detonating	1.4B	UN0257	II	1.4B	116	114	EXPLOSIVES 1.4
	Fuzes, detonating	1.4S	UN0367	II	1.4S	116	114	EXPLOSIVES 1.4
	Fuzes, detonating, *with protective features*	1.1D	UN0408	II	1.1D		112	EXPLOSIVES 1.1*
	Fuzes, detonating, *with protective features*	1.2D	UN0409	II	1.2D		112	EXPLOSIVES 1.2*
	Fuzes, detonating, *with protective features*	1.4D	UN0410	II	1.4D	116	114	EXPLOSIVES 1.4
	Fuzes, igniting	1.3G	UN0316	II	1.3G		112	EXPLOSIVES 1.3*
	Fuzes, igniting	1.4G	UN0317	II	1.4G		114	EXPLOSIVES 1.4
	Fuzes, igniting	1.4S	UN0368	II	1.4S		114	EXPLOSIVES 1.4
	Galactsan trinitrate	Forbidden						

Sym-bols	Hazardous materials descriptions and proper shipping names	Hazard class or Division	Identifica-tion Numbers	PG	Label Codes	Special provisions (§172.102)	ERG Guide No.	Placard Advisory Consult §172.504 & §172.505 *Placard any quantity
(1)	(2)	(3)	(4)	(5)	(6)	(7)		
	Gallium	8	UN2803	III	8	T1, TP33	172	CORROSIVE
	Gas cartridges, *(flammable) wihout a release device, non-refillable*	2.1	UN2037		2.1		115	FLAMMABLE GAS
	Gas generator assemblies (aircraft), *containing a non-flammable non-toxic gas and a propellant cartridge*	2.2			2.2		171	NONFLAMMABLE GAS
D	**Gas identification set**	2.3	NA9035		2.3	6	123	POISON GAS*
	Gas oil	3	UN1202	III	3	144, B1, IB3, T2, TP1	128	FLAMMABLE
G	**Gas, refrigerated liquid, flammable, n.o.s.** *(cryogenic liquid)*	2.1	UN3312		2.1	T75, TP5	115	FLAMMABLE GAS
G	**Gas, refrigerated liquid, n.o.s.** *(cryogenic liquid)*	2.2	UN3158		2.2	T75, TP5	120	NONFLAMMABLE GAS
G	**Gas, refrigerated liquid, oxidizing, n.o.s.** *(cryogenic liquid)*	2.2	UN3311		2.2, 5.1	T75, TP5, TP22	122	NONFLAMMABLE GAS
	Gas sample, non-pressurized, flammable, n.o.s., *not refrigerated liquid*	2.1	UN3167		2.1		115	FLAMMABLE GAS
	Gas sample, non-pressurized, toxic, flammable, n.o.s., *not refrigerated liquid*	2.3	UN3168		2.3, 2.1	6	119	POISON GAS*
	Gas sample, non-pressurized, toxic, n.o.s., *not refrigerated liquid*	2.3	UN3169		2.3	6	123	POISON GAS*

Sym-bols	Hazardous materials descriptions and proper shipping names	Hazard class or Division	Identifica-tion Numbers	PG	Label Codes	Special provisions (§172.102)	ERG Guide No.	Placard Advisory Consult §172.504 & §172.505 *Placard any quantity
(1)	(2)	(3)	(4)	(5)	(6)	(7)		
D	**Gasohol** *gasoline mixed with ethyl alcohol*, **with not more than 20 percent** *alcohol*	3	NA1203	II	3	144	128	FLAMMABLE
	Gasoline	3	UN1203	II	3	144, B33, T8	128	FLAMMABLE
	Gasoline, casinghead, see **Gasoline**							
	Gelatine, blasting, see **Explosive, blasting, type A**							
	Gelatine dynamites, see **Explosive, blasting, type A**							
	Germane	2.3	UN2192		2.3, 2.1	2	119	POISON GAS*
	Glycerol-1,3-dinitrate	Forbidden						
	Glycerol gluconate trinitrate	Forbidden						
	Glycerol lactate trinitrate	Forbidden						
	Glycerol alpha-monochlorohydrin	6.1	UN2689	III	6.1	IB3, T4, TP1	153	POISON
	Glyceryl trinitrate, see **Nitroglycerin,** *etc.*							
	Glycidaldehyde	3	UN2622	II	3, 6.1	IB2, IP8, T7, TP1	131P	FLAMMABLE
	Grenades, *hand or rifle, with bursting charge*	1.1D	UN0284	II	1.1D		112	EXPLOSIVES 1.1*
	Grenades, *hand or rifle, with bursting charge*	1.2D	UN0285	II	1.2D		112	EXPLOSIVES 1.2*
	Grenades, *hand or rifle, with bursting charge*	1.1F	UN0292	II	1.1F		112	EXPLOSIVES 1.1*

Symbols	Hazardous materials descriptions and proper shipping names	Hazard class or Division	Identification Numbers	PG	Label Codes	Special provisions (§172.102)	ERG Guide No.	Placard Advisory Consult §172.504 & §172.505 *Placard any quantity
(1)	(2)	(3)	(4)	(5)	(6)	(7)		
	Grenades, *hand or rifle, with bursting charge*	1.1F	UN0292	II	1.1F		112	EXPLOSIVES 1.1*
	Grenades, *hand or rifle, with bursting charge*	1.2F	UN0293	II	1.2F		112	EXPLOSIVES 1.2*
	Grenades, illuminating, see **Ammunition, illuminating,** *etc.*							
	Grenades, practice, *hand or rifle*	1.4S	UN0110	II	1.4S		114	EXPLOSIVES 1.4
	Grenades, practice, *hand or rifle*	1.3G	UN0318	II	1.3G		112	EXPLOSIVES 1.3*
	Grenades, practice, *hand or rifle*	1.2G	UN0372	II	1.2G		112	EXPLOSIVES 1.2*
	Grenades practice *Hand or rifle*	1.4G	UN0452	II	1.4G		114	EXPLOSIVES 1.4
	Grenades, smoke, see **Ammunition, smoke,** *etc.*							
	Guanidine nitrate	5.1	UN1467	III	5.1	A1, IB8, IP3, T1, TP33	143	OXIDIZER
	Guanyl nitrosaminoguanylidene hydrazine (dry)	Forbidden						
	Guanyl nitrosaminoguanylidene hydrazine, wetted *with not less than 30 percent water, by mass*	1.1A	UN0113	II	1.1A	111, 117	112	EXPLOSIVES 1.1*
	Guanyl nitrosaminoguanyltetrazene (dry)	Forbidden						

Symbols	Hazardous materials descriptions and proper shipping names	Hazard class or Division	Identification Numbers	PG	Label Codes	Special provisions (§172.102)	ERG Guide No.	Placard Advisory Consult §172.504 & §172.505 *Placard any quantity
(1)	(2)	(3)	(4)	(5)	(6)	(7)		
	Guanyl nitrosaminoguanyltetrazene, wetted *or* **Tetrazene, wetted** *with not less than 30 percent water or mixture of alcohol and water, by mass*	1.1A	UN0114	II	1.1A	111, 117	112	EXPLOSIVES 1.1*
	Gunpowder, compressed *or* **Gunpowder in pellets,** *see* **Black powder** *(UN 0028)*							
	Gunpowder, *granular or as a meal, see* **Black powder** *(UN 0027)*							
	Hafnium powder, dry	4.2	UN2545	I	4.2		135	SPONTANEOUSLY COMBUSTIBLE
				II	4.2	A19, A20, IB6, IP2, N34, T3, TP33	135	SPONTANEOUSLY COMBUSTIBLE
				III	4.2	IB8, IP3, T1, TP33	135	SPONTANEOUSLY COMBUSTIBLE
	Hafnium powder, wetted *with not less than 25 percent water (a visible excess of water must be present) (a) mechanically produced, particle size less than 53 microns; (b) chemically produced, particle size less than 840 microns*	4.1	UN1326	II	4.1	A6, A19, A20, IB6, IP2, N34, T3, TP33	170	FLAMMABLE SOLID
	Hand signal device, see **Signal devices, hand**							

Sym-bols	Hazardous materials descriptions and proper shipping names	Hazard class or Division	Identifica-tion Numbers	PG	Label Codes	Special provisions (§172.102)	ERG Guide No.	Placard Advisory Consult §172.504 & §172.505 *Placard any quantity
(1)	(2)	(3)	(4)	(5)	(6)	(7)		
	Hazardous substances, liquid or solid, n.o.s., see **Environmentally hazardous substances,** *etc.*							
D G	**Hazardous waste, liquid, n.o.s.**	9	NA3082	III	9	IB3, T2, TP1	171	CLASS 9
D G	**Hazardous waste, solid, n.o.s.**	9	NA3077	III	9	B54, IB8, IP2, T1, TP33	171	CLASS 9
	Heating oil, light	3	UN1202	III	3	B1, IB3, T2, TP1	128	FLAMMABLE
	Helium, compressed	2.2	UN1046		2.2		121	NONFLAMMABLE GAS
	Helium-oxygen mixture, see **Rare gases and oxygen mixtures**							
	Helium, refrigerated liquid *(cryogenic liquid)*	2.2	UN1963		2.2	T75, TP5	120	NONFLAMMABLE GAS
	Heptafluoropropane *or* **Refrigerant gas R 227**	2.2	UN3296		2.2	T50	126	NONFLAMMABLE GAS
	n-Heptaldehyde	3	UN3056	III	3	B1, IB3, T2, TP1	129	FLAMMABLE
	Heptanes	3	UN1206	II	3	IB2, T4, TP1	128	FLAMMABLE
	n-Heptene	3	UN2278	II	3	IB2, T4, TP1	128	FLAMMABLE
	Hexachloroacetone	6.1	UN2661	III	6.1	IB3, T4, TP1	153	POISON
	Hexachlorobenzene	6.1	UN2729	III	6.1	B3, IB8, IP3, T1, TP33	152	POISON
	Hexachlorobutadiene	6.1	UN2279	III	6.1	IB3, T4, TP1	151	POISON

Sym-bols	Hazardous materials descriptions and proper shipping names	Hazard class or Division	Identification Numbers	PG	Label Codes	Special provisions (§172.102)	ERG Guide No.	Placard Advisory Consult §172.504 & §172.505 *Placard any quantity
(1)	(2)	(3)	(4)	(5)	(6)	(7)		
	Hexachlorocyclopentadiene	6.1	UN2646	I	6.1	2, B9, B14, B32, B74, B77, T20, TP2, TP13, TP38, TP45	151	POISON INHALATION HAZARD*
	Hexachlorophene	6.1	UN2875	III	6.1	IB8, IP3, T1, TP33	151	POISON
	Hexadecyltrichlorosilane	8	UN1781	II	8	A7, B2, B6, IB2, N34, T7, TP2	156	CORROSIVE
	Hexadienes	3	UN2458	II	3	IB2, T4, TP1	130	FLAMMABLE
	Hexaethyl tetraphosphate and compressed gas mixtures	2.3	UN1612		2.3	3	123	POISON GAS*
	Hexaethyl tetraphosphate, *liquid*	6.1	UN1611	II	6.1	IB2, N76, T7, TP2	151	POISON
	Hexaethyl tetraphosphate, *solid*	6.1	UN1611	II	6.1	IB8, IP2, IP4, N76	151	POISON
	Hexafluoroacetone	2.3	UN2420		2.3, 8	2, B9, B14	125	POISON GAS*
	Hexafluoroacetone hydrate, liquid	6.1	UN2552	II	6.1	IB2, T7, TP2	151	POISON
	Hexafluoroacetone hydrate, solid	6.1	UN3436	II	6,1	IB8, IP2, IP4, T3, TP33	151	POISON
	Hexafluoroethane, *or* **Refrigerant gas R 116**	2.2	UN2193		2.2		126	NONFLAMMABLE GAS
	Hexafluorophosphoric acid	8	UN1782	II	8	A6, A7, B2, IB2, N3, N34, T8, TP2, TP12	154	CORROSIVE
	Hexafluoropropylene, compressed *or* **Refrigerant gas R 1216**	2.2	UN1858		2.2	T50	126	NONFLAMMABLE GAS

Sym-bols	Hazardous materials descriptions and proper shipping names	Hazard class or Division	Identifica-tion Numbers	PG	Label Codes	Special provisions (§172.102)	ERG Guide No.	Placard Advisory Consult §172.504 & §172.505 *Placard any quantity
(1)	(2)	(3)	(4)	(5)	(6)	(7)		
	Hexaldehyde	3	UN1207	III	3	B1, IB3, T2, TP1	130	FLAMMABLE
	Hexamethylene diisocyanate	6.1	UN2281	II	6.1	IB2, T7, TP2, TP13	156	POISON
	Hexamethylene triperoxide diamine (dry)	Forbidden						
	Hexamethylenediamine, solid	8	UN2280	III	8	IB8, IP3, T1, TP33	153	CORROSIVE
	Hexamethylenediamine solution	8	UN1783	II	8	IB2, T7, TP2	153	CORROSIVE
				III	8	IB3, T4, TP1	153	CORROSIVE
	Hexamethyleneimine	3	UN2493	II	3, 8	IB2, T7, TP1	132	FLAMMABLE
	Hexamethylenetetramine	4.1	UN1328	III	4.1	A1, IB8, IP3, T1, TP33	133	FLAMMABLE SOLID
	Hexamethylol benzene hexanitrate	Forbidden						
	Hexanes	3	UN1208	II	3	IB2, T4, TP1	128	FLAMMABLE
	2,2′,4,4′,6,6′-Hexanitro-3, 3′-dihydroxyazobenzene (dry)	Forbidden						
	Hexanitroazoxy benzene	Forbidden						
	N,N′-(hexanitrodiphenyl) ethylene dinitramine (dry)	Forbidden						
	Hexanitrodiphenyl urea	Forbidden						
	2,2′,3′,4,4′,6-Hexanitrodiphenylamine	Forbidden						
	Hexanitrodiphenylamine *or* **Dipicrylamine** *or* **Hexyl**	1.1D	UN0079	II	1.1D		112	EXPLOSIVES 1.1*

Symbols	Hazardous materials descriptions and proper shipping names	Hazard class or Division	Identification Numbers	PG	Label Codes	Special provisions (§172.102)	ERG Guide No.	Placard Advisory Consult §172.504 & §172.505 *Placard any quantity
(1)	(2)	(3)	(4)	(5)	(6)	(7)		
	2,3',4,4',6,6'-Hexanitrodiphenylether	Forbidden						
	Hexanitroethane	Forbidden						
	Hexanitrooxanilide	Forbidden						
	Hexanitrostilbene	1.1D	UN0392	II	1.1D		112	EXPLOSIVES 1.1*
	Hexanoic acid, see **Corrosive liquids, n.o.s.**							
	Hexanols	3	UN2282	III	3	B1, IB3, T2, TP1	129	FLAMMABLE
	1-Hexene	3	UN2370	II	3	IB2, T4, TP1	128	FLAMMABLE
	Hexogen and cyclotetramethylenetetranitramine mixtures, wetted *or* **desensitized** *see* **RDX and HMX mixtures, wetted** *or* **desensitized** *etc.*							
	Hexogen and HMX mixtures, wetted *or* **desensitized** *see* **RDX and HMX mixtures, wetted** *or* **desensitized** *etc.*							
	Hexogen and octogen mixtures, wetted *or* **desensitized** *see* **RDX and HMX mixtures, wetted** *or* **desensitized** *etc.*							
	Hexogen, *see* **Cyclotrimethylenetrinitramine,** *etc.*							

Symbols	Hazardous materials descriptions and proper shipping names	Hazard class or Division	Identification Numbers	PG	Label Codes	Special provisions (§172.102)	ERG Guide No.	Placard Advisory Consult §172.504 & §172.505 *Placard any quantity
(1)	(2)	(3)	(4)	(5)	(6)	(7)		
	Hexolite, *or* **Hexotol** *dry or wetted with less than 15 percent water, by mass*	1.1D	UN0118	II	1.1D		112	EXPLOSIVES 1.1*
	Hexotonal	1.1D	UN0393	II	1.1D		112	EXPLOSIVES 1.1*
	Hexyl, *see* **Hexanitrodiphenylamine**							
	Hexyltrichlorosilane	8	UN1784	II	8	A7, B2, B6, IB2, N34, T7, TP2, TP13	156	CORROSIVE
	High explosives, see individual explosives' entries							
	HMX, *see* **Cyclotetramethylenetetranitramine,** *etc.*							
	Hydrazine, anhydrous	8	UN2029	I	8, 3, 6.1	A3, A6, A7, A10, B7, B16, B53	132	CORROSIVE
	Hydrazine, aqueous solution *with not more than 37 percent hydrazine, by mass*	6.1	UN3293	III	6.1	IB3, T4, TP1	152	POISON
	Hydrazine aqueous solution, *with more than 37% hydrazine, by mass*	8	UN2030	I	8, 6.1	151, B16, B53, T10, TP2, TP13	153	CORROSIVE
				II	8, 6.1	B16, B53, IB2, T7, TP2, TP13	153	CORROSIVE
				III	8, 6.1	B16, B53, IB3, T4, TP1	153	CORROSIVE
	Hydrazine azide	Forbidden						

Symbols	Hazardous materials descriptions and proper shipping names	Hazard class or Division	Identification Numbers	PG	Label Codes	Special provisions (§172.102)	ERG Guide No.	Placard Advisory Consult §172.504 & §172.505 *Placard any quantity
(1)	(2)	(3)	(4)	(5)	(6)	(7)		
	Hydrazine chlorate	Forbidden						
	Hydrazine dicarbonic acid diazide	Forbidden						
	Hydrazine perchlorate	Forbidden						
	Hydrazine selenate	Forbidden						
	Hydriodic acid, anhydrous, see **Hydrogen iodide, anhydrous**							
	Hydriodic acid	8	UN1787	II	8	A3, A6, B2, IB2, N41, T7, TP2	154	CORROSIVE
				III	8	IB3, T4, TP1	154	CORROSIVE
	Hydrobromic acid, anhydrous, see **Hydrogen bromide, anhydrous**							
	Hydrobromic acid, *with more than 49 percent hydrobromic acid*	8	UN1788	II	8	B2, B15, IB2, N41, T7, TP2	154	CORROSIVE
				III	8	IB3, T4, TP1	154	CORROSIVE
	Hydrobromic acid, *with not more than 49 percent hydrobromic acid*	8	UN1788	II	8	A3, A6, B2, B15, IB2, N41, T7, TP2	154	CORROSIVE
				III	8	A3, IB3, T4, TP1	154	CORROSIVE
	Hydrocarbon gas mixture, compressed, n.o.s.	2.1	UN1964		2.1		115	FLAMMABLE GAS
	Hydrocarbon gas mixture, liquefied, n.o.s.	2.1	UN1965		2.1	T50	115	FLAMMABLE GAS

Sym-bols	Hazardous materials descriptions and proper shipping names	Hazard class or Division	Identifica-tion Numbers	PG	Label Codes	Special provisions (§172.102)	ERG Guide No.	Placard Advisory Consult §172.504 & §172.505 *Placard any quantity
(1)	(2)	(3)	(4)	(5)	(6)	(7)		
	Hydrocarbons, liquid, n.o.s.	3	UN3295	I	3	144, T11, TP1, TP8, TP28	128	FLAMMABLE
				II	3	144, IB2, T7, TP1, TP8, TP28	128	FLAMMABLE
				III	3	144, B1, IB3, T4, TP1, TP29	128	FLAMMABLE
	Hydrochloric acid, anhydrous, see **Hydrogen chloride, anhydrous**							
	Hydrochloric acid	8	UN1789	II	8	A3, A6, B3, B15, IB2, N41, T8, TP2, TP12	157	CORROSIVE
				III	8	A3, IB3, T4, TP1, TP12	157	CORROSIVE
	Hydrocyanic acid, anhydrous, see **Hydrogen cyanide** *etc.*							
	Hydrocyanic acid, aqueous solutions *or* **Hydrogen cyanide, aqueous solutions** *with not more than 20 percent hydrogen cyanide*	6.1	UN1613	I	6.1	2, B61, B65, B77, B82, T20, TP2, TP13	154	POISON INHALATION HAZARD*
D	**Hydrocyanic acid, aqueous solutions** *with less than 5 percent hydrogen canide*	6.1	NA1613	II	6.1	IB1, T14, TP2, TP13, TP27	154	POISON
	Hydrocyanic acid, liquefied, see **Hydrogen cyanide,** *etc.*							

Sym-bols	Hazardous materials descriptions and proper shipping names	Hazard class or Division	Identifica-tion Numbers	PG	Label Codes	Special provisions (§172.102)	ERG Guide No.	Placard Advisory Consult §172.504 & §172.505 *Placard any quantity
(1)	(2)	(3)	(4)	(5)	(6)	(7)		
	Hydrocyanic acid (prussic), unstabilized	Forbidden						
	Hydrofluoric acid and Sulfuric acid mixtures	8	UN1786	I	8, 6.1	A6, A7, B15, B23, N5, N34, T10, TP2, TP12, TP13	157	CORROSIVE
	Hydrofluoric acid, anhydrous, see **Hydrogen fluoride, anhydrous**							
	Hydrofluoric acid, *with more than 60 percent strength*	8	UN1790	I	8, 6.1	A6, A7, B4, B15, B23, N5, N34, T10, TP2, TP12, TP13	157	CORROSIVE
	Hydrofluoric acid, *with not more than 60 percent strength*	8	UN1790	II	8, 6.1	A6, A7, B15, IB2, N5, N34, T8, TP2, TP12	157	CORROSIVE
	Hydrofluoroboric acid, see **Fluoroboric acid**							
	Hydrofluorosilicic acid, see **Fluorosilicic acid**							
	Hydrogen and Methane mixtures, compressed	2.1	UN2034		2.1		115	FLAMMABLE GAS
	Hydrogen bromide, anhydrous	2.3	UN1048		2.3, 8	3, B14	125	POISON GAS*
	Hydrogen chloride, anhydrous	2.3	UN1050		2.3, 8	3	125	POISON GAS*
	Hydrogen chloride, refrigerated liquid	2.3	UN2186		2.3, 8	3, B6	125	POISON GAS*
	Hydrogen, compressed	2.1	UN1049		2.1		115	FLAMMABLE GAS

Symbols	Hazardous materials descriptions and proper shipping names	Hazard class or Division	Identification Numbers	PG	Label Codes	Special provisions (§172.102)	ERG Guide No.	Placard Advisory Consult §172.504 & §172.505 *Placard any quantity
(1)	(2)	(3)	(4)	(5)	(6)	(7)		
	Hydrogen cyanide, solution in alcohol *with not more than 45 percent hydrogen cyanide*	6.1	UN3294	I	6.1, 3	2, B9, B14, B32, B74, T20, TP2, TP13, TP38, TP45	131	POISON INHALATION HAZARD*
	Hydrogen cyanide, stabilized *with less than 3 percent water*	6.1	UN1051	I	6.1, 3	1, B35, B61, B65, B77, B82	117	POISON INHALATION HAZARD*
	Hydrogen cyanide, stabilized, *with less than 3 percent water and absorbed in a porous inert material*	6.1	UN1614	I	6.1	5	152	POISON
	Hydrogen fluoride, anhydrous	8	UN1052	I	8, 6.1	3, B7, B46, B71, B77, T10, TP2	125	CORROSIVE, POISON INHALATION HAZARD*
	Hydrogen in a metal hydride storage system	2.1	UN3468		2.1	167	115	FLAMMABLE GAS
	Hydrogen iodide, anhydrous	2.3	UN2197		2.3	3, B14	125	POISON GAS*
	Hydrogen iodide solution, see **Hydriodic acid**							
	Hydrogen peroxide and peroxyacetic acid mixtures, stabilized *with acids, water and not more than 5 percent peroxyacetic acid*	5.1	UN3149	II	5.1, 8	145, A2, A3, A6, B53, IB2, T7, TP2, TP6, TP24	140	OXIDIZER

Symbols	Hazardous materials descriptions and proper shipping names	Hazard class or Division	Identification Numbers	PG	Label Codes	Special provisions (§172.102)	ERG Guide No.	Placard Advisory Consult §172.504 & §172.505 *Placard any quantity
(1)	(2)	(3)	(4)	(5)	(6)	(7)		
	Hydrogen peroxide, aqueous solutions *with more than 40 percent but not more than 60 percent hydrogen peroxide (stabilized as necessary)*	5.1	UN2014	II	5.1, 8	12, B53, B80, B81, B85, IB2, T7, TP2, TP6, TP24, TP37	140	OXIDIZER
	Hydrogen peroxide, aqueous solutions *with not less than 20 percent but not more than 40 percent hydrogen peroxide (stabilized as necessary)*	5.1	UN2014	II	5.1, 8	A2, A3, A6, B53, IB2, T7, TP2, TP6, TP24, TP37	140	OXIDIZER
	Hydrogen peroxide, aqueous solutions *with not less than 8 percent but less than 20 percent hydrogen peroxide (stabilized as necessary)*	5.1	UN2984	III	5.1	A1, IB2, T4, TP1, TP6, TP24, TP37	140	OXIDIZER
	Hydrogen peroxide, stabilized *or* **Hydrogen peroxide aqueous solutions, stabilized** *with more than 60 percent hydrogen peroxide*	5.1	UN2015	I	5.1, 8	12, B53, B80, B81, B85, T10, TP2, TP6, TP24, TP37	143	OXIDIZER
	Hydrogen, refrigerated liquid *(cryogenic liquid)*	2.1	UN1966		2.1	T75, TP5	115	FLAMMABLE GAS
	Hydrogen selenide, anhydrous	2.3	UN2202		2.3, 2.1	1	117	POISON GAS*
	Hydrogen sulfate, see **Sulfuric acid**							
	Hydrogen sulfide	2.3	UN1053		2.3, 2.1	2, B9, B14	117	POISON GAS*
	Hydrogendifluorides, n.o.s.	8	UN1740	II	8	IB8, IP2, IP4, N3, N34, T3, TP33	154	CORROSIVE

Sym-bols	Hazardous materials descriptions and proper shipping names	Hazard class or Division	Identifica-tion Numbers	PG	Label Codes	Special provisions (§172.102)	ERG Guide No.	Placard Advisory Consult §172.504 & §172.505 *Placard any quantity
(1)	(2)	(3)	(4)	(5)	(6)	(7)		
				III	8	IB8, IP3, N3, N34, T1, TP33	154	CORROSIVE
	Hydroquinone, solid	6.1	UN2662	III	6.1	IB8, IP3, T1, TP33	153	POISON
	Hydroquinone solution	6.1	UN3435	III	6.1	IB3, T4, TP1	153	POISON
	Hydrosilicofluoric acid, see **Fluorosilicic acid**							
	Hydroxyl amine iodide	Forbidden						
	Hydroxylamine sulfate	8	UN2865	III	8	IB8, IP3, T1, TP33	154	CORROSIVE
	Hypochlorite solutions	8	UN1791	II	8	A7, B2, B15, IB2, N34, T7, TP2, TP24	154	CORROSIVE
				III	8	IB3, N34, T4, TP2, TP24	154	CORROSIVE
	Hypochlorites, inorganic, n.o.s.	5.1	UN3212	II	5.1	A9, IB8, IP2, IP4, T3, TP33	140	OXIDIZER
	Hyponitrous acid	Forbidden						
	Igniter fuse, metal clad, see **Fuse,** *igniter, tubular, metal clad*							
	Igniters	1.1G	UN0121	II	1.1G		112	EXPLOSIVES 1.1*
	Igniters	1.2G	UN0314	II	1.2G		112	EXPLOSIVES 1.2*
	Igniters	1.3G	UN0315	II	1.3G		112	EXPLOSIVES 1.3*
	Igniters	1.4G	UN0325	II	1.4G		114	EXPLOSIVES 1.4

Symbols	Hazardous materials descriptions and proper shipping names	Hazard class or Division	Identification Numbers	PG	Label Codes	Special provisions (§172.102)	ERG Guide No.	Placard Advisory Consult §172.504 & §172.505 *Placard any quantity
(1)	(2)	(3)	(4)	(5)	(6)	(7)		
	Igniters	1.4S	UN0454	II	1.4S		114	EXPLOSIVES 1.4
	3,3′-Iminodipropylamine	8	UN2269	III	8	IB3, T4, TP2	153	CORROSIVE
G	**Infectious substances, affecting animals** *only*	6.2	UN2900		6.2	A81, A82	158	NONE
G	**Infectious substances, affecting humans**	6.2	UN2814		6.2	A81, A82	158	NONE
	Inflammable, see Flammable							
	Initiating explosives (dry)	Forbidden						
	Inositol hexanitrate (dry)	Forbidden						
G	**Insecticide gases, n.o.s.**	2.2	UN1968		2.2		126	NONFLAMMABLE GAS
G	**Insecticide gases, flammable, n.o.s.**	2.1	UN3354		2.1	T50	115	FLAMMABLE GAS
G	**Insecticide gases, toxic, flammable, n.o.s.** *Inhalation hazard Zone A*	2.3	UN3355		2.3, 2.1	1	119	POISON GAS*
G	**Insecticide gases, toxic, flammable, n.o.s.** *Inhalation hazard Zone B*	2.3	UN3355		2.3, 2.1	2, B9, B14	119	POISON GAS*
G	**Insecticide gases, toxic, flammable, n.o.s.** *Inhalation hazard Zone C*	2.3	UN3355		2.3, 2.1	3, B14	119	POISON GAS*
G	**Insecticide gases toxic, flammable, n.o.s.** *Inhalation hazard Zone D*	2.3	UN3355		2.3, 2.1	4	119	POISON GAS*
G	**Insecticide gases, toxic, n.o.s.**	2.3	UN1967		2.3	3	123	POISON GAS*
	Inulin trinitrate (dry)	Forbidden						

Symbols	Hazardous materials descriptions and proper shipping names	Hazard class or Division	Identification Numbers	PG	Label Codes	Special provisions (§172.102)	ERG Guide No.	Placard Advisory Consult §172.504 & §172.505 *Placard any quantity
(1)	(2)	(3)	(4)	(5)	(6)	(7)		
	Iodine azide (dry)	Forbidden						
	Iodine monochloride	8	UN1792	II	8	B6, IB8, IP2, IP4, N41, T7, TP2	157	CORROSIVE
	Iodine pentafluoride	5.1	UN2495	I	5.1, 6.1, 8		144	OXIDIZER
	2-Iodobutane	3	UN2390	II	3	IB2, T4, TP1	129	FLAMMABLE
	Iodomethylpropanes	3	UN2391	II	3	IB2, T4, TP1	129	FLAMMABLE
	Iodopropanes	3	UN2392	III	3	B1, IB3, T2, TP1	129	FLAMMABLE
	Iodoxy compounds (dry)	Forbidden						
	Iridium nitratopentamine iridium nitrate	Forbidden						
	Iron chloride, see **Ferric chloride**							
	Iron oxide, spent, *or* **Iron sponge, spent** *obtained from coal gas purification*	4.2	UN1376	III	4.2	B18, IB8, IP3, T1, TP33	135	SPONTANEOUSLY COMBUSTIBLE
	Iron pentacarbonyl	6.1	UN1994	I	6.1, 3	1, B9, B14, B30, B72, B77, T22, TP2, TP13, TP38, TP44	131	POISON INHALATION HAZARD*
	Iron sesquichloride, see **Ferric chloride**							
	Irritating material, see **Tear gas substances,** *etc.*							
	Isobutane *see also* **Petroleum gases, liquefied**	2.1	UN1969		2.1	19, T50	115	FLAMMABLE GAS

Symbols	Hazardous materials descriptions and proper shipping names	Hazard class or Division	Identification Numbers	PG	Label Codes	Special provisions (§172.102)	ERG Guide No.	Placard Advisory Consult §172.504 & §172.505 *Placard any quantity
(1)	(2)	(3)	(4)	(5)	(6)	(7)		
	Isobutanol *or* **Isobutyl alcohol**	3	UN1212	III	3	B1, IB3, T2, TP1	129	FLAMMABLE
	Isobutyl acetate	3	UN1213	II	3	IB2, T4, TP1	129	FLAMMABLE
	Isobutyl acrylate, inhibited	3	UN2527	III	3	B1, IB3, T2, TP1	130P	FLAMMABLE
	Isobutyl alcohol, *see* **Isobutanol**							
	Isobutyl aldehyde, *see* **Isobutyraldehyde**							
D	**Isobutyl chloroformate**	6.1	NA2742	I	6.1, 3, 8	2, B9, B14, B32, B74, T20, TP4, TP12, TP13, TP38, TP45	155	POISON INHALATION HAZARD*
	Isobutyl formate	3	UN2393	II	3	IB2, T4, TP1	129	FLAMMABLE
	Isobutyl isobutyrate	3	UN2528	III	3	B1, IB3, T2, TP1	130	FLAMMABLE
+	**Isobutyl isocyanate**	3	UN2486	I	3, 6.1	1, B9, B14, B30, B72, T22, TP2, TP13, TP27	155	FLAMMABLE, POISON INHALATION HAZARD*
	Isobutyl methacrylate, stabilized	3	UN2283	III	3	B1, IB3, T2, TP1	130P	FLAMMABLE
	Isobutyl propionate	3	UN2394	III	3	B1, IB3, T2, TP1	129	FLAMMABLE
	Isobutylamine	3	UN1214	II	3, 8	IB2, T7, TP1	132	FLAMMABLE
	Isobutylene *see also* **Petroleum gases, liquefied**	2.1	UN1055		2.1	19, T50	115	FLAMMABLE GAS
	Isobutyraldehyde *or* **Isobutyl aldehyde**	3	UN2045	II	3	IB2, T4, TP1	130	FLAMMABLE

Sym-bols	Hazardous materials descriptions and proper shipping names	Hazard class or Division	Identification Numbers	PG	Label Codes	Special provisions (§172.102)	ERG Guide No.	Placard Advisory Consult §172.504 & §172.505 *Placard any quantity
(1)	(2)	(3)	(4)	(5)	(6)	(7)		
	Isobutyric acid	3	UN2529	III	3, 8	B1, IB3, T4, TP1	132	FLAMMABLE
	Isobutyronitrile	3	UN2284	II	3, 6.1	IB2, T7, TP2, TP13	131	FLAMMABLE
	Isobutyryl chloride	3	UN2395	II	3, 8	IB1, T7, TP2	132	FLAMMABLE
G	**Isocyanates, flammable, toxic, n.o.s.** *or* **Isocyanate solutions, flammable, toxic, n.o.s.** *flash point less than 23 degrees C*	3	UN2478	II	3, 6.1	5, A3, A7, IB2, T11, TP2, TP13, TP27	155	FLAMMABLE, POISON INHALATION HAZARD*
				III	3, 6.1	5, A3, A7, IB3, T7, TP1, TP13, TP28	155	FLAMMABLE, POISON INHALATION HAZARD*
G	**Isocyanates, toxic, flammable, n.o.s.** *or* **Isocyanate solutions, toxic, flammable, n.o.s.,** *flash point not less than 23 degrees C but not more than 61 degrees C and boiling point less than 300 degrees C*	6.1	UN3080	II	6.1, 3	IB2, T11, TP2, TP13, TP27	155	POISON
G	**Isocyanates, toxic, n.o.s.** *or* **Isocyanate, solutions, toxic, n.o.s.,** *flash point more than 61 degrees C and boiling point less than 300 degrees C*	6.1	UN2206	II	6.1	IB2, T11, TP2, TP13, TP27	155	POISON
				III	6.1	IB3, T7, TP1, TP13, TP28	155	POISON

Symbols	Hazardous materials descriptions and proper shipping names	Hazard class or Division	Identification Numbers	PG	Label Codes	Special provisions (§172.102)	ERG Guide No.	Placard Advisory Consult §172.504 & §172.505 *Placard any quantity
(1)	(2)	(3)	(4)	(5)	(6)	(7)		
	Isocyanatobenzotrifluorides	6.1	UN2285	II	6.1, 3	5, IB2, T7, TP2	156	POISON INHALATION HAZARD*
	Isoheptenes	3	UN2287	II	3	IB2, T4, TP1	128	FLAMMABLE
	Isohexenes	3	UN2288	II	3	IB2, IP8, T11, TP1	128	FLAMMABLE
	Isooctane, see **Octanes**							
	Isooctenes	3	UN1216	II	3	IB2, T4, TP1	128	FLAMMABLE
	Isopentane, see **Pentane**							
	Isopentanoic acid, see **Corrosive liquids, n.o.s.**							
	Isopentenes	3	UN2371	I	3	T11, TP2	128	FLAMMABLE
	Isophorone diisocyanate	6.1	UN2290	III	6.1	IB3, T4, TP2	156	POISON
	Isophoronediamine	8	UN2289	III	8	IB3, T4, TP1	153	CORROSIVE
	Isoprene, stabilized	3	UN1218	I	3	T11, TP2	130P	FLAMMABLE
	Isopropanol *or* **Isopropyl alcohol**	3	UN1219	II	3	IB2, T4, TP1	129	FLAMMABLE
	Isopropenyl acetate	3	UN2403	II	3	IB2, T4, TP1	129P	FLAMMABLE
	Isopropenylbenzene	3	UN2303	III	3	B1, IB3, T2, TP1	128	FLAMMABLE
	Isopropyl acetate	3	UN1220	II	3	IB2, T4, TP1	129	FLAMMABLE
	Isopropyl acid phosphate	8	UN1793	III	8	IB2, T4, TP1	153	CORROSIVE
	Isopropyl alcohol, *see* **Isopropanol**							
	Isopropyl butyrate	3	UN2405	III	3	B1, IB3, T2, TP1	129	FLAMMABLE

Sym-bols	Hazardous materials descriptions and proper shipping names	Hazard class or Division	Identifica-tion Numbers	PG	Label Codes	Special provisions (§172.102)	ERG Guide No.	Placard Advisory Consult §172.504 & §172.505 *Placard any quantity
(1)	(2)	(3)	(4)	(5)	(6)	(7)		
	Isopropyl chloroacetate	3	UN2947	III	3	B1, IB3, T2, TP1	155	FLAMMABLE
	Isopropyl chloroformate	6.1	UN2407	I	6.1, 3, 8	2, B9, B14, B32, B74, B77, T20, TP2, TP13, TP38, TP44	155	POISON INHALATION HAZARD*
	Isopropyl 2-chloropropionate	3	UN2934	III	3	B1, IB3, T2, TP1	129	FLAMMABLE
	Isopropyl isobutyrate	3	UN2406	II	3	IB2, T4, TP1	127	FLAMMABLE
+	**Isopropyl isocyanate**	3	UN2483	I	3, 6.1	1, B9, B14, B30, B72, T22, TP2, TP13, TP38, TP44	155	FLAMMABLE, POISON INHALATION HAZARD*
	Isopropyl mercaptan, see **Propanethiols**							
	Isopropyl nitrate	3	UN1222	II	3	IB9	130	FLAMMABLE
	Isopropyl phosphoric acid, see **Isopropyl acid phosphate**							
	Isopropyl propionate	3	UN2409	II	3	IB2, T4, TP1	129	FLAMMABLE
	Isopropylamine	3	UN1221	I	3, 8	T11, TP2	132	FLAMMABLE
	Isopropylbenzene	3	UN1918	III	3	B1, IB3, T2, TP1	130	FLAMMABLE
	Isopropylcumyl hydroperoxide, with more than 72 percent in solution	Forbidden						

Symbols	Hazardous materials descriptions and proper shipping names	Hazard class or Division	Identification Numbers	PG	Label Codes	Special provisions (§172.102)	ERG Guide No.	Placard Advisory Consult §172.504 & §172.505 *Placard any quantity
(1)	(2)	(3)	(4)	(5)	(6)	(7)		
	Isosorbide dinitrate mixture *with not less than 60 percent lactose, mannose, starch or calcium hydrogen phosphate*	4.1	UN2907	II	4.1	IB6, IP2, N85	133	FLAMMABLE SOLID
	Isosorbide-5-mononitrate	4.1	UN3251	III	4.1	66, IB8	133	FLAMMABLE SOLID
	Isothiocyanic acid	Forbidden						
	Jet fuel, see **Fuel aviation, turbine engine**							
D	**Jet perforating guns, charged oil well, with detonator**	1.1D	NA0124	II	1.1D	55, 56	112	EXPLOSIVES 1.1*
D	**Jet perforating guns, charged oil well, with detonator**	1.4D	NA0494	II	1.4D	55, 56	114	EXPLOSIVES 1.4
	Jet perforating guns, charged *oil well, without detonator*	1.1D	UN0124	II	1.1D	55	112	EXPLOSIVES 1.1*
	Jet perforating guns, charged, *oil well, without detonator*	1.4D	UN0494	II	1.4D	55, 114	114	EXPLOSIVES 1.4
	Jet perforators, see **Charges, shaped,** *etc.*							
	Jet tappers, without detonator, see **Charges, shaped,** *etc.*							
	Jet thrust igniters, for rocket motors or Jato, see **Igniters**							

Sym-bols	Hazardous materials descriptions and proper shipping names	Hazard class or Division	Identifica-tion Numbers	PG	Label Codes	Special provisions (§172.102)	ERG Guide No.	Placard Advisory Consult §172.504 & §172.505 *Placard any quantity
(1)	(2)	(3)	(4)	(5)	(6)	(7)		
	Jet thrust unit (Jato), see **Rocket motors**							
	Kerosene	3	UN1223	III	3	144, B1, IB3, T2, TP2	128	FLAMMABLE
G	**Ketones, liquid, n.o.s.**	3	UN1224	I	3	T11, TP1, TP8, TP27	127	FLAMMABLE
				II	3	IB2, T7, TP1, TP8, TP28	127	FLAMMABLE
				III	3	B1, IB3, T4, TP1, TP29	127	FLAMMABLE
	Krypton, compressed	2.2	UN1056		2.2		121	NONFLAMMABLE GAS
	Krypton, refrigerated liquid *(cryogenic liquid)*	2.2	UN1970		2.2	T75, TP5	120	NONFLAMMABLE GAS
	Lacquer base or lacquer chips, nitrocellulose, dry, see **Nitrocellulose,** *etc. (UN 2557)*							
	Lacquer base or lacquer chips, plastic, wet with alcohol or solvent, see **Nitrocellulose** *(UN2059, UN2555, UN2556, UN2557) or* **Paint** *etc. (UN1263)*							
	Lead acetate	6.1	UN1616	III	6.1	IB8, IP3, T1, TP33	151	POISON

Sym-bols	Hazardous materials descriptions and proper shipping names	Hazard class or Division	Identifica-tion Numbers	PG	Label Codes	Special provisions (§172.102)	ERG Guide No.	Placard Advisory Consult §172.504 & §172.505 *Placard any quantity
(1)	(2)	(3)	(4)	(5)	(6)	(7)		
	Lead arsenates	6.1	UN1617	II	6.1	IB8, IP2, IP4, T3, TP33	151	POISON
	Lead arsenites	6.1	UN1618	II	6.1	IB8, IP2, IP4, T3, TP33	151	POISON
	Lead azide (dry)	Forbidden						
	Lead azide, wetted *with not less than 20 percent water or mixture of alcohol and water, by mass*	1.1A	UN0129	II	1.1A	111, 117	112	EXPLOSIVES 1.1*
	Lead compounds, soluble, n.o.s.	6.1	UN2291	III	6.1	138, IB8, IP3, T1, TP33	151	POISON
	Lead cyanide	6.1	UN1620	II	6.1	IB8, IP2, IP4, T3, TP33	151	POISON
	Lead dioxide	5.1	UN1872	III	5.1	A1, IB8, IP3, T1, TP33	141	OXIDIZER
	Lead dross, see **Lead sulfate,** *with more than 3 percent free acid*							
	Lead nitrate	5.1	UN1469	II	5.1, 6.1	IB8, IP2, IP4, T3, TP33	141	OXIDIZER
	Lead nitroresorcinate (dry)	Forbidden						
	Lead perchlorate, solid	5.1	UN1470	II	5.1, 6.1	IB6, IP2, T3, TP33	141	OXIDIZER
	Lead perchlorate, solution	5.1	UN3408	II	5.1, 6.1	IB2, T4, TP1	141	OXIDIZER

Sym-bols	Hazardous materials descriptions and proper shipping names	Hazard class or Division	Identification Numbers	PG	Label Codes	Special provisions (§172.102)	ERG Guide No.	Placard Advisory Consult §172.504 & §172.505 *Placard any quantity
(1)	(2)	(3)	(4)	(5)	(6)	(7)		
				III	5.1, 6.1	IB2, T4, TP1	141	OXIDIZER
	Lead peroxide, see **Lead dioxide**							
	Lead phosphite, dibasic	4.1	UN2989	II	4.1	IB8, IP2, IP4, T3, TP33	133	FLAMMABLE SOLID
				III	4.1	IB8, IP3, T1, TP33	133	FLAMMABLE SOLID
	Lead picrate (dry)	Forbidden						
	Lead styphnate (dry)	Forbidden						
	Lead styphnate, wetted *or* **Lead trinitroresorcinate, wetted** *with not less than 20 percent water or mixture of alcohol and water, by mass*	1.1A	UN0130	II	1.1A	111, 117	112	EXPLOSIVES 1.1*
	Lead sulfate *with more than 3 percent free acid*	8	UN1794	II	8	IB8, IP2, IP4, T3, TP33	154	CORROSIVE
	Lead trinitroresorcinate, *see* **Lead styphnate,** *etc.*							
	Life-saving appliances, not self inflating *containing dangerous goods as equipment*	9	UN3072		None		171	CLASS 9
	Life-saving appliances, self inflating	9	UN2990		None		171	CLASS 9

Sym-bols	Hazardous materials descriptions and proper shipping names	Hazard class or Division	Identifica-tion Numbers	PG	Label Codes	Special provisions (§172.102)	ERG Guide No.	Placard Advisory Consult §172.504 & §172.505 *Placard any quantity
(1)	(2)	(3)	(4)	(5)	(6)	(7)		
	Lighter replacement cartridges containing liquefied petroleum gases (and similar devices, each not exceeding 65 grams), see **Lighters** *or* **lighter refills** *etc. containing flammable gas*							
	Lighters, fuse	1.4S	UN0131	II	1.4S		114	EXPLOSIVES 1.4
	Lighters *or* **Lighter refills** *containing flammable gas*	2.1	UN1057		2.1	N10	115	FLAMMABLE GAS
	Lime, unslaked, see **Calcium oxide**							
G	**Liquefied gas, flammable, n.o.s.**	2.1	UN3161		2.1	T50	115	FLAMMABLE GAS
G	**Liquefied gas, n.o.s.**	2.2	UN3163		2.2	T50	126	NONFLAMMABLE GAS
G	**Liquefied gas, oxidizing, n.o.s.**	2.2	UN3157		2.2, 5.1	A14	122	NONFLAMMABLE GAS
G I	**Liquefied gas, toxic, corrosive, n.o.s.** *Inhalation Hazard Zone A*	2.3	UN3308		2.3, 8	1	123	POISON GAS*
G I	**Liquefied gas, toxic, corrosive, n.o.s.** *Inhalation Hazard Zone B*	2.3	UN3308		2.3, 8	2, B9, B14	123	POISON GAS*
G I	**Liquefied gas, toxic, corrosive, n.o.s.** *Inhalation Hazard Zone C*	2.3	UN3308		2.3, 8	3, B14	123	POISON GAS*
G I	**Liquefied gas, toxic, corrosive, n.o.s.** *Inhalation Hazard Zone D*	2.3	UN3308		2.3, 8	4	123	POISON GAS*

Symbols	Hazardous materials descriptions and proper shipping names	Hazard class or Division	Identification Numbers	PG	Label Codes	Special provisions (§172.102)	ERG Guide No.	Placard Advisory Consult §172.504 & §172.505 *Placard any quantity
(1)	(2)	(3)	(4)	(5)	(6)	(7)		
G I	**Liquefied gas, toxic, flammable, corrosive, n.o.s.** *Inhalation Hazard Zone A*	2.3	UN3309		2.3, 2.1, 8	1	119	POISON GAS*
G I	**Liquefied gas, toxic, flammable, corrosive, n.o.s.** *Inhalation Hazard Zone B*	2.3	UN3309		2.3, 2.1, 8	2, B9, B14	119	POISON GAS*
G I	**Liquefied gas, toxic, flammable, corrosive, n.o.s.** *Inhalation Hazard Zone C*	2.3	UN3309		2.3, 2.1, 8	3, B14	119	POISON GAS*
G I	**Liquefied gas, toxic, flammable, corrosive, n.o.s.** *Inhalation Hazard Zone D*	2.3	UN3309		2.3, 2.1, 8	4	119	POISON GAS*
G	**Liquefied gas, toxic, flammable, n.o.s.** *Inhalation Hazard Zone A*	2.3	UN3160		2.3, 2.1	1	119	POISON GAS*
G	**Liquefied gas, toxic, flammable, n.o.s.** *Inhalation Hazard Zone B*	2.3	UN3160		2.3, 2.1	2, B9, B14	119	POISON GAS*
G	**Liquefied gas, toxic, flammable, n.o.s.** *Inhalation Hazard Zone C*	2.3	UN3160		2.3, 2.1	3, B14	119	POISON GAS*
G	**Liquefied gas, toxic, flammable, n.o.s.** *Inhalation Hazard Zone D*	2.3	UN3160		2.3, 2.1	4	119	POISON GAS*
G	**Liquefied gas, toxic, n.o.s.** *Inhalation Hazard Zone A*	2.3	UN3162		2.3	1	123	POISON GAS*
G	**Liquefied gas, toxic, n.o.s.** *Inhalation Hazard Zone B*	2.3	UN3162		2.3	2, B9, B14	123	POISON GAS*

Symbols	Hazardous materials descriptions and proper shipping names	Hazard class or Division	Identification Numbers	PG	Label Codes	Special provisions (§172.102)	ERG Guide No.	Placard Advisory Consult §172.504 & §172.505 *Placard any quantity
(1)	(2)	(3)	(4)	(5)	(6)	(7)		
G	**Liquefied gas, toxic, n.o.s.** *Inhalation Hazard Zone C*	2.3	UN3162		2.3	3, B14	123	POISON GAS*
G	**Liquefied gas, toxic, n.o.s.** *Inhalation Hazard Zone D*	2.3	UN3162		2.3	4	123	POISON GAS*
G I	**Liquefied gas, toxic, oxidizing, corrosive, n.o.s.** *Inhalation Hazard Zone A*	2.3	UN3310		2.3, 5.1, 8	1	124	POISON GAS*
G I	**Liquefied gas, toxic, oxidizing, corrosive, n.o.s.** *Inhalation Hazard Zone B*	2.3	UN3310		2.3, 5.1, 8	2, B9, B14	124	POISON GAS*
G I	**Liquefied gas, toxic, oxidizing, corrosive, n.o.s.** *Inhalation Hazard Zone C*	2.3	UN3310		2.3, 5.1, 8	3, B14	124	POISON GAS*
G I	**Liquefied gas, toxic, oxidizing, corrosive, n.o.s.** *Inhalation Hazard Zone D*	2.3	UN3310		2.3, 5.1, 8	4	124	POISON GAS*
G	**Liquefied gas, toxic, oxidizing, n.o.s.** *Inhalation Hazard Zone A*	2.3	UN3307		2.3, 5.1	1	124	POISON GAS*
G	**Liquefied gas, toxic, oxidizing, n.o.s.** *Inhalation Hazard Zone B*	2.3	UN3307		2.3, 5.1	2, B9, B14	124	POISON GAS*
G	**Liquefied gas, toxic, oxidizing, n.o.s.** *Inhalation Hazard Zone C*	2.3	UN3307		2.3, 5.1	3, B14	124	POISON GAS*
G	**Liquefied gas, toxic, oxidizing, n.o.s.** *Inhalation Hazard Zone D*	2.3	UN3307		2.3, 5.1	4	124	POISON GAS*
	Liquefied gases, *non-flammable charged with nitrogen, carbon dioxide or air*	2.2	UN1058		2.2		120	NONFLAMMABLE GAS

Sym-bols	Hazardous materials descriptions and proper shipping names	Hazard class or Division	Identifica-tion Numbers	PG	Label Codes	Special provisions (§172.102)	ERG Guide No.	Placard Advisory Consult §172.504 & §172.505 *Placard any quantity
(1)	(2)	(3)	(4)	(5)	(6)	(7)		
	Liquefied hydrocarbon gas, see **Hydrocarbon gas mixture, liquefied, n.o.s.**							
	Liquefied natural gas, see **Methane,** *etc. (UN 1972)*							
	Liquefied petroleum gas *see* **Petroleum gases, liquefied**							
	Lithium	4.3	UN1415	I	4.3	A7, A19, IB4, IP1, N45	138	DANGEROUS WAHEN WET*
	Lithium acetylide ethylenediamine complex, see **Water reactive solid** *etc.*							
	Lithium alkyls, liquid	4.2	UN2445	I	4.2, 4.3	173, B11, T21, TP2, TP7	135	SPONTANEOUSLY COMBUSTIBLE, DANGEROUS WHEN WET*
	Lithium alkyls, solid	4.2	UN3433	I	4.2, 4.3	173, B11, T21, TP7, TP33	135	SPONTANEOUSLY COMBUSTIBLE, DANGEROUS WHEN WET*
	Lithium aluminum hydride	4.3	UN1410	I	4.3	A19	138	DANGEROUS WHEN WET*
	Lithium aluminum hydride, ethereal	4.3	UN1411	I	4.3, 3	A2, A3, A11, N34	138	DANGEROUS WHEN WET*
	Lithium batteries, contained in equipment	9	UN3091	II	9	29, A54, A55, A102, A104	138	CLASS 9

Symbols	Hazardous materials descriptions and proper shipping names	Hazard class or Division	Identification Numbers	PG	Label Codes	Special provisions (§172.102)	ERG Guide No.	Placard Advisory Consult §172.504 & §172.505 *Placard any quantity
(1)	(2)	(3)	(4)	(5)	(6)	(7)		
	Lithium batteries packed with equipment	9	UN3091	II	9	29, A54, A55, A101, A103	138	CLASS 9
	Lithium battery	9	UN3090	II	9	29, A54, A55, A100	138	CLASS 9
	Lithium borohydride	4.3	UN1413	I	4.3	A19, N40	138	DANGEROUS WHEN WET*
	Lithium ferrosilicon	4.3	UN2830	II	4.3	A19, IB7, IP2, T3, TP33	139	DANGEROUS WHEN WET*
	Lithium hydride	4.3	UN1414	I	4.3	A19, N40	138	DANGEROUS WHEN WET*
	Lithium hydride, fused solid	4.3	UN2805	II	4.3	A8, A19, A20, IB4, T3, TP33	138	DANGEROUS WHEN WET*
	Lithium hydroxide	8	UN2680	II	8	IB8, IP2, IP4, T3, TP33	154	CORROSIVE
	Lithium hydroxide, solution	8	UN2679	II	8	B2, IB2, T7, TP2	154	CORROSIVE
				III	8	IB3, T4, TP2	154	CORROSIVE
	Lithium hypochlorite, dry *with more than 39% available chlorine (8.8% available oxygen) or* **Lithium hypochlorite mixtures, dry** *with more than 39% available chlorine (8.8% available oxygen)*	5.1	UN1471	II	5.1	A9, IB8, IP2, IP4, N34	140	OXIDIZER
	Lithium in cartridges, see **Lithium**							

Sym-bols	Hazardous materials descriptions and proper shipping names	Hazard class or Division	Identifica-tion Numbers	PG	Label Codes	Special provisions (§172.102)	ERG Guide No.	Placard Advisory Consult §172.504 & §172.505 *Placard any quantity
(1)	(2)	(3)	(4)	(5)	(6)	(7)		
	Lithium nitrate	5.1	UN2722	III	5.1	A1, IB8, IP3, T1, TP33	140	OXIDIZER
	Lithium nitride	4.3	UN2806	I	4.3	A19, IB4, IP1, N40	138	DANGEROUS WHEN WET*
	Lithium peroxide	5.1	UN1472	II	5.1	A9, IB6, IP2, N34, T3, TP33	143	OXIDIZER
	Lithium silicon	4.3	UN1417	II	4.3	A19, A20, IB7, IP2, T3, TP33	138	DANGEROUS WHEN WET*
	LNG, see **Methane** *etc. (UN 1972)*							
	London purple	6.1	UN1621	II	6.1	IB8, IP2, IP4, T3, TP33	151	POISON
	LPG, see **Petroleum gases, liquefied**							
	Lye, see **Sodium hydroxide, solutions**							
	Magnesium alkyls	4.2	UN3053	I	4.2, 4.3	B11, T21, TP2, TP7	135	SPONTANEOUSLY COMBUSTIBLE, DANGEROUS WHEN WET*
	Magnesium aluminum phosphide	4.3	UN1419	I	4.3, 6.1	A19, N34, N40	139	DANGEROUS WHEN WET*
+	**Magnesium arsenate**	6.1	UN1622	II	6.1	IB8, IP2, IP4, T3, TP33	151	POISON
	Magnesium bisulfite solution, see **Bisulfites, aqueous solutions, n.o.s.**							

Sym-bols	Hazardous materials descriptions and proper shipping names	Hazard class or Division	Identifica-tion Numbers	PG	Label Codes	Special provisions (§172.102)	ERG Guide No.	Placard Advisory Consult §172.504 & §172.505 *Placard any quantity
(1)	(2)	(3)	(4)	(5)	(6)	(7)		
	Magnesium bromate	5.1	UN1473	II	5.1	A1, IB8, IP4, T3, TP33	140	OXIDIZER
	Magnesium chlorate	5.1	UN2723	II	5.1	IB8, IP2, IP4, T3, TP33	140	OXIDIZER
	Magnesium diamide	4.2	UN2004	II	4.2	A8, A19, A20, IB6, T3, TP33	135	SPONTANEOUSLY COMBUSTIBLE
	Magnesium diphenyl	4.2	UN2005	I	4.2	173, T21, TP7, TP33	135	SPONTANEOUSLY COMBUSTIBLE
	Magnesium dross, wet or hot	Forbidden						
	Magnesium fluorosilicate	6.1	UN2853	III	6.1	IB8, IP3, T1, TP33	151	POISON
	Magnesium granules, coated, *particle size not less than 149 microns*	4.3	UN2950	III	4.3	A1, A19, IB8, IP4, T1, TP33	138	DANGEROUS WHEN WET*
	Magnesium hydride	4.3	UN2010	I	4.3	A19, N40	138	DANGEROUS WHEN WET*
	Magnesium *or* **Magnesium alloys** *with more than 50 percent magnesium in pellets, turnings or ribbons*	4.1	UN1869	III	4.1	A1, IB8, IP3, T1, TP33	138	FLAMMABLE SOLID
	Magnesium nitrate	5.1	UN1474	III	5.1	A1, IB8, IP3, T1, TP33	140	OXIDIZER
	Magnesium perchlorate	5.1	UN1475	II	5.1	IB6, IP2, T3, TP33	140	OXIDIZER
	Magnesium peroxide	5.1	UN1476	II	5.1	IB6, IP2, T3, TP33	140	OXIDIZER
	Magnesium phosphide	4.3	UN2011	I	4.3, 6.1	A19, N40	139	DANGEROUS WHEN WET*

Sym-bols	Hazardous materials descriptions and proper shipping names	Hazard class or Division	Identifica-tion Numbers	PG	Label Codes	Special provisions (§172.102)	ERG Guide No.	Placard Advisory Consult §172.504 & §172.505 *Placard any quantity
(1)	(2)	(3)	(4)	(5)	(6)	(7)		
	Magnesium, powder *or* **Magnesium alloys, powder**	4.3	UN1418	I	4.3, 4.2	A19, B56	138	DANGEROUS WHEN WET*
				II	4.3, 4.2	A19, B56, IB5, IP2, T3, TP33	138	DANGEROUS WHEN WET*
				III	4.3, 4.2	A19, B56, IB8, IP4, T1, TP33	138	DANGEROUS WHEN WET*
	Magnesium scrap, see **Magnesium,** *etc. (UN 1869)*							
	Magnesium silicide	4.3	UN2624	II	4.3	A19, A20, IB7, IP2, T3, TP33	138	DANGEROUS WHEN WET*
	Magnetized material, see §173.21							
	Maleic anhydride	8	UN2215	III	8	IB8, IP3, T1, TP33	156	CORROSIVE
	Maleic anhydride, molten	8	UN2215	III	8	T4, TP3	156	CORROSIVE
	Malononitrile	6.1	UN2647	II	6.1	IB8, IP2, IP4, T3, TP33	153	POISON
	Mancozeb (manganese ethylenebis-dithiocarbamate complex with zinc) see **Maneb**							
	Maneb *or* **Maneb preparations** *with not less than 60 percent maneb*	4.2	UN2210	III	4.2, 4.3	57, A1, A19, IB6, T1, TP33	135	SPONTANEOUSLY COMBUSTIBLE, DANGEROUS WHEN WET*
	Maneb stabilized *or* **Maneb preparations, stabilized** *against self-heating*	4.3	UN2968	III	4.3	54, A1, A19, IB8, IP4, T1, TP33	135	DANGEROUS WHEN WET*

Sym-bols	Hazardous materials descriptions and proper shipping names	Hazard class or Division	Identifica-tion Numbers	PG	Label Codes	Special provisions (§172.102)	ERG Guide No.	Placard Advisory Consult §172.504 & §172.505 *Placard any quantity
(1)	(2)	(3)	(4)	(5)	(6)	(7)		
	Manganese nitrate	5.1	UN2724	III	5.1	A1, IB8, IP3, T1, TP33	140	OXIDIZER
	Manganese resinate	4.1	UN1330	III	4.1	A1, IB6, T1, TP33	133	FLAMMABLE SOLID
	Mannitan tetranitrate	Forbidden						
	Mannitol hexanitrate (dry)	Forbidden						
	Mannitol hexanitrate, wetted *or* **Nitromannite, wetted** *with not less than 40 percent water, or mixture of alcohol and water, by mass*	1.1D	UN0133	II	1.1D	121	112	EXPLOSIVES 1.1*
	Marine pollutants, liquid or solid, n.o.s., see **Environmentally hazardous substances, liquid** *or* **solid, n.o.s.**							
	Matches, block, see **Matches, 'strike anywhere'**							
	Matches, fusee	4.1	UN2254	III	4.1		133	FLAMMABLE SOLID
	Matches, safety *(book, card or strike on box)*	4.1	UN1944	III	4.1		133	FLAMMABLE SOLID
	Matches, strike anywhere	4.1	UN1331	III	4.1		133	FLAMMABLE SOLID
	Matches, wax, Vesta	4.1	UN1945	III	4.1		133	FLAMMABLE SOLID
	Matting acid, see **Sulfuric acid**							

Symbols	Hazardous materials descriptions and proper shipping names	Hazard class or Division	Identification Numbers	PG	Label Codes	Special provisions (§172.102)	ERG Guide No.	Placard Advisory Consult §172.504 & §172.505 *Placard any quantity
(1)	(2)	(3)	(4)	(5)	(6)	(7)		
	Medicine, liquid, flammable, toxic, n.o.s.	3	UN3248	II	3, 6.1	36, IB2	131	FLAMMABLE
				III	3, 6.1	36, IB3	131	FLAMMABLE
	Medicine, liquid, toxic, n.o.s.	6.1	UN1851	II	6.1	36	151	POISON
				III	6.1	36	151	POISON
	Medicine, solid, toxic, n.o.s.	6.1	UN3249	II	6.1	36, T3, TP33	151	POISON
				III	6.1	36, T1, TP33	151	POISON
	Memtetrahydrophthalic anhydride, see **Corrosive liquids, n.o.s.**							
	Mercaptans, liquid, flammable, n.o.s. *or* **Mercaptan mixture, liquid, flammable, n.o.s.**	3	UN3336	I	3	T11, TP2	130	FLAMMABLE
				II	3	IB2, T7, TP1, TP8, TP28	130	FLAMMABLE
				III	3	B1, B52, IB3, T4, TP1, TP29	130	FLAMMABLE
	Mercaptans, liquid, flammable, toxic, n.o.s. *or* **Mercaptan mixtures, liquid, flammable, toxic, n.o.s.**	3	UN1228	II	3, 6.1	IB2, T11, TP2, TP27	131	FLAMMABLE
				III	3, 6.1	A6, B1, IB3, T7, TP1, TP28	131	FLAMMABLE

Sym-bols	Hazardous materials descriptions and proper shipping names	Hazard class or Division	Identification Numbers	PG	Label Codes	Special provisions (§172.102)	ERG Guide No.	Placard Advisory Consult §172.504 & §172.505 *Placard any quantity
(1)	(2)	(3)	(4)	(5)	(6)	(7)		
	Mercaptans, liquid, toxic, flammable, n.o.s. *or* **Mercaptan mixtures, liquid, toxic, flammable, n.o.s.,** *flash point not less than 23 degrees C*	6.1	UN3071	II	6.1, 3	A6, IB2, T11, TP2, TP13, TP27	131	POISON
	5-Mercaptotetrazol-1-acetic acid	1.4C	UN0448	II	1.4C		114	EXPLOSIVES 1.4
	Mercuric arsenate	6.1	UN1623	II	6.1	IB8, IP2, IP4, T3, TP33	151	POISON
	Mercuric chloride	6.1	UN1624	II	6.1	IB8, IP2, IP4, T3, TP33	154	POISON
	Mercuric compounds, see **Mercury compounds,** *etc.*							
	Mercuric nitrate	6.1	UN1625	II	6.1	IB8, IP2, IP4, N73, T3, TP33	141	POISON
+	**Mercuric potassium cyanide**	6.1	UN1626	I	6.1	IB7, IP1, N74, N75, T6, TP33	157	POISON
	Mercuric sulfocyanate, see **Mercury thiocyanate**							
	Mercurol, see **Mercury nucleate**							
	Mercurous azide	Forbidden						
	Mercurous compounds, see **Mercury compounds,** *etc.*							
	Mercurous nitrate	6.1	UN1627	II	6.1	IB8, IP2, IP4, T3, TP33	141	POISON

Sym-bols	Hazardous materials descriptions and proper shipping names	Hazard class or Division	Identifica-tion Numbers	PG	Label Codes	Special provisions (§172.102)	ERG Guide No.	Placard Advisory Consult §172.504 & §172.505 *Placard any quantity
(1)	(2)	(3)	(4)	(5)	(6)	(7)		
A W	**Mercury**	8	UN2809	III	8		172	CORROSIVE
	Mercury acetate	6.1	UN1629	II	6.1	IB8, IP2, IP4, T3, TP33	151	POISON
	Mercury acetylide	Forbidden						
	Mercury ammonium chloride	6.1	UN1630	II	6.1	IB8, IP2, IP4, T3, TP33	151	POISON
	Mercury based pesticides, liquid, flammable, toxic, *flash point less than 23 degrees C*	3	UN2778	I	3, 6.1	T14, TP2, TP13, TP27	131	FLAMMABLE
				II	3, 6.1	IB2, T11, TP2, TP13, TP27	131	FLAMMABLE
	Mercury based pesticides, liquid, toxic	6.1	UN3012	I	6.1	T14, TP2, TP13, TP27	151	POISON
				II	6.1	IB2, T11, TP2, TP13, TP27	151	POISON
				III	6.1	IB3, T7, TP2, TP28	151	POISON
	Mercury based pesticides, liquid, toxic, flammable, *flash point not less than 23 degrees C*	6.1	UN3011	I	6.1, 3	T14, TP2, TP13, TP27	131	POISON
				II	6.1, 3	IB2, T11, TP2, TP13, TP27	131	POISON
				III	6.1, 3	IB3, T7, TP2, TP28	131	POISON

Sym-bols	Hazardous materials descriptions and proper shipping names	Hazard class or Division	Identifica-tion Numbers	PG	Label Codes	Special provisions (§172.102)	ERG Guide No.	Placard Advisory Consult §172.504 & §172.505 *Placard any quantity
(1)	(2)	(3)	(4)	(5)	(6)	(7)		
	Mercury based pesticides, solid, toxic	6.1	UN2777	I	6.1	IB7, IP1, T6, TP33	151	POISON
				II	6.1	IB8, IP2, IP4, T3, TP33	151	POISON
				III	6.1	IB8, IP3. T1, TP33	151	POISON
	Mercury benzoate	6.1	UN1631	II	6.1	IB8, IP2, IP4, T3, TP33	154	POISON
	Mercury bromides	6.1	UN1634	II	6.1	IB8, IP2, IP4, T3, TP33	154	POISON
	Mercury compounds, liquid, n.o.s.	6.1	UN2024	I	6.1		151	POISON
				II	6.1	IB2	151	POISON
				III	6.1	IB3	151	POISON
	Mercury compounds, solid, n.o.s.	6.1	UN2025	I	6.1	IB7, IP1, T6, TP33	151	POISON
				II	6.1	IB8, IP2, IP4, T3, TP33	151	POISON
				III	6.1	IB8, IP3, T1, TP33	151	POISON
A	**Mercury** *contained in manufactured articles*	8	UN2809	III	8		172	CORROSIVE
	Mercury cyanide	6.1	UN1636	II	6.1	IB8, IP2, IP4, N74, N75, T3, TP33	154	POISON
	Mercury fulminate, wetted *with not less than 20 percent water, or mixture of alcohol and water, by mass*	1.1A	UN0135	II	1.1A	111, 117	112	EXPLOSIVES 1.1*

Symbols	Hazardous materials descriptions and proper shipping names	Hazard class or Division	Identification Numbers	PG	Label Codes	Special provisions (§172.102)	ERG Guide No.	Placard Advisory Consult §172.504 & §172.505 *Placard any quantity
(1)	(2)	(3)	(4)	(5)	(6)	(7)		
	Mercury gluconate	6.1	UN1637	II	6.1	IB8, IP2, IP4, T3, TP33	151	POISON
	Mercury iodide	6.1	UN1638	II	6.1	IB2, IP2, IP4, T3, TP33	151	POISON
	Mercury iodide aquabasic ammonobasic (Iodide of Millon's base)	Forbidden						
	Mercury nitride	Forbidden						
	Mercury nucleate	6.1	UN1639	II	6.1	IB8, IP2, IP4, T3, TP33	151	POISON
	Mercury oleate	6.1	UN1640	II	6.1	IB8, IP2, IP4, T3, TP33	151	POISON
	Mercury oxide	6.1	UN1641	II	6.1	IB8, IP2, IP4, T3, TP33	151	POISON
	Mercury oxycyanide	Forbidden						
	Mercury oxycyanide, desensitized	6.1	UN1642	II	6.1	IB8, IP2, IP4, T3, TP33	151	POISON
	Mercury potassium iodide	6.1	UN1643	II	6.1	IB8, IP2, IP4, T3, TP33	151	POISON
	Mercury salicylate	6.1	UN1644	II	6.1	IB8, IP2, IP4, T3, TP33	151	POISON
+	**Mercury sulfates**	6.1	UN1645	II	6.1	IB8, IP2, IP4, T3, TP33	151	POISON

Symbols	Hazardous materials descriptions and proper shipping names	Hazard class or Division	Identification Numbers	PG	Label Codes	Special provisions (§172.102)	ERG Guide No.	Placard Advisory Consult §172.504 & §172.505 *Placard any quantity
(1)	(2)	(3)	(4)	(5)	(6)	(7)		
	Mercury thiocyanate	6.1	UN1646	II	6.1	IB8, IP2, IP4, T3, TP33	151	POISON
	Mesityl oxide	3	UN1229	III	3	B1, IB3, T2, TP1	129	FLAMMABLE
G	**Metal carbonyls, liquid, n.o.s.**	6.1	UN3281	I	6.1	5, T14, TP2, TP13, TP27	151	POISON
				II	6.1	IB2, T11, TP2, TP27	151	POISON
				III	6.1	IB3, T7, TP1, TP28	151	POISON
G	**Metal carbonyls, solid, n.o.s.**	6.1	UN3466	I	6.1	IB7, IP1, T6, TP33	151	POISON
				II	6.1	IB8, IP2, IP4, T3, TP33	151	POISON
				III	6.1	IB8, IP3, T1, TP33	151	POISON
	Metal catalyst, dry	4.2	UN2881	I	4.2	N34, T21, TP7, TP33	135	SPONTANEOUSLY COMBUSTIBLE
				II	4.2	IB6, IP2, N34, T3, TP33	135	SPONTANEOUSLY COMBUSTIBLE
				III	4.2	IB8, IP3, N34, T1, TP33	135	SPONTANEOUSLY COMBUSTIBLE
	Metal catalyst, wetted *with a visible excess of liquid*	4.2	UN1378	II	4.2	A2, A8, IB1, N34, T3, TP33	170	SPONTANEOUSLY COMBUSTIBLE
	Metal hydrides, flammable, n.o.s.	4.1	UN3182	II	4.1	A1, IB4, T3, TP33	170	FLAMMABLE SOLID

Sym-bols	Hazardous materials descriptions and proper shipping names	Hazard class or Division	Identifica-tion Numbers	PG	Label Codes	Special provisions (§172.102)	ERG Guide No.	Placard Advisory Consult §172.504 & §172.505 *Placard any quantity
(1)	(2)	(3)	(4)	(5)	(6)	(7)		
				III	4.1	A1, IB4, T1, TP33	170	FLAMMABLE SOLID
	Metal hydrides, water reactive, n.o.s.	4.3	UN1409	I	4.3	A19, N34, N40	138	DANGEROUS WHEN WET*
				II	4.3	A19, IB4, N34, N40, T3, TP33	138	DANGEROUS WHEN WET*
	Metal powder, self-heating, n.o.s.	4.2	UN3189	II	4.2	IB6, IP2, T3, TP33	135	SPONTANEOUSLY COMBUSTIBLE
				III	4.2	IB8, IP3, T1, TP33	135	SPONTANEOUSLY COMBUSTIBLE
	Metal powders, flammable, n.o.s.	4.1	UN3089	II	4.1	IB8, IP2, IP4, T3, TP33	170	FLAMMABLE SOLID
				III	4.1	IB6, T1, TP33	170	FLAMMABLE SOLID
	Metal salts of methyl nitramine (dry)	Forbidden						
G	**Metal salts of organic compounds, flammable, n.o.s.**	4.1	UN3181	II	4.1	A1, IB8, IP2, IP4, T3, TP33	133	FLAMMABLE SOLID
				III	4.1	A1, IB8, IP3, T1, TP33	133	FLAMMABLE SOLID
	Metaldehyde	4.1	UN1332	III	4.1	A1, IB8, IP3, T1, TP33	133	FLAMMABLE SOLID
G	**Metallic substance, water-reactive, n.o.s.**	4.3	UN3208	I	4.3	A7, IB4	138	DANGEROUS WHEN WET*

Sym-bols	Hazardous materials descriptions and proper shipping names	Hazard class or Division	Identification Numbers	PG	Label Codes	Special provisions (§172.102)	ERG Guide No.	Placard Advisory Consult §172.504 & §172.505 *Placard any quantity
(1)	(2)	(3)	(4)	(5)	(6)	(7)		
				II	4.3	A7, IB7, IP2, T3, TP33	138	DANGEROUS WHEN WET*
				III	4.3	A7, IB8, IP4, T1, TP33	138	DANGEROUS WHEN WET*
G	**Metallic substance, water-reactive, self-heating, n.o.s.**	4.3	UN3209	I	4.3, 4.2	A7	138	DANGEROUS WHEN WET*
				II	4.3, 4.2	A7, IB5, IP2, T3, TP33	138	DANGEROUS WHEN WET*
				III	4.3, 4.2	A7, IB8, IP4, T1, TP33	138	DANGEROUS WHEN WET*
	Methacrylaldehyde, stabilized	3	UN2396	II	3, 6.1	45, IB2, T7, TP1, TP13	131P	FLAMMABLE
	Methacrylic acid, stabilized	8	UN2531	II	8	IB2, T7, TP1, TP18, TP30	153P	CORROSIVE
+	**Methacrylonitrile, stabilized**	3	UN3079	I	3, 6.1	2, B9, B14, B32, B74,T20, TP2, TP13, TP38, TP45	131P	FLAMMABLE, POISON INHALATION HAZARD*
	Methallyl alcohol	3	UN2614	III	3	B1, IB3, T2, TP1	129	FLAMMABLE
	Methane and hydrogen, mixtures, see **Hydrogen and methane, mixtures,** *etc.*							

Symbols	Hazardous materials descriptions and proper shipping names	Hazard class or Division	Identification Numbers	PG	Label Codes	Special provisions (§172.102)	ERG Guide No.	Placard Advisory Consult §172.504 & §172.505 *Placard any quantity
(1)	(2)	(3)	(4)	(5)	(6)	(7)		
	Methane, compressed or **Natural gas, compressed** *(with high methane content)*	2.1	UN1971		2.1		115	FLAMMABLE GAS
	Methane, refrigerated liquid *(cryogenic liquid) or* **Natural gas, refrigerated liquid** *(cryogenic liquid), with high methane content)*	2.1	UN1972		2.1	T75, TP5	115	FLAMMABLE GAS
	Methanesulfonyl chloride	6.1	UN3246	I	6.1, 8	2, B9, B14, B32, B74, T20, TP2, TP12, TP13, TP38, TP45	156	POISON INHALATION HAZARD*
+ I	**Methanol**	3	UN1230	II	3, 6.1	IB2, T7,TP2	131	FLAMMABLE
D	**Methanol**	3	UN1230	II	3	IB2, T7,TP2	131	FLAMMABLE
	Methazoic acid	Forbidden						
	4-Methoxy-4-methylpentan-2-one	3	UN2293	III	3	B1, IB3, T2, TP1	128	FLAMMABLE
	1-Methoxy-2-propanol	3	UN3092	III	3	B1, IB3, T2, TP1	129	FLAMMABLE
+	**Methoxymethyl isocyanate**	3	UN2605	I	3, 6.1	1, B9, B14, B30, B72, T22, TP2, TP13, TP38, TP44	155	FLAMMABLE, POISON INHALATION HAZARD*
	Methyl acetate	3	UN1231	II	3	IB2, T4, TP1	129	FLAMMABLE
	Methyl acetylene and propadiene mixtures, stabilized	2.1	UN1060		2.1	T50	116P	FLAMMABLE GAS
	Methyl acrylate, stabilized	3	UN1919	II	3	IB2, T4, TP1, TP13	129P	FLAMMABLE

Symbols	Hazardous materials descriptions and proper shipping names	Hazard class or Division	Identification Numbers	PG	Label Codes	Special provisions (§172.102)	ERG Guide No.	Placard Advisory Consult §172.504 & §172.505 *Placard any quantity
(1)	(2)	(3)	(4)	(5)	(6)	(7)		
	Methyl alcohol, see **Methanol**							
	Methyl allyl chloride	3	UN2554	II	3	IB2, T4, TP1, TP13	130P	FLAMMABLE
	Methyl amyl ketone, see **Amyl methyl ketone**							
	Methyl bromide	2.3	UN1062		2.3	3, B14, T50	123	POISON GAS*
	Methyl bromide and chloropicrin mixtures with more than 2 percent chloropicrin, see **Chloropicrin and methyl bromide mixtures**							
	Methyl bromide and chloropicrin mixtures with not more than 2 percent chloropicrin, see **Methyl bromide**							
	Methyl bromide and ethylene dibromide mixtures, liquid	6.1	UN1647	I	6.1	2, B9, B14, B32, B74, N65, T20, TP2, TP13, TP38, TP44	151	POISON INHALATION HAZARD*
	Methyl bromoacetate	6.1	UN2643	II	6.1	IB2, T7, TP2	155	POISON
	2-Methylbutanal	3	UN3371	II	3	IB2, T4, TP1	129	FLAMMABLE
	2-Methyl-1-butene	3	UN2459	I	3	T11, TP2	128	FLAMMABLE
	2-Methyl-2-butene	3	UN2460	II	3	IB2, IP8, T7, TP1	128	FLAMMABLE
	3-Methyl-1-butene	3	UN2561	I	3	T11, TP2	128	FLAMMABLE
	Methyl tert-butyl ether	3	UN2398	II	3	IB2, T7, TP1	127	FLAMMABLE
	Methyl butyrate	3	UN1237	II	3	IB2, T4, TP1	129	FLAMMABLE

Symbols	Hazardous materials descriptions and proper shipping names	Hazard class or Division	Identification Numbers	PG	Label Codes	Special provisions (§172.102)	ERG Guide No.	Placard Advisory Consult §172.504 & §172.505 *Placard any quantity
(1)	(2)	(3)	(4)	(5)	(6)	(7)		
	Methyl chloride *or* **Refrigerant gas R 40**	2.1	UN1063		2.1	T50	115	FLAMMABLE GAS
	Methyl chloride and chloropicrin mixtures, see **Chloropicrin and methyl chloride mixtures**							
	Methyl chloride and methylene chloride mixtures	2.1	UN1912		2.1	T50	115	FLAMMABLE GAS
	Methyl chloroacetate	6.1	UN2295	I	6.1, 3	T14, TP2, TP13	155	POISON
	Methyl chlorocarbonate, see **Methyl chloroformate**							
	Methyl chloroform, see **1,1, 1-Trichloroethane**							
	Methyl chloroformate	6.1	UN1238	I	6.1, 3, 8	1, B9, B14, B30, B72, N34, T22, TP2, TP13, TP38, TP44	155	POISON INHALATION HAZARD*
	Methyl chloromethyl ether	6.1	UN1239	I	6.1, 3	1, B9, B14, B30, B72, T22, TP2, TP38, TP44	131	POISON INHALATION HAZARD*
	Methyl 2-chloropropionate	3	UN2933	III	3	B1, IB3, T2, TP1	129	FLAMMABLE
	Methyl dichloroacetate	6.1	UN2299	III	6.1	IB3, T4, TP1	155	POISON
	Methyl ethyl ether, see **Ethyl methyl ether**							

Sym-bols	Hazardous materials descriptions and proper shipping names	Hazard class or Division	Identification Numbers	PG	Label Codes	Special provisions (§172.102)	ERG Guide No.	Placard Advisory Consult §172.504 & §172.505 *Placard any quantity
(1)	(2)	(3)	(4)	(5)	(6)	(7)		
	Methyl ethyl ketone, *see* **Ethyl methyl ketone**							
	Methyl ethyl ketone peroxide, in solution with more than 9 percent by mass active oxygen	Forbidden						
	2-Methyl-5-ethylpyridine	6.1	UN2300	III	6.1	IB3, T4, TP1	153	POISON
	Methyl fluoride *or* **Refrigerant gas R 41**	2.1	UN2454		2.1		115	FLAMMABLE GAS
	Methyl formate	3	UN1243	I	3	T11, TP2	129	FLAMMABLE
	2-Methyl-2-heptanethiol	6.1	UN3023	I	6.1, 3	2, B9, B14, B32, B74, T20, TP2, TP13, TP38, TP45	131	POISON INHALATION HAZARD*
	Methyl iodide	6.1	UN2644	I	6.1	2, B9, B14, B32, B74, T20, TP2, TP13, TP38, TP45	151	POISON INHALATION HAZARD*
	Methyl isobutyl carbinol	3	UN2053	III	3	B1, IB3, T2, TP1	129	FLAMMABLE
	Methyl isobutyl ketone	3	UN1245	II	3	IB2, T4, TP1	127	FLAMMABLE
	Methyl isobutyl ketone peroxide, in solution with more than 9 percent by mass active oxygen	Forbidden						
	Methyl isocyanate	6.1	UN2480	I	6.1, 3	1, B9, B14, B30, B72, T22, TP2, TP13, TP38, TP44	155	POISON INHALATION HAZARD*
	Methyl isopropenyl ketone, stabilized	3	UN1246	II	3	IB2, T4, TP1	127P	FLAMMABLE

Symbols	Hazardous materials descriptions and proper shipping names	Hazard class or Division	Identification Numbers	PG	Label Codes	Special provisions (§172.102)	ERG Guide No.	Placard Advisory Consult §172.504 & §172.505 *Placard any quantity
(1)	(2)	(3)	(4)	(5)	(6)	(7)		
	Methyl isothiocyanate	6.1	UN2477	I	6.1, 3	2, B9, B14, B32, B74, T20, TP2, TP13, TP38, TP45	131	POISON INHALATION HAZARD*
	Methyl isovalerate	3	UN2400	II	3	IB2, T4, TP1	130	FLAMMABLE
	Methyl magnesium bromide, in ethyl ether	4.3	UN1928	I	4.3, 3		135	DANGEROUS WHEN WET*
	Methyl mercaptan	2.3	UN1064		2.3, 2.1	3, B7, B9, B14, T50	117	POISON GAS*
	Methyl mercaptopropionaldehyde, see **4-Thiapentanal**							
	Methyl methacrylate monomer, stabilized	3	UN1247	II	3	IB2, T4,TP1	129P	FLAMMABLE
	Methyl nitramine (dry)	Forbidden						
	Methyl nitrate	Forbidden						
	Methyl nitrite	Forbidden						
	Methyl norbornene dicarboxylic anhydride, see **Corrosive liquids, n.o.s.**							
	Methyl orthosilicate	6.1	UN2606	I	6.1, 3	2, B9, B14, B32, B74, T20, TP2, TP13, TP38, TP45	155	POISON INHALATION HAZARD*
D	**Methyl phosphonic dichloride**	6.1	NA9206	I	6.1, 8	2, B9, B14, B32, B74, N34, N43, T20, TP4,TP12, TP13, TP38, TP45	137	POISON INHALATION HAZARD*

Sym-bols	Hazardous materials descriptions and proper shipping names	Hazard class or Division	Identifica-tion Numbers	PG	Label Codes	Special provisions (§172.102)	ERG Guide No.	Placard Advisory Consult §172.504 & §172.505 *Placard any quantity
(1)	(2)	(3)	(4)	(5)	(6)	(7)		
	Methyl phosphonothioic dichloride, anhydrous, see **Corrosive liquid, n.o.s.**							
D	**Methyl phosphonous dichloride,** *pyrophoric liquid*	6.1	NA2845	I	6.1, 4.2	2, B9, B14, B16, B32, B74, T20, TP4, TP12, TP13, TP38, TP45	135	POISON INHALATION HAZARD*
	Methyl picric acid (heavy metal salts of)	Forbidden						
	Methyl propionate	3	UN1248	II	3	IB2, T4, TP1	129	FLAMMABLE
	Methyl propyl ether	3	UN2612	II	3	IB2, IP8, T7, TP2	127	FLAMMABLE
	Methyl propyl ketone	3	UN1249	II	3	IB2, T4, TP1	127	FLAMMABLE
	Methyl sulfate, see **Dimethyl sulfate**							
	Methyl sulfide, see **Dimethyl sulfide**							
	Methyl trichloroacetate	6.1	UN2533	III	6.1	IB3, T4, TP1	156	POISON
	Methyl trimethylol methane trinitrate	Forbidden						
	Methyl vinyl ketone, stabilized	6.1	UN1251	I	6.1, 3, 8	1, B9, B14, B30, B72, T22, TP2, TP13, TP38, TP44	131P	POISON INHALATION HAZARD*
	Methylal	3	UN1234	II	3	IB2, IP8, T7, TP2	127	FLAMMABLE
	Methylamine, anhydrous	2.1	UN1061		2.1	T50	118	FLAMMABLE GAS
	Methylamine, aqueous solution	3	UN1235	II	3, 8	B1, IB2, T7, TP1	132	FLAMMABLE

Symbols	Hazardous materials descriptions and proper shipping names	Hazard class or Division	Identification Numbers	PG	Label Codes	Special provisions (§172.102)	ERG Guide No.	Placard Advisory Consult §172.504 & §172.505 *Placard any quantity
(1)	(2)	(3)	(4)	(5)	(6)	(7)		
	Methylamine dinitramine and dry salts thereof	Forbidden						
	Methylamine nitroform	Forbidden						
	Methylamine perchlorate (dry)	Forbidden						
	Methylamyl acetate	3	UN1233	III	3	B1, IB3, T2, TP1	130	FLAMMABLE
	N-Methylaniline	6.1	UN2294	III	6.1	IB3, T4, TP1	153	POISON
	alpha-Methylbenzyl alcohol, liquid	6.1	UN2937	III	6.1	IB3, T4, TP1	153	POISON
	alpha-Methylbenzyl alcohol, solid	6.1	UN3438	III	6.1	IB8, IP3, T1, TP33	153	POISON
	3-Methylbutan-2-one	3	UN2397	II	3	IB2, T4, TP1	127	FLAMMABLE
	N-Methylbutylamine	3	UN2945	II	3, 8	IB2, T7, TP1	132	FLAMMABLE
	Methylchlorosilane	2.3	UN2534		2.3, 2.1, 8	2, B9, B14, N34	119	POISON GAS*
	Methylcyclohexane	3	UN2296	II	3	B1, IB2, T4, TP1	128	FLAMMABLE
	Methylcyclohexanols, *flammable*	3	UN2617	III	3	B1, IB3, T2, TP1	129	FLAMMABLE
	Methylcyclohexanone	3	UN2297	III	3	B1, IB3, T2, TP1	128	FLAMMABLE
	Methylcyclopentane	3	UN2298	II	3	IB2, T4, TP1	128	FLAMMABLE
D	**Methyldichloroarsine**	6.1	NA1556	I	6.1	2, T20, TP4, TP12, TP13, TP38, TP45	152	POISON INHALATION HAZARD*
	Methyldichlorosilane	4.3	UN1242	I	4.3, 8, 3	A2, A3, A7, B6, B77, N34, T10, TP2, TP7, TP13	139	DANGEROUS WHEN WET*

Sym-bols	Hazardous materials descriptions and proper shipping names	Hazard class or Division	Identification Numbers	PG	Label Codes	Special provisions (§172.102)	ERG Guide No.	Placard Advisory Consult §172.504 & §172.505 *Placard any quantity
(1)	(2)	(3)	(4)	(5)	(6)	(7)		
	Methylene chloride, see **Dichloromethane**							
	Methylene glycol dinitrate	Forbidden						
	2-Methylfuran	3	UN2301	II	3	IB2, T4, TP1	128	FLAMMABLE
	a-Methylglucoside tetranitrate	Forbidden						
	a-Methylglycerol trinitrate	Forbidden						
	5-Methylhexan-2-one	3	UN2302	III	3	B1, IB3, T2, TP1	127	FLAMMABLE
	Methylhydrazine	6.1	UN1244	I	6.1, 3, 8	1, B7, B9, B14, B30, B72, B77, N34, T22, TP2, TP13, TP38, TP44	131	POISON INHALATION HAZARD*
	4-Methylmorpholine *or* **n-methylmorpholine**	3	UN2535	II	3, 8	B6, IB2, T7, TP1	132	FLAMMABLE
	Methylpentadienes	3	UN2461	II	3	IB2, T4, TP1	128	FLAMMABLE
	2-Methylpentan-2-ol	3	UN2560	III	3	B1, IB3, T2, TP1	129	FLAMMABLE
	Methylpentanes, see **Hexanes**							
	Methylphenyldichlorosilane	8	UN2437	II	8	IB2, T7, TP2, TP13	156	CORROSIVE
	1-Methylpiperidine	3	UN2399	II	3, 8	IB2, T7, TP1	132	FLAMMABLE
	Methyltetrahydrofuran	3	UN2536	II	3	IB2, T4, TP1	127	FLAMMABLE
	Methyltrichlorosilane	3	UN1250	I	3, 8	A7, B6, B77, N34, T11, TP2, TP13	155	FLAMMABLE
	alpha-Methylvaleraldehyde	3	UN2367	II	3	B1, IB2, T4, TP1	130	FLAMMABLE

Sym-bols	Hazardous materials descriptions and proper shipping names	Hazard class or Division	Identifica-tion Numbers	PG	Label Codes	Special provisions (§172.102)	ERG Guide No.	Placard Advisory Consult §172.504 & §172.505 *Placard any quantity
(1)	(2)	(3)	(4)	(5)	(6)	(7)		
	Mine rescue equipment containing carbon dioxide, see **Carbon dioxide**							
	Mines *with bursting charge*	1.1F	UN0136	II	1.1F		112	EXPLOSIVES 1.1*
	Mines *with bursting charge*	1.1D	UN0137	II	1.1D		112	EXPLOSIVES 1.1*
	Mines *with bursting charge*	1.2D	UN0138	II	1.2D		112	EXPLOSIVES 1.2*
	Mines *with bursting charge*	1.2F	UN0294	II	1.2F		112	EXPLOSIVES 1.2*
	Mixed acid, see **Nitrating acid, mixtures** *etc.*							
	Mobility aids, see **Battery powered equipment** *or* **Battery powered vehicle**							
D	**Model rocket motor**	1.4C	NA0276	II	1.4C	51	114	EXPLOSIVES 1.4*
D	**Model rocket motor**	1.4S	NA0323	II	1.4S	51	114	EXPLOSIVES 1.4*
	Molybdenum pentachloride	8	UN2508	III	8	IB8, IP3, T1, TP33	156	CORROSIVE
	Monochloroacetone (unstabilized)	Forbidden						
	Monochloroethylene, see **Vinyl chloride, stabilized**							
	Monoethanolamine, see **Ethanolamine, solutions**							
	Monoethylamine, see **Ethylamine**							
	Morpholine	8	UN2054	I	8, 3	A6, T10, TP2	132	CORROSIVE

Symbols	Hazardous materials descriptions and proper shipping names	Hazard class or Division	Identification Numbers	PG	Label Codes	Special provisions (§172.102)	ERG Guide No.	Placard Advisory Consult §172.504 & §172.505 *Placard any quantity
(1)	(2)	(3)	(4)	(5)	(6)	(7)		
	Morpholine, aqueous, mixture, see **Corrosive liquids, n.o.s.**							
	Motor fuel anti-knock compounds *see* **Motor fuel anti-knock mixtures**							
+	**Motor fuel anti-knock mixtures**	6.1	UN1649	I	6.1, 3	14, 151, B9, B90, T14, TP2, TP13	131	POISON
	Motor spirit, *see* **Gasoline**							
	Muriatic acid, see **Hydrochloric acid**							
	Musk xylene, *see* **5-tert-Butyl-2,4, 6-trinitro-m-xylene**							
	Naphtha see **Petroleum distallate n.o.s.**							
	Naphthalene, crude *or* **Naphthalene, refined**	4.1	UN1334	III	4.1	A1, IB8, IP3, T1, TP33	133	FLAMMABLE SOLID
	Naphthalene diozonide	Forbidden						
	beta-Naphthylamine, solid	6.1	UN1650	II	6.1	IB8, IP2, IP4, T3, TP33	153	POISON
	beta-Naphthylamine solution	6.1	UN3411	II	6.1	IB2, T7, TP2	153	POISON
				III	6.1	IB2, T7, TP2	153	POISON
	alpha-Naphthylamine	6.1	UN2077	III	6.1	IB8, IP3, T1, TP33	153	POISON
	Naphthalene, molten	4.1	UN2304	III	4.1	IB1, T1, TP3	133	FLAMMABLE SOLID

Symbols	Hazardous materials descriptions and proper shipping names	Hazard class or Division	Identification Numbers	PG	Label Codes	Special provisions (§172.102)	ERG Guide No.	Placard Advisory Consult §172.504 & §172.505 *Placard any quantity
(1)	(2)	(3)	(4)	(5)	(6)	(7)		
	Naphthylamineperchlorate	Forbidden						
	Naphthylthiourea	6.1	UN1651	II	6.1	IB8, IP2, IP4, T3, TP33	153	POISON
	Naphthylurea	6.1	UN1652	II	6.1	IB8, IP2, IP4, T3, TP33	153	POISON
	Natural gases (with high methane content), see **Methane,** *etc. (UN 1971, UN 1972)*							
	Neohexane, see **Hexanes**							
	Neon, compressed	2.2	UN1065		2.2		121	NONFLAMMABLE GAS
	Neon, refrigerated liquid *(cryogenic liquid)*	2.2	UN1913		2.2	T75, TP5	120	NONFLAMMABLE GAS
	New explosive or explosive device, see §§173.51 and 173.56							
	Nickel carbonyl	6.1	UN1259	I	6.1, 3	1	131	POISON INHALATION HAZARD*
	Nickel cyanide	6.1	UN1653	II	6.1	IB8, IP2, IP4, N74, N75, T3, TP33	151	POISON
	Nickel nitrate	5.1	UN2725	III	5.1	A1, IB8, IP3, T1, TP33	140	OXIDIZER
	Nickel nitrite	5.1	UN2726	III	5.1	A1, IB8, IP3, T1, TP33	140	OXIDIZER

Sym-bols	Hazardous materials descriptions and proper shipping names	Hazard class or Division	Identifica-tion Numbers	PG	Label Codes	Special provisions (§172.102)	ERG Guide No.	Placard Advisory Consult §172.504 & §172.505 *Placard any quantity
(1)	(2)	(3)	(4)	(5)	(6)	(7)		
	Nickel picrate	Forbidden						
	Nicotine	6.1	UN1654	II	6.1	IB2	151	POISON
	Nicotine compounds, liquid, n.o.s. *or* **Nicotine preparations, liquid, n.o.s.**	6.1	UN3144	I	6.1	A4	151	POISON
				II	6.1	IB2, T11, TP2, TP27	151	POISON
				III	6.1	IB3, T7, TP1, TP28	151	POISON
	Nicotine compounds, solid, n.o.s. *or* **Nicotine preparations, solid, n.o.s.**	6.1	UN1655	I	6.1	IB7, IP1, T6, TP33	151	POISON
				II	6.1	IB8, IP2, IP4, T3, TP33	151	POISON
				III	6.1	IB8, IP3, T1, TP33	151	POISON
	Nicotine hydrochloride liquid *or* **solution**	6.1	UN1656	II	6.1	IB2	151	POISON
				III	6.1	IB3	151	POISON
	Nicotine hydrochloride, solid	6.1	UN3444	II	6.1	IB8, IP2, IP4, T3, TP33	151	POISON
	Nicotine salicylate	6.1	UN1657	II	6.1	IB8, IP2, IP4, T3, TP33	151	POISON
	Nicotine sulfate solution	6.1	UN1658	II	6.1	IB2, T7, TP2	151	POISON
				III	6.1	IB3, T7, TP2	151	POISON

Sym-bols	Hazardous materials descriptions and proper shipping names	Hazard class or Division	Identifica-tion Numbers	PG	Label Codes	Special provisions (§172.102)	ERG Guide No.	Placard Advisory Consult §172.504 & §172.505 *Placard any quantity
(1)	(2)	(3)	(4)	(5)	(6)	(7)		
	Nicotine sulphate, solid	6.1	UN3445	II	6.1	IB8, IP2, IP4, T3, TP33	151	POISON
	Nicotine tartrate	6.1	UN1659	II	6.1	IB8, IP2, IP4, T3, TP33	151	POISON
	Nitrated paper (unstable)	Forbidden						
	Nitrates, inorganic, aqueous solution, n.o.s.	5.1	UN3218	II	5.1	58, IB2, T4, TP1	140	OXIDIZER
				III	5.1	58, IB2, T4, TP1	140	OXIDIZER
	Nitrates, inorganic, n.o.s.	5.1	UN1477	II	5.1	IB8, IP2, IP4, T3, TP33	140	OXIDIZER
				III	5.1	IB8, IP3, T1, TP33	140	OXIDIZER
	Nitrates of diazonium compounds	Forbidden						OXIDIZER
	Nitrating acid mixtures, spent *with more than 50 percent nitric acid*	8	UN1826	I	8, 5.1	A7, T10, TP2, TP12, TP13	157	
	Nitrating acid mixtures spent *with not more than 50 percent nitric acid*	8	UN1826	II	8	A7, B2, IB2, T8, TP2, TP12	157	CORROSIVE
	Nitrating acid mixtures *with more than 50 percent nitric acid*	8	UN1796	I	8, 5.1	A7, T10, TP2, TP12, TP13	157	CORROSIVE
	Nitrating acid mixtures *with not more than 50 percent nitric acid*	8	UN1796	II	8	A7, B2, IB2, T8, TP2, TP12, TP13	157	CORROSIVE
	Nitric acid *other than red fuming, with more than 70 percent nitric acid*	8	UN2031	I	8, 5.1	A3, B47, B53, T10, TP2, TP12, TP13	157	CORROSIVE

Symbols	Hazardous materials descriptions and proper shipping names	Hazard class or Division	Identification Numbers	PG	Label Codes	Special provisions (§172.102)	ERG Guide No.	Placard Advisory Consult §172.504 & §172.505 *Placard any quantity
(1)	(2)	(3)	(4)	(5)	(6)	(7)		
	Nitric acid *other than red fuming, with not more than 70 percent nitric acid*	8	UN2031	II	8	A6, B2, B47, B53, IB2, T8, TP2, TP12	157	CORROSIVE
+	**Nitric acid, red fuming**	8	UN2032	I	8, 5.1, 6.1	2, B9, B32, B74, T20, TP2, TP12, TP13, TP38, TP45	157	CORROSIVE, POISON INHALATION HAZARD*
	Nitric oxide, compressed	2.3	UN1660		2.3, 5.1, 8	1, B37, B46, B50, B60, B77	124	POISON GAS*
	Nitric oxide and dinitrogen tetroxide mixtures *or* **Nitric oxide and nitrogen dioxide mixtures**	2.3	UN1975		2.3, 5.1, 8	1, B7, B9, B14, B45, B46, B61, B66, B67, B77	124	POISON GAS*
G	**Nitriles, flammable, toxic, n.o.s.**	3	UN3273	I	3, 6.1	T14, TP2, TP13, TP27	131	FLAMMABLE
				II	3, 6.1	IB2, T11, TP2, TP13, TP27	131	FLAMMABLE
G	**Nitriles, toxic, flammable, n.o.s.**	6.1	UN3275	I	6.1, 3	5, T14, TP2, TP13, TP27	131	POISON
				II	6.1, 3	IB2, T11, TP2, TP13, TP27	131	POISON
G	**Nitriles, toxic, liquid, n.o.s.**	6.1	UN3276	I	6.1	5, T14, TP2, TP13, TP27	151	POISON
				II	6.1	IB2, T11, TP2, TP27	151	POISON
				III	6.1	IB3, T7, TP1, TP28	151	POISON

Symbols	Hazardous materials descriptions and proper shipping names	Hazard class or Division	Identification Numbers	PG	Label Codes	Special provisions (§172.102)	ERG Guide No.	Placard Advisory Consult §172.504 & §172.505 *Placard any quantity
(1)	(2)	(3)	(4)	(5)	(6)	(7)		
G	**Nitriles, toxic, solid, n.o.s.**	6.1	UN3439	I	6.1	IB7, IP1, T6, TP33	151	POISON
				II	6.1	IB8, IP2, IP4, T3, TP33	151	POISON
				III	6.1	IB8, IP3, T1, TP33	151	POISON
	Nitrites, inorganic, aqueous solution, n.o.s.	5.1	UN3219	II	5.1	IB1, T4, TP1	140	OXIDIZER
				III	5.1	IB2, T4, TP1	140	OXIDIZER
	Nitrites, inorganic, n.o.s.	5.1	UN2627	II	5.1	33, IB8, IP4, T3, TP33	140	OXIDIZER
	3-Nitro-4-chlorobenzotrifluoride	6.1	UN2307	II	6.1	IB2, T7, TP2	152	POISON
	6-Nitro-4-diazotoluene-3-sulfonic acid (dry)	Forbidden						
	Nitro isobutane triol trinitrate	Forbidden						
	N-Nitro-N-methylglycolamide nitrate	Forbidden						
	2-Nitro-2-methylpropanol nitrate	Forbidden						
	Nitro urea	1.1D	UN0147	II	1.1D		112	EXPLOSIVES 1.1*
	N-Nitroaniline	Forbidden						
+	**Nitroanilines** *(o-; m-; p-;)*	6.1	UN1661	II	6.1	IB8, IP2, IP4, T3, TP33	153	POISON
	Nitroanisole, liquid	6.1	UN2730	III	6.1	IB3, T4, TP1	152	POISON
	Nitroanisoles, solid	6.1	UN3458	III	6.1	IB8, IP3, T1, TP33	152	POISON

Sym-bols	Hazardous materials descriptions and proper shipping names	Hazard class or Division	Identifica-tion Numbers	PG	Label Codes	Special provisions (§172.102)	ERG Guide No.	Placard Advisory Consult §172.504 & §172.505 *Placard any quantity
(1)	(2)	(3)	(4)	(5)	(6)	(7)		
+	**Nitrobenzene**	6.1	UN1662	II	6.1	IB2, T7, TP2	152	POISON
	m-Nitrobenzene diazonium perchlorate	Forbidden						
	Nitrobenzenesulfonic acid	8	UN2305	II	8	B2, B4, IB8, IP2, IP4, T3, TP33	153	CORROSIVE
	Nitrobenzol, see **Nitrobenzene**							
	5-Nitrobenzotriazol	1.1D	UN0385	II	1.1D		112	EXPLOSIVES 1.1*
	Nitrobenzotrifluorides, liquid	6.1	UN2306	II	6.1	IB2, T7, TP2	152	POISON
	Nitrobenzotrifluorides, solid	6.1	UN3431	II	6.1	IB8, IP2, IP4, T3, TP33	152	POISON
	Nitrobromobenzenes, liquid	6.1	UN2732	III	6.1	IB3, T4, TP1	152	POISON
	Nitrobromobenzenes, solid	6.1	UN3459	III	6.1	IB8, IP3, T1, TP33	152	POISON
	Nitrocellulose, *dry or wetted with less than 25 percent water (or alcohol), by mass*	1.1D	UN0340	II	1.1D		112	EXPLOSIVES 1.1*
	Nitrocellulose membrane filters, *with not more than 12.6% nitrogen, by dry mass*	4.1	UN3270	II	4.1	43, A1	133	FLAMMABLE SOLID
	Nitrocellulose, plasticized *with not less than 18 percent plasticizing substance, by mass*	1.3C	UN0343	II	1.3C		112	EXPLOSIVES 1.3*

Symbols	Hazardous materials descriptions and proper shipping names	Hazard class or Division	Identification Numbers	PG	Label Codes	Special provisions (§172.102)	ERG Guide No.	Placard Advisory Consult §172.504 & §172.505 *Placard any quantity
(1)	(2)	(3)	(4)	(5)	(6)	(7)		
	Nitrocellulose, solution, flammable *with not more than 12.6 percent nitrogen, by mass, and not more than 55 percent nitrocellulose*	3	UN2059	I	3	T11. TP1, TP8, TP27	127	FLAMMABLE
				II	3	IB2, T4, TP1, TP8	127	FLAMMABLE
				III	3	B1, IB3, T2, TP1	127	FLAMMABLE
	Nitrocellulose, *unmodified or plasticized with less than 18 percent plasticizing substance, by mass*	1.1D	UN0341	II	1.1D		112	EXPLOSIVES 1.1*
	Nitrocellulose, wetted *with not less than 25 percent alcohol, by mass*	1.3C	UN0342	II	1.3C		112	EXPLOSIVES 1.3*
	Nitrocellulose with alcohol *with not less than 25 percent alcohol by mass, and with not more than 12.6 percent nitrogen, by dry mass*	4.1	UN2556	II	4.1		113	FLAMMABLE SOLID
	Nitrocellulose, *with not more than 12.6 percent nitrogen, by dry mass, or* **Nitrocellulose mixture with pigment** *or* **Nitrocellulose mixture with plasticizer** *or* **Nitrocellulose mixture with pigment and plasticizer**	4.1	UN2557	II	4.1	44	133	FLAMMABLE SOLID
	Nitrocellulose with water *with not less than 25 percent water, by mass*	4.1	UN2555	II	4.1		113	FLAMMABLE SOLID
	Nitrochlorobenzene, see **Chloronitrobenzenes** *etc.*							

Sym-bols	Hazardous materials descriptions and proper shipping names	Hazard class or Division	Identification Numbers	PG	Label Codes	Special provisions (§172.102)	ERG Guide No.	Placard Advisory Consult §172.504 & §172.505 *Placard any quantity
(1)	(2)	(3)	(4)	(5)	(6)	(7)		
	Nitrocresols, solid	6.1	UN2446	III	6.1	IB8, IP3, T1, TP33	153	POISON
	Nitrocresols, liquid	6.1	UN3434	III	6.1	IB3, T4, TP1	153	POISON
	Nitroethane	3	UN2842	III	3	B1, IB3, T2, TP1	129	FLAMMABLE
	Nitroethyl nitrate	Forbidden						
	Nitroethylene polymer	Forbidden						
	Nitrogen, compressed	2.2	UN1066		2.2		121	NONFLAMMABLE GAS
	Nitrogen dioxide *see* **Dinitrogen tetroxide**							
	Nitrogen fertilizer solution, see **Fertilizer ammoniating solution** *etc.*							
	Nitrogen, mixtures with rare gases, see **Rare gases and nitrogen mixtures**							
	Nitrogen peroxide, see **Dinitrogen tetroxide**							
	Nitrogen, refrigerated liquid *cryogenic liquid*	2.2	UN1977		2.2	T75, TP5	120	NONFLAMMABLE GAS
	Nitrogen tetroxide and nitric oxide mixtures, see **Nitric oxide and nitrogen tetroxide mixtures**							
	Nitrogen tetroxide, see **Dinitrogen tetroxide**							
	Nitrogen trichloride	Forbidden						

Sym-bols	Hazardous materials descriptions and proper shipping names	Hazard class or Division	Identifica-tion Numbers	PG	Label Codes	Special provisions (§172.102)	ERG Guide No.	Placard Advisory Consult §172.504 & §172.505 *Placard any quantity
(1)	(2)	(3)	(4)	(5)	(6)	(7)		
	Nitrogen trifluoride	2.2	UN2451		2.2, 5.1		122	NONFLAMMABLE GAS
	Nitrogen triiodide	Forbidden						
	Nitrogen triiodide monoamine	Forbidden						
	Nitrogen trioxide	2.3	UN2421		2.3, 5.1, 8	1	124	POISON GAS*
	Nitroglycerin, desensitized *with not less than 40 percent non-volatile water insoluble phlegmatizer, by mass*	1.1D	UN0143	II	1.1D, 6.1	125	112	EXPLOSIVES 1.1*
	Nitroglycerin, liquid, not desensitized	Forbidden						
	Nitroglycerin mixture, desensitized, liquid, flammable, n.o.s. *with not more than 30 percent nitroglycerin, by mass*	3	UN3343		3	129	113	FLAMMABLE
	Nitroglycerin mixture, desensitized, liquid, n.o.s. *with not more than 30% nitroglycer in, by mass*	3	UN3357	II	3	142	113	FLAMMABLE
	Nitroglycerin mixture, desensitized, solid, n.o.s. *with more than 2 percent but not more than 10 percent nitro-glycerin, by mass*	4.1	UN3319	II	4.1	118	113	FLAMMABLE SOLID
	Nitroglycerin, solution in alcohol, *with more than 1 percent but not more than 5 percent nitroglycerin*	3	UN3064	II	3	N8	127	FLAMMABLE

Sym-bols	Hazardous materials descriptions and proper shipping names	Hazard class or Division	Identifica-tion Numbers	PG	Label Codes	Special provisions (§172.102)	ERG Guide No.	Placard Advisory Consult §172.504 & §172.505 *Placard any quantity
(1)	(2)	(3)	(4)	(5)	(6)	(7)		
	Nitroglycerin, solution in alcohol, *with more than 1 percent but not more than 10 percent nitrogylcerin*	1.1D	UN0144	II	1.1D		112	EXPLOSIVES 1.1*
	Nitroglycerin solution in alcohol *with not more than 1 percent nitroglycerin*	3	UN1204	II	3	IB2, N34	127	FLAMMABLE
	Nitroguanidine nitrate	Forbidden						
	Nitroguanidine *or* **Picrite,** *dry or wetted with less than 20 percent water, by mass*	1.1D	UN0282	II	1.1D		112	EXPLOSIVES 1.1*
	Nitroguanidine, wetted *or* **Picrite, wetted** *with not less than 20 percent water, by mass*	4.1	UN1336	I	4.1	23, A8, A19, A20, N41	113	FLAMMABLE SOLID
	1-Nitrohydantoin	Forbidden						
	Nitrohydrochloric acid	8	UN1798	I	8	A3, B10, N41, T10, TP2, TP12, TP13	157	CORROSIVE
	Nitromannite (dry)	Forbidden						
	Nitromannite, wetted, *see* **Mannitol hexanitrate,** *etc.*							
	Nitromethane	3	UN1261	II	3		129	FLAMMABLE
	Nitromuriatic acid, see **Nitrohydrochloric acid**							
	Nitronaphthalene	4.1	UN2538	III	4.1	A1, IB8, IP3, T1, TP33	133	FLAMMABLE SOLID

Sym-bols	Hazardous materials descriptions and proper shipping names	Hazard class or Division	Identification Numbers	PG	Label Codes	Special provisions (§172.102)	ERG Guide No.	Placard Advisory Consult §172.504 & §172.505 *Placard any quantity
(1)	(2)	(3)	(4)	(5)	(6)	(7)		
+	**Nitrophenols** *(o-; m-; p-;)*	6.1	UN1663	III	6.1	IB8, IP3, T1, TP33	153	POISON
	m-Nitrophenyldinitro methane	Forbidden						
	4-Nitrophenylhydrazine, *with not less than 30% water, by mass*	4.1	UN3376	I	4.1	164, A8, A19, A20, N41	113	FLAMMABLE SOLID
	Nitropropanes	3	UN2608	III	3	B1, IB3, T2, TP1	129	FLAMMABLE
	p-Nitrosodimethylaniline	4.2	UN1369	II	4.2	A19, A20, IB6, IP2, N34, T3, TP33	135	SPONTANEOUSLY COMBUSTIBLE
	Nitrostarch, *dry or wetted with less than 20 percent water, by mass*	1.1D	UN0146	II	1.1D		112	EXPLOSIVES 1.1*
	Nitrostarch, wetted *with not less than 20 percent water, by mass*	4.1	UN1337	I	4.1	23, A8, A19, A20, N41	113	FLAMMABLE SOLID
	Nitrosugars (dry)	Forbidden						
	Nitrosyl chloride	2.3	UN1069		2.3, 8	3, B14	125	POISON GAS*
	Nitrosylsulfuric acid, liquid	8	UN2308	II	8	A3, A6, A7, B2, IB2, N34, T8, TP2, TP12	157	CORROSIVE
	Nitrosylsulphuric acid, solid	8	UN3456	II	8	IB8, IP2, IP4, T3, TP33	157	CORROSIVE
	Nitrotoluenes, liquid	6.1	UN1664	II	6.1	IB2, T7, TP2	152	POISON
	Nitrotoluenes, solid	6.1	UN3446	II	6.1	IB8, IP2, IP4, T3, TP33	152	POISON
	Nitrotoluidines (mono)	6.1	UN2660	III	6.1	IB8, IP3, T1, TP33	153	POISON

Symbols	Hazardous materials descriptions and proper shipping names	Hazard class or Division	Identification Numbers	PG	Label Codes	Special provisions (§172.102)	ERG Guide No.	Placard Advisory Consult §172.504 & §172.505 *Placard any quantity
(1)	(2)	(3)	(4)	(5)	(6)	(7)		
	Nitrotriazolone *or* **NTO**	1.1D	UN0490	II	1.1D		112	EXPLOSIVES 1.1*
	Nitrous oxide and carbon dioxide mixtures, see **Carbon dioxide and nitrous oxide mixtures**							
	Nitrous oxide	2.2	UN1070		2.2, 5.1	A14	122	NONFLAMMABLE GAS
	Nitrous oxide, refrigerated liquid	2.2	UN2201		2.2, 5.1	B6, T75, TP5, TP22	122	NONFLAMMABLE GAS
	Nitroxylenes, liquid	6.1	UN1665	II	6.1	IB2, T7, TP2	152	POISON
	Nitroxylenes, solid	6.1	UN3447	II	6.1	IB8, IP2, IP4, T3, TP33	152	POISON
	Nitroxylol, see **Nitroxylenes**							
	Nonanes	3	UN1920	III	3	B1, IB3, T2, TP1	128	FLAMMABLE
	Nonflammable gas, n.o.s., see **Compressed gas,** *etc. or* **Liquefied gas,** *etc.*							
	Nonliquefied gases, see **Compressed gases,** *etc.*							
	Nonliquefied hydrocarbon gas, see **Hydrocarbon gas mixture, compressed, n.o.s.**							
	Nonyltrichlorosilane	8	UN1799	II	8	A7, B2, B6, IB2, N34, T7, TP2, TP13	156	CORROSIVE

Sym-bols	Hazardous materials descriptions and proper shipping names	Hazard class or Division	Identification Numbers	PG	Label Codes	Special provisions (§172.102)	ERG Guide No.	Placard Advisory Consult §172.504 & §172.505 *Placard any quantity
(1)	(2)	(3)	(4)	(5)	(6)	(7)		
	2,5-Norbornadiene, stabilized, see **Bicyclo 2,2,1 hepta-2,5-diene, stabilized**							
	Nordhausen acid, see **Sulfuric acid, fuming** *etc.*							
	Octadecyltrichlorosilane	8	UN1800	II	8	A7, B2, B6, IB2, N34, T7, TP2, TP13	156	CORROSIVE
	Octadiene	3	UN2309	II	3	B1, IB2, T4, TP1	128P	FLAMMABLE
	1,7-Octadine-3,5-diyne-1,8-dimethoxy-9-octa decynoic acid	Forbidden						
	Octafluorobut-2-ene *or* **Refrigerant gas R 1318**	2.2	UN2422		2.2		126	NONFLAMMABLE GAS
	Octafluorocyclobutane *or* **Refrigerant gas RC 318**	2.2	UN1976		2.2	T50	126	NONFLAMMABLE GAS
	Octafluoropropane *or* **Refrigerant gas R 218**	2.2	UN2424		2.2	T50	126	NONFLAMMABLE GAS
	Octanes	3	UN1262	II	3	IB2, T4, TP1	128	FLAMMABLE
	Octogen, *etc. see* **Cyclotetramethylene tetranitramine,** *etc.*							
	Octolite *or* **Octol,** *dry or wetted with less than 15 percent water, by mass*	1.1D	UN0266	II	1.1D		112	EXPLOSIVES 1.1*
	Octonal	1.1D	UN0496		1.1D		112	EXPLOSIVES 1.1*

Symbols (1)	Hazardous materials descriptions and proper shipping names (2)	Hazard class or Division (3)	Identification Numbers (4)	PG (5)	Label Codes (6)	Special provisions (§172.102) (7)	ERG Guide No.	Placard Advisory Consult §172.504 & §172.505 *Placard any quantity
	Octyl aldehydes	3	UN1191	III	3	B1, IB3, T2, TP1	129	FLAMMABLE
	Octyltrichlorosilane	8	UN1801	II	8	A7, B2, B6, IB2, N34, T7, TP2, TP13	156	CORROSIVE
	Oil gas, compressed	2.3	UN1071		2.3, 2.1	6	119	POISON GAS*
	Oleum, see **Sulfuric acid, fuming**							
	Organic peroxide type A, liquid or solid	Forbidden						
G	**Organic peroxide type B, liquid**	5.2	UN3101	II	5.2, 1	53	146	ORGANIC PEROXIDE
G	**Organic peroxide type B, liquid, temperature controlled**	5.2	UN3111	II	5.2, 1	53	148	ORGANIC PEROXIDE*
G	**Organic peroxide type B, solid**	5.2	UN3102	II	5.2, 1	53	146	ORGANIC PEROXIDE
G	**Organic peroxide type B, solid, temperature controlled**	5.2	UN3112	II	5.2, 1	53	148	ORGANIC PEROXIDE*
G	**Organic peroxide type C, liquid**	5.2	UN3103	II	5.2		146	ORGANIC PEROXIDE
G	**Organic peroxide type C, liquid, temperature controlled**	5.2	UN3113	II	5.2		148	ORGANIC PEROXIDE
G	**Organic peroxide type C, solid**	5.2	UN3104	II	5.2		146	ORGANIC PEROXIDE

Symbols	Hazardous materials descriptions and proper shipping names	Hazard class or Division	Identification Numbers	PG	Label Codes	Special provisions (§172.102)	ERG Guide No.	Placard Advisory Consult §172.504 & §172.505 *Placard any quantity
(1)	(2)	(3)	(4)	(5)	(6)	(7)		
G	**Organic peroxide type C, solid, temperature controlled**	5.2	UN3114	II	5.2		148	ORGANIC PEROXIDE
G	**Organic peroxide type D, liquid**	5.2	UN3105	II	5.2		145	ORGANIC PEROXIDE
G	**Organic peroxide type D, liquid, temperature controlled**	5.2	UN3115	II	5.2		148	ORGANIC PEROXIDE
G	**Organic peroxide type D, solid**	5.2	UN3106	II	5.2		145	ORGANIC PEROXIDE
G	**Organic peroxide type D, solid, temperature controlled**	5.2	UN3116	II	5.2		148	ORGANIC PEROXIDE
G	**Organic peroxide type E, liquid**	5.2	UN3107	II	5.2		145	ORGANIC PEROXIDE
G	**Organic peroxide type E, liquid, temperature controlled**	5.2	UN3117	II	5.2		148	ORGANIC PEROXIDE
G	**Organic peroxide type E, solid**	5.2	UN3108	II	5.2		145	ORGANIC PEROXIDE
G	**Organic peroxide type E, solid, temperature controlled**	5.2	UN3118	II	5.2		148	ORGANIC PEROXIDE
G	**Organic peroxide type F, liquid**	5.2	UN3109	II	5.2	IP5	145	ORGANIC PEROXIDE
G	**Organic peroxide type F, liquid, temperature controlled**	5.2	UN3119	II	5.2	IP5	148	ORGANIC PEROXIDE
G	**Organic peroxide type F, solid**	5.2	UN3110	II	5.2	TP33	145	ORGANIC PEROXIDE

Sym-bols	Hazardous materials descriptions and proper shipping names	Hazard class or Division	Identifica-tion Numbers	PG	Label Codes	Special provisions (§172.102)	ERG Guide No.	Placard Advisory Consult §172.504 & §172.505 *Placard any quantity
(1)	(2)	(3)	(4)	(5)	(6)	(7)		
G	**Organic peroxide type F, solid, temperature controlled**	5.2	UN3120	II	5.2	TP33	148	ORGANIC PEROXIDE
D	**Organic phosphate, mixed with compressed gas** *or* **Organic phosphate compound, mixed with compressed gas** *or* **Organic phosphorus compound, mixed with compressed gas**	2.3	NA1955		2.3	3	123	POISON GAS*
	Organic pigments, self-heating	4.2	UN3313	II	4.2	IB8, IP2, IP4, T3, TP33	135	SPONTANEOUSLY COMBUSTIBLE
				III	4.2	IB8, IP3, T1, TP33	135	SPONTANEOUSLY COMBUSTIBLE
G	**Organoarsenic compound, liquid, n.o.s.**	6.1	UN3280	I	6.1	5, T14, TP2, TP13, TP27	151	POISON
				II	6.1	IB2, T11, TP2, TP27	151	POISON
				III	6.1	IB3, T7, TP1, TP28	151	POISON
G	**Organoarsenic compound, solid, n.o.s.**	6.1	UN3465	I	6.1	IB7, IP1, T6, TP33	151	POISON
				II	6.1	IB8, IP2, IP4, T3, TP33	151	POISON
				III	6.1	IB8, IP3, T1, TP33	151	POISON

Symbols	Hazardous materials descriptions and proper shipping names	Hazard class or Division	Identification Numbers	PG	Label Codes	Special provisions (§172.102)	ERG Guide No.	Placard Advisory Consult §172.504 & §172.505 *Placard any quantity
(1)	(2)	(3)	(4)	(5)	(6)	(7)		
	Organochlorine pesticides liquid, flammable, toxic, *flash point less than 23 degrees C*	3	UN2762	I	3, 6.1	T14, TP2, TP13, TP27	131	FLAMMABLE
				II	3, 6.1	IB2, T11, TP2, TP13, TP27	131	FLAMMABLE
	Organochlorine pesticides, liquid, toxic	6.1	UN2996	I	6.1	T14, TP2, TP13, TP27	151	POISON
				II	6.1	IB2, T11, TP2, TP13, TP27	151	POISON
				III	6.1	IB3, T7, TP2, TP28	151	POISON
	Organochlorine pesticides, liquid, toxic, flammable, *flash point not less than 23 degrees C*	6.1	UN2995	I	6.1, 3	T14, TP2, TP13, TP27	131	POISON
				II	6.1, 3	IB2, T11, TP2, TP13, TP27	131	POISON
				III	6.1, 3	B1, IB3, T7, TP2, TP28	131	POISON
	Organochlorine, pesticides, solid, toxic	6.1	UN2761	I	6.1	IB7, IP1, T6, TP33	151	POISON
				II	6.1	IB8, IP2, IP4, T3, TP33	151	POISON
				III	6.1	IB8, IP3, T1, TP33	151	POISON
G	**Organometallic compound, toxic, liquid, n.o.s.**	6.1	UN3282	I	6.1	T14, TP2, TP13, TP27	151	POISON

Sym-bols	Hazardous materials descriptions and proper shipping names	Hazard class or Division	Identification Numbers	PG	Label Codes	Special provisions (§172.102)	ERG Guide No.	Placard Advisory Consult §172.504 & §172.505 *Placard any quantity
(1)	(2)	(3)	(4)	(5)	(6)	(7)		
				II	6.1	IB2, T11, TP2, TP27	151	POISON
				III	6.1	IB3, T7, TP1, TP28	151	POISON
G	**Organometallic compound, toxic, solid, n.o.s.**	6.1	UN3467	I	6.1	IB7, IP1, T6, TP33	151	POISON
				II	6.1	IB8, IP2, IP4, T3, TP33	151	POISON
				III	6.1	IB8, IP3, T1, TP33	151	POISON
G	**Organometallic substance, liquid, pyrophoric**	4.2	UN3392	I	4.2	B11, T21, TP2, TP7	135	SPONTANEOUSLY COMBUSTIBLE
G	**Organometallic substance, liquid, pyrophoric, water-reactive**	4.2	UN3394	I	4.2, 4.3	B11, T21, TP2, TP7	135	SPONTANEOUSLY COMBUSTIBLE DANGEROUS WHEN WET*
G	**Organometallic substance, liquid, water-reactive**	4.3	UN3398	I	4.3	T13, TP2, TP7	135	DANGEROUS WHEN WET*
				II	4.3	IB1, T7, TP2, TP7	135	DANGEROUS WHEN WET*
				III	4.3	IB2, T7, TP2, TP7	135	DANGEROUS WHEN WET*
G	**Organometallic substance, liquid, water-reactive, flammable**	4.3	UN3399	I	4.3, 3	T13, TP2, TP7	138	DANGEROUS WHEN WET*
				II	4.3, 3	IB1, IP2, T7, TP2, TP7	138	DANGEROUS WHEN WET*

Sym-bols	Hazardous materials descriptions and proper shipping names	Hazard class or Division	Identification Numbers	PG	Label Codes	Special provisions (§172.102)	ERG Guide No.	Placard Advisory Consult §172.504 & §172.505 *Placard any quantity
(1)	(2)	(3)	(4)	(5)	(6)	(7)		
				III	4.3, 3	IB2, IP4, T7, TP2, TP7	138	DANGEROUS WHEN WET*
G	**Organometallic substance, solid, pyrophoric**	4.2	UN3391	I	4.2	T21, TP7, TP33	135	SPONTANEOUSLY COMBUSTIBLE
G	**Organometallic substance, solid, pyrophoric, water-reactive**	4.2	UN3393	I	4.2, 4.3	B11, T21, TP7, TP33	135	SPONTANEOUSLY COMBUSTIBLE DANGEROUS WHEN WET*
G	**Organometallic substance, solid, self-heating**	4.2	UN3400	II	4.2	IB6, T3, TP33	138	SPONTANEOUSLY COMBUSTIBLE
				III	4.2	IB8, T1, TP33	138	SPONTANEOUSLY COMBUSTIBLE
G	**Organometallic substance, solid, water-reactive**	4.3	UN3395	I	4.3	N40, T9, TP7, TP33	135	DANGEROUS WHEN WET*
				II	4.3	IB4, T3, TP33	135	DANGEROUS WHEN WET*
				III	4.3	IB6, T1, TP33	135	DANGEROUS WHEN WET*
G	**Organometallic substance, solid, water-reactive, flammable**	4.3	UN3396	I	4.3, 4.1	N40, T9, TP7, TP33	138	DANGEROUS WHEN WET*
				II	4.3, 4.1	IB4, T3, TP33	138	DANGEROUS WHEN WET*
				III	4.3, 4.1	IB6, T1, TP33	138	DANGEROUS WHEN WET*

Symbols	Hazardous materials descriptions and proper shipping names	Hazard class or Division	Identification Numbers	PG	Label Codes	Special provisions (§172.102)	ERG Guide No.	Placard Advisory Consult §172.504 & §172.505 *Placard any quantity
(1)	(2)	(3)	(4)	(5)	(6)	(7)		
G	**Organometallic substance, solid, water-reactive, self-heating**	4.3	UN3397	I	4.3, 4.2	N40, T9, TP7, TP33	138	DANGEROUS WHEN WET*
				II	4.3, 4.2	IB4, T3, TP33	138	DANGEROUS WHEN WET*
				III	4.3, 4.2	IB6, T1, TP33	138	DANGEROUS WHEN WET*
	Organophosphorus compound, toxic, flammable, n.o.s.	6.1	UN3279	I	6.1, 3	5, T14, TP2, TP13, TP27	131	POISON
				II	6.1, 3	IB2, T11, TP2, TP13, TP27	131	POISON
G	**Organophosphorus compound, toxic, liquid, n.o.s.**	6.1	UN3278	I	6.1	5, T14, TP2, TP13, TP27	151	POISON
				II	6.1	IB2, T11, TP2, TP27	151	POISON
				III	6.1	IB3, T7, TP1, TP28	151	POISON
G	**Organophosphorus compound, toxic, solid, n.o.s.**	6.1	UN3464	I	6.1	IB7, IP1, T6, TP33	151	POISON
				II	6.1	IB8, IP2, IP4, T3, TP33	151	POISON
				III	6.1	IB8, IP3, T1, TP33	151	POISON
	Organophosphorus pesticides, liquid, flammable, toxic, *flash point less than 23 degrees C*	3	UN2784	I	3, 6.1	T14, TP2, TP13, TP27	131	FLAMMABLE

Sym-bols	Hazardous materials descriptions and proper shipping names	Hazard class or Division	Identification Numbers	PG	Label Codes	Special provisions (§172.102)	ERG Guide No.	Placard Advisory Consult §172.504 & §172.505 *Placard any quantity
(1)	(2)	(3)	(4)	(5)	(6)	(7)		
				II	3, 6.1	IB2, T11, TP2, TP13, TP27	131	FLAMMABLE
	Organophosphorus pesticides, liquid, toxic	6.1	UN3018	I	6.1	N76, T14, TP2, TP13, TP27	152	POISON
				II	6.1	IB2, N76, T11, TP2, TP13, TP27	152	POISON
				III	6.1	IB3, N76, T7, TP2, TP28	152	POISON
	Organophosphorus pesticides, liquid, toxic, flammable, *flashpoint not less than 23 degrees C*	6.1	UN3017	I	6.1, 3	N76, T14, TP2, TP13, TP27	131	POISON
				II	6.1, 3	IB2, N76, T11, TP2, TP13, TP27	131	POISON
				III	6.1, 3	B1, IB3, N76, T7, TP2, TP28	131	POISON
	Organophosphorus pesticides, solid, toxic	6.1	UN2783	I	6.1	IB7, IP1, N77, T6, TP33	152	POISON
				II	6.1	IB8, IP2, IP4, N77, T3, TP33	152	POISON
				III	6.1	IB8, IP3, N77, T1, TP33	152	POISON
	Organotin compounds, liquid, n.o.s.	6.1	UN2788	I	6.1	A3, N33, N34, T14, TP2, TP13, TP27	153	POISON

Sym-bols	Hazardous materials descriptions and proper shipping names	Hazard class or Division	Identifica-tion Numbers	PG	Label Codes	Special provisions (§172.102)	ERG Guide No.	Placard Advisory Consult §172.504 & §172.505 *Placard any quantity
(1)	(2)	(3)	(4)	(5)	(6)	(7)		
				II	6.1	A3, IB2, N33, N34, T11, TP2, TP13, TP27	153	POISON
				III	6.1	IB3, T7, TP2, TP28	153	POISON
	Organotin compounds, solid, n.o.s.	6.1	UN3146	I	6.1	A5, IB7, IP1, T6, TP33	153	POISON
				II	6.1	IB8, IP2, IP4, T3, TP33	153	POISON
				III	6.1	IB8, IP3, T1, TP33	153	POISON
	Organotin pesticides, liquid, flammable, toxic, *flash point less than 23 degrees C*	3	UN2787	I	3, 6.1	T14, TP2, TP13, TP27	131	FLAMMABLE
				II	3, 6.1	IB2, T11, TP2, TP13, TP27	131	FLAMMABLE
	Organotin pesticides, liquid, toxic	6.1	UN3020	I	6.1	T14, TP2, TP13, TP27	153	POISON
				II	6.1	IB2, T11, TP2, TP13, TP27	153	POISON
				III	6.1	IB3, T7, TP2, TP28	153	POISON
	Organotin pesticides, liquid, toxic, flammable, *flashpoint not less than 23 degrees C*	6.1	UN3019	I	6.1, 3	T14, TP2, TP13, TP27	131	POISON
				II	6.1, 3	IB2, T11, TP2, TP13, TP27	131	POISON

Sym-bols	Hazardous materials descriptions and proper shipping names	Hazard class or Division	Identifica-tion Numbers	PG	Label Codes	Special provisions (§172.102)	ERG Guide No.	Placard Advisory Consult §172.504 & §172.505 *Placard any quantity
(1)	(2)	(3)	(4)	(5)	(6)	(7)		
				III	6.1, 3	B1, IB3, T7, TP2, TP28	131	POISON
	Organotin pesticides, solid, toxic	6.1	UN2786	I	6.1	IB7, IP1, T6, TP33	153	POISON
				II	6.1	IB8, IP2, IP4, T3, TP33	153	POISON
				III	6.1	IB8, IP3, T1, TP33	153	POISON
	Orthonitroaniline, see **Nitroanilines** *etc.*							
	Osmium tetroxide	6.1	UN2471	I	6.1	A8, IB7, IP1, N33, N34, T6, TP33	154	POISON
D G	**Other regulated substances, liquid, n.o.s.**	9	NA3082	III	9	IB3, T2, TP1	171	CLASS 9
D G	**Other regulated substances, solid, n.o.s.**	9	NA3077	III	9	B54, IB8, IP2	171	CLASS 9
G	**Oxidizing liquid, corrosive, n.o.s.**	5.1	UN3098	I	5.1, 8	A6	140	OXIDIZER
				II	5.1, 8	IB1	140	OXIDIZER
				III	5.1, 8	IB2	140	OXIDIZER
G	**Oxidizing liquid, n.o.s.**	5.1	UN3139	I	5.1	127, A2, A6	140	OXIDIZER
				II	5.1	127, A2, IB2	140	OXIDIZER
				III	5.1	127, A2, IB2	140	OXIDIZER
G	**Oxidizing liquid, toxic, n.o.s.**	5.1	UN3099	I	5.1, 6.1	A6	142	OXIDIZER

Sym-bols	Hazardous materials descriptions and proper shipping names	Hazard class or Division	Identifica-tion Numbers	PG	Label Codes	Special provisions (§172.102)	ERG Guide No.	Placard Advisory Consult §172.504 & §172.505 *Placard any quantity
(1)	(2)	(3)	(4)	(5)	(6)	(7)		
				II	5.1, 6.1	IB1	142	OXIDIZER
				III	5.1, 6.1	IB2	142	OXIDIZER
G	**Oxidizing solid, corrosive, n.o.s.**	5.1	UN3085	I	5.1, 8		140	OXIDIZER
				II	5.1, 8	IB6, IP2, T3, TP33	140	OXIDIZER
				III	5.1, 8	IB8, IP3, T1, TP33	140	OXIDIZER
G	**Oxidizing solid, flammable, n.o.s.**	5.1	UN3137	I	5.1, 4.1		140	OXIDIZER
G	**Oxidizing solid, n.o.s.**	5.1	UN1479	I	5.1	IB5, IP1	140	OXIDIZER
				II	5.1	IB8, IP2, IP4, T3, TP33	140	OXIDIZER
				III	5.1	IB8, IP3, T1, TP33	140	OXIDIZER
G	**Oxidizing solid, self-heating, n.o.s.**	5.1	UN3100	I	5.1, 4.2		135	OXIDIZER
				II	5.1, 4.2		135	OXIDIZER
G	**Oxidizing solid, toxic, n.o.s.**	5.1	UN3087	I	5.1, 6.1		141	OXIDIZER
				II	5.1, 6.1	IB6, IP2, T3, TP33	141	OXIDIZER
				III	5.1, 6.1	IB8, IP3, T1, TP33	141	OXIDIZER

Symbols	Hazardous materials descriptions and proper shipping names	Hazard class or Division	Identification Numbers	PG	Label Codes	Special provisions (§172.102)	ERG Guide No.	Placard Advisory Consult §172.504 & §172.505 *Placard any quantity
(1)	(2)	(3)	(4)	(5)	(6)	(7)		
G	**Oxidizing solid, water-reactive, n.o.s.**	5.1	UN3121		5.1, 4.3		144	OXIDIZER, DANGEROUS WHEN WET*
	Oxygen and carbon dioxide mixtures, see **Carbon dioxide and oxygen mixtures**							
	Oxygen, compressed	2.2	UN1072		2.2, 5.1	A14, A52	122	NONFLAMMABLE GAS
	Oxygen difluoride, compressed	2.3	UN2190		2.3, 5.1, 8	1	124	POISON GAS*
	Oxygen generator, chemical *(including when contained in associated equipment, e.g., passenger service units (PSUs), portable breathing equipment (PBE), etc.)*	5.1	UN3356	II	5.1	60, A51	140	OXIDIZER
+	**Oxygen generator, chemical, spent**	9	NA3356	III	9	61	140	CLASS 9
	Oxygen, mixtures with rare gases, see **Rare gases and oxygen mixtures**							
	Oxygen, refrigerated liquid *(cryogenic liquid)*	2.2	UN1073		2.2, 5.1	T75, TP5, TP22	122	NONFLAMMABLE GAS
	Paint *including paint, lacquer, enamel, stain, shellac solutions, varnish, polish, liquid filler, and liquid lacquer base*	3	UN1263	I	3	T11, TP1, TP8	128	FLAMMABLE
				II	3	149, B52, IB2, T4, TP1, TP8	128	FLAMMABLE

Sym-bols	Hazardous materials descriptions and proper shipping names	Hazard class or Division	Identifica-tion Numbers	PG	Label Codes	Special provisions (§172.102)	ERG Guide No.	Placard Advisory Consult §172.504 & §172.505 *Placard any quantity
(1)	(2)	(3)	(4)	(5)	(6)	(7)		
				III	3	B1, B52, IB3, T2, TP1	128	FLAMMABLE
	Paint *or* **Paint related material**	8	UN3066	II	8	B2, IB2, T7, TP2	153	CORROSIVE
				III	8	B52, IB3, T4, TP1	153	CORROSIVE
	Paint related material *including paint thinning, drying, removing, or reducing compound*	3	UN1263	I	3	T11, TP1, TP8	128	FLAMMABLE
				II	3	149, B52, IB2, T4, TP1, TP8	128	FLAMMABLE
				III	3	B1, B52, IB3, T2, TP1	128	FLAMMABLE
	Paper, unsaturated oil treated *incompletely dried (including carbon paper)*	4.2	UN1379	III	4.2	IB8, IP3	133	SPONTANEOUSLY COMBUSTIBLE
	Paraformaldehyde	4.1	UN2213	III	4.1	A1, IB8, IP3, T1, TP33	133	FLAMMABLE SOLID
	Paraldehyde	3	UN1264	III	3	B1, IB3, T2, TP1	129	FLAMMABLE
	Paranitroaniline, solid, see **Nitroanilines** *etc.*							
D	**Parathion and compressed gas mixture**	2.3	NA1967		2.3	3	123	POISON GAS*
	Paris green, solid, see **Copper acetoarsenite**							
A W	**PCB,** *see* **Polychlorinated biphenyls**							

Symbols	Hazardous materials descriptions and proper shipping names	Hazard class or Division	Identification Numbers	PG	Label Codes	Special provisions (§172.102)	ERG Guide No.	Placard Advisory Consult §172.504 & §172.505 *Placard any quantity
(1)	(2)	(3)	(4)	(5)	(6)	(7)		
+	**Pentaborane**	4.2	UN1380	I	4.2, 6.1	1	135	SPONTANEOUSLY COMBUSTIBLE, POISON INHALATION HAZARD*
	Pentachloroethane	6.1	UN1669	II	6.1	IB2, T7, TP2	151	POISON
	Pentachlorophenol	6.1	UN3155	II	6.1	IB8, IP2, IP4, T3, TP33	154	POISON
	Pentaerythrite tetranitrate (dry)	Forbidden						
	Pentaerythrite tetranitrate mixture, desensitized, solid, n.o.s. *with more than 10 percent but not more than 20 percent PETN, by mass*	4.1	UN3344	II	4.1	118, N85	113	FLAMMABLE SOLID
	Pentaerythrite tetranitrate *or* **Pentaerythritol tetranitrate** *or* **PETN,** *with not less than 7 percent wax by mass*	1.1D	UN0411	II	1.1D		112	EXPLOSIVES 1.1*
	Pentaerythrite tetranitrate, wetted *or* **Pentaerythritol tetranitrate, wetted,** *or* **PETN, wetted** *with not less than 25 percent water, by mass, or* **Pentaerythrite tetranitrate,** *or* **Pentaerythritol tetranitrate** *or* **PETN, desensitized** *with not less than 15 percent phlegmatizer by mass*	1.1D	UN0150	II	1.1D	121	112	EXPLOSIVES 1.1*

Symbols	Hazardous materials descriptions and proper shipping names	Hazard class or Division	Identification Numbers	PG	Label Codes	Special provisions (§172.102)	ERG Guide No.	Placard Advisory Consult §172.504 & §172.505 *Placard any quantity
(1)	(2)	(3)	(4)	(5)	(6)	(7)		
	Pentaerythritol tetranitrate, *see* **Pentaerythrite tetranitrate,** *etc.*							
	Pentafluoroethane *or* **Refrigerant gas R 125**	2.2	UN3220		2.2	T50	126	NONFLAMMABLE GAS
	Pentamethylheptane	3	UN2286	III	3	B1, IB3, T2, TP1	128	FLAMMABLE
	Pentane-2,4-dione	3	UN2310	III	3, 6.1	B1, IB3, T4, TP1	131	FLAMMABLE
	Pentanes	3	UN1265	I	3	T11, TP2	128	FLAMMABLE
				II	3	IB2, IP8, T4, TP1	128	FLAMMABLE
	Pentanitroaniline (dry)	Forbidden						
	Pentanols	3	UN1105	II	3	IB2, T4, TP1, TP29	129	FLAMMABLE
				III	3	B1, B3, IB3, T2, TP1	129	FLAMMABLE
	1-Pentene (*n-amylene*)	3	UN1108	I	3	T11, TP2	128	FLAMMABLE
	1-Pentol	8	UN2705	II	8	B2, IB2, T7, TP2	153P	CORROSIVE
	Pentolite, *dry or wetted with less than 15 percent water, by mass*	1.1D	UN0151	II	1.1D		112	EXPLOSIVES 1.1*
	Pepper spray, see **Aerosols,** *etc. or* **Self-defense spray, non-pressurized**							
	Perchlorates, inorganic, aqueous solution, n.o.s.	5.1	UN3211	II	5.1	IB2, T4, TP1	140	OXIDIZER
				III	5.1	IB2, T4, TP1	140	OXIDIZER

Sym-bols	Hazardous materials descriptions and proper shipping names	Hazard class or Division	Identifica-tion Numbers	PG	Label Codes	Special provisions (§172.102)	ERG Guide No.	Placard Advisory Consult §172.504 & §172.505 *Placard any quantity
(1)	(2)	(3)	(4)	(5)	(6)	(7)		
	Perchlorates, inorganic, n.o.s.	5.1	UN1481	II	5.1	IB6, IP2, T3, TP33	140	OXIDIZER
				III	5.1	IB8, IP3, T1, TP33	140	OXIDIZER
	Perchloric acid, with more than 72 percent acid by mass	Forbidden						
	Perchloric acid *with more than 50 percent but not more than 72 percent acid, by mass*	5.1	UN1873	I	5.1, 8	A2, A3, N41, T10, TP1, TP12	143	OXIDIZER
	Perchloric acid *with not more than 50 percent acid by mass*	8	UN1802	II	8, 5.1	IB2, N41, T7, TP2	140	CORROSIVE
	Perchloroethylene, see **Tetrachloroethylene**							
	Perchloromethyl mercaptan	6.1	UN1670	I	6.1	2, B9, B14, B32, B74, N34, T20, TP2, TP13, TP38, TP45	157	POISON INHALATION HAZARD*
	Perchloryl fluoride	2.3	UN3083		2.3, 5.1	2, B9, B14	124	POISON GAS*
	Percussion caps, see **Primers, cap type**							
	Perfluoro-2-butene, see **Octafluorobut-2-ene**							
	Perfluoro(ethyl vinyl ether)	2.1	UN3154		2.1		115	FLAMMABLE GAS
	Perfluoro(methyl vinyl ether)	2.1	UN3153		2.1	T50	115	FLAMMABLE GAS

Sym-bols	Hazardous materials descriptions and proper shipping names	Hazard class or Division	Identifica-tion Numbers	PG	Label Codes	Special provisions (§172.102)	ERG Guide No.	Placard Advisory Consult §172.504 & §172.505 *Placard any quantity
(1)	(2)	(3)	(4)	(5)	(6)	(7)		
	Perfumery products *with flammable solvents*	3	UN1266	II	3	149, IB2, T4, TP1, TP8	127	FLAMMABLE
				III	3	B1, IB3, T2, TP1	127	FLAMMABLE
	Permanganates, inorganic, aqueous solution, n.o.s.	5.1	UN3214	II	5.1	26, IB2, T4, TP1	140	OXIDIZER
	Permanganates, inorganic, n.o.s.	5.1	UN1482	II	5.1	26, A30, IB6, IP2, T3, TP33	140	OXIDIZER
				III	5.1	26, A30, IB8, IP3, T1, TP33	140	OXIDIZER
	Peroxides, inorganic, n.o.s.	5.1	UN1483	II	5.1	A7, A20, IB6, IP2, N34, T3, TP33	140	OXIDIZER
				III	5.1	A7, A20, IB8, IP3, N34, T1, TP33	140	OXIDIZER
	Peroxyacetic acid, with more than 43 percent and with more than 6 percent hydrogen peroxide	Forbidden						
	Persulfates, inorganic, aqueous solution, n.o.s.	5.1	UN3216	III	5.1	IB2, T4, TP1, TP29	140	OXIDIZER
	Persulfates, inorganic, n.o.s.	5.1	UN3215	III	5.1	IB8, IP3, T1, TP33	140	OXIDIZER
G	**Pesticides, liquid, flammable, toxic,** *flash point less than 23 degrees C*	3	UN3021	I	3, 6.1	B5, T14, TP2, TP13, TP27	131	FLAMMABLE
				II	3, 6.1	IB2, T11, TP2, TP13, TP27	131	FLAMMABLE

Sym-bols	Hazardous materials descriptions and proper shipping names	Hazard class or Division	Identifica-tion Numbers	PG	Label Codes	Special provisions (§172.102)	ERG Guide No.	Placard Advisory Consult §172.504 & §172.505 *Placard any quantity
(1)	(2)	(3)	(4)	(5)	(6)	(7)		
G	**Pesticides, liquid, toxic, flammable, n.o.s.** *flash point not less than 23 degrees C*	6.1	UN2903	I	6.1, 3	T14, TP2, TP13, TP27	131	POISON
				II	6.1, 3	IB2, T11, TP2, TP13, TP27	131	POISON
				III	6.1, 3	B1, IB3, T7, TP2	131	POISON
G	**Pesticides, liquid, toxic, n.o.s.**	6.1	UN2902	I	6.1	T14, TP2, TP13, TP27	151	POISON
				II	6.1	IB2, T11, TP2, TP13, TP27	151	POISON
				III	6.1	IB3, T7, TP2, TP28	151	POISON
G	**Pesticides, solid, toxic, n.o.s.**	6.1	UN2588	I	6.1	IB7, T6, TP33	151	POISON
				II	6.1	IB8, IP2, IP4, T3, TP33	151	POISON
				III	6.1	IB8, IP3, T1, TP33	151	POISON
	PETN, *see* **Pentaerythrite tetranitrate**							
	PETN/TNT, *see* **Pentolite,** *etc.*							
	Petrol, *see* **Gasoline**							
	Petroleum crude oil	3	UN1267	I	3	144, T11, TP1, TP8	128	FLAMMABLE
				II	3	144, IB2, T4, TP1, TP8	128	FLAMMABLE

Sym-bols	Hazardous materials descriptions and proper shipping names	Hazard class or Division	Identifica-tion Numbers	PG	Label Codes	Special provisions (§172.102)	ERG Guide No.	Placard Advisory Consult §172.504 & §172.505 *Placard any quantity
(1)	(2)	(3)	(4)	(5)	(6)	(7)		
				III	3	144, B1, IB3, T2, TP1	128	FLAMMABLE
	Petroleum distillates, n.o.s. *or* **Petroleum products, n.o.s.**	3	UN1268	I	3	144, T11, TP1, TP8	128	FLAMMABLE
				II	3	144, IB2, T7, TP1, TP8, TP28	128	FLAMMABLE
				III	3	144, B1, IB3, T4, TP1, TP29	128	FLAMMABLE
	Petroleum gases, liquefied *or* **Liquefied petroleum gas**	2.1	UN1075		2.1	T50	115	FLAMMABLE GAS
D	**Petroleum oil**	3	NA1270	I	3	144, T11, TP1	128	FLAMMABLE
				II	3	144, IB2, T7, TP1, TP8, TP28	128	FLAMMABLE
				III	3	144, B1, IB3, T4, TP1, TP29	128	FLAMMABLE
	Phenacyl bromide	6.1	UN2645	II	6.1	IB8, IP2, IP4, T3, TP33	153	POISON
+	**Phenetidines**	6.1	UN2311	III	6.1	IB3, T4, TP1	153	POISON
	Phenol, molten	6.1	UN2312	II	6.1	B14, T7, TP3	153	POISON
+	**Phenol, solid**	6.1	UN1671	II	6.1	IB8, IP2, IP4, N78, T3, TP33	153	POISON
	Phenol solutions	6.1	UN2821	II	6.1	IB2, T7, TP2	153	POISON
				III	6.1	IB3, T4, TP1	153	POISON

Sym-bols	Hazardous materials descriptions and proper shipping names	Hazard class or Division	Identifica-tion Numbers	PG	Label Codes	Special provisions (§172.102)	ERG Guide No.	Placard Advisory Consult §172.504 & §172.505 *Placard any quantity
(1)	(2)	(3)	(4)	(5)	(6)	(7)		
	Phenolsulfonic acid, liquid	8	UN1803	II	8	B2, IB2, N41, T7, TP2	153	CORROSIVE
	Phenoxyacetic acid derivative pesticide, liquid, flammable, toxic, *flash point less than 23 degrees C*	3	UN3346	I	3, 6.1	T14, TP2, TP13, TP27	131	FLAMMABLE
				II	3, 6.1	IB2, T11, TP2, TP13, TP27	131	FLAMMABLE
	Phenoxyacetic acid derivative pesticide, liquid, toxic	6.1	UN3348	I	6.1	T14, TP2, TP13, TP27	153	POISON
				II	6.1	IB2, T11, TP2, TP27	153	POISON
				III	6.1	IB3, T7, TP2, TP28	153	POISON
	Phenoxyacetic acid derivative pesticide, liquid, toxic, flammable, *flash point not less than 23 degrees C*	6.1	UN3347	I	6.1, 3	T14, TP2, TP13, TP27	131	POISON
				II	6.1, 3	IB2, T11, TP2, TP13, TP27	131	POISON
				III	6.1, 3	IB3, T7, TP2, TP28	131	POISON
	Phenoxyacetic acid derivative pesticide, solid, toxic	6.1	UN3345	I	6.1	IB7, IP1, T6, TP33	153	POISON
				II	6.1	IB8, IP2, IP4, T3, TP33	153	POISON
				III	6.1	IB8, IP3, T1, TP33	153	POISON

Symbols	Hazardous materials descriptions and proper shipping names	Hazard class or Division	Identification Numbers	PG	Label Codes	Special provisions (§172.102)	ERG Guide No.	Placard Advisory Consult §172.504 & §172.505 *Placard any quantity
(1)	(2)	(3)	(4)	(5)	(6)	(7)		
	Phenyl chloroformate	6.1	UN2746	II	6.1, 8	IB2, T7, TP2, TP13	156	POISON
	Phenyl isocyanate	6.1	UN2487	I	6.1, 3	2, B9, B14, B32, B74, B77, N33, N34, T20, TP2, TP13, TP38, TP45	155	POISON INHALATION HAZARD*
	Phenyl mercaptan	6.1	UN2337	I	6.1, 3	2, B9, B14, B32, B74, B77, T20, TP2, TP13, TP38, TP45	131	POISON INHALATION HAZARD*
	Phenyl phosphorus dichloride	8	UN2798	II	8	B2, B15, IB2, T7, TP2	137	CORROSIVE
	Phenyl phosphorus thiodichloride	8	UN2799	II	8	B2, B15, IB2, T7, TP2	137	CORROSIVE
	Phenyl urea pesticides, liquid, toxic	6.1	UN3002	I	6.1	T14, TP2, TP27	151	POISON
				II	6.1	T7, TP2	151	POISON
				III	6.1	T4, TP1	151	POISON
	Phenylacetonitrile, liquid	6.1	UN2470	III	6.1	IB3, T4, TP1	152	POISON
	Phenylacetyl chloride	8	UN2577	II	8	B2, IB2, T7, TP2	156	CORROSIVE
	Phenylcarbylamine chloride	6.1	UN1672	I	6.1	2, B9, B14, B32, B74, T20, TP2, TP13, TP38, TP45	151	POISON INHALATION HAZARD*
	m-Phenylene diaminediperchlorate (dry)	Forbidden						
+	**Phenylenediamines** *(o-; m-; p-;)*	6.1	UN1673	III	6.1	IB8, IP3, T1, TP33	153	POISON
	Phenylhydrazine	6.1	UN2572	II	6.1	IB2, T7, TP2	153	POISON

Symbols	Hazardous materials descriptions and proper shipping names	Hazard class or Division	Identification Numbers	PG	Label Codes	Special provisions (§172.102)	ERG Guide No.	Placard Advisory Consult §172.504 & §172.505 *Placard any quantity
(1)	(2)	(3)	(4)	(5)	(6)	(7)		
	Phenylmercuric acetate	6.1	UN1674	II	6.1	IB8, IP2, IP4, T3, TP33	151	POISON
	Phenylmercuric compounds, n.o.s.	6.1	UN2026	I	6.1	IB7, IP1, T6, TP33	151	POISON
				II	6.1	IB8, IP2, IP4, T3, TP33	151	POISON
				III	6.1	IB8, IP3, T1, TP33	151	POISON
	Phenylmercuric hydroxide	6.1	UN1894	II	6.1	IB8, IP2, IP4, T3, TP33	151	POISON
	Phenylmercuric nitrate	6.1	UN1895	II	6.1	IB8, IP2, IP4, T3, TP33	151	POISON
	Phenyltrichlorosilane	8	UN1804	II	8	A7, B6, IB2, N34, T7, TP2	156	CORROSIVE
	Phosgene	2.3	UN1076		2.3, 8	1, B7, B46	125	POISON GAS*
	9-Phosphabicyclononanes *or* **Cyclooctadiene phosphines**	4.2	UN2940	II	4.2	A19, IB6, IP2, T3, TP33	135	SPONTANEOUSLY COMBUSTIBLE
	Phosphine	2.3	UN2199		2.3, 2.1	1	119	POISON GAS*
	Phosphoric acid solution	8	UN1805	III	8	A7, IB3, N34, T4, TP1	154	CORROSIVE
	Phosphoric acid, solid	8	UN3453	III	8	IB8, IP3, T1, TP33	154	CORROSIVE
	Phosphoric acid triethyleneimine, see **Tris-(1-aziridiyl)phosphine oxide, solution**							
	Phosphoric anhydride, see **Phosphorus pentoxide**							

Sym-bols	Hazardous materials descriptions and proper shipping names	Hazard class or Division	Identifica-tion Numbers	PG	Label Codes	Special provisions (§172.102)	ERG Guide No.	Placard Advisory Consult §172.504 & §172.505 *Placard any quantity
(1)	(2)	(3)	(4)	(5)	(6)	(7)		
	Phosphorous acid	8	UN2834	III	8	IB8, IP3, T1, TP33	154	CORROSIVE
	Phosphorus, amorphous	4.1	UN1338	III	4.1	A1, A19, B1, B9, B26, IB8, IP3, T1, TP33	133	FLAMMABLE SOLID
	Phosphorus bromide, see **Phosphorus tribromide**							
	Phosphorus chloride, see **Phosphorus trichloride**							
	Phosphorus heptasulfide, *free from yellow or white phosphorus*	4.1	UN1339	II	4.1	A20, IB4, N34, T3, TP33	139	FLAMMABLE SOLID
	Phosphorus oxybromide	8	UN1939	II	8	B8, IB8, IP2, IP4, N41, N43, T3, TP33	137	CORROSIVE
	Phosphorus oxybromide, molten	8	UN2576	II	8	B2, B8, IB1, N41, N43, T7, TP3, TP13	137	CORROSIVE
+	**Phosphorus oxychloride**	8	UN1810	II	8, 6.1	2, B9, B14, B32, B74, B77, N34, T20, TP2, TP38, TP45	137	CORROSIVE, POISON INHALATION HAZARD*
	Phosphorus pentabromide	8	UN2691	II	8	A7, IB8, IP2, IP4, N34, T3, TP33	137	CORROSIVE
	Phosphorus pentachloride	8	UN1806	II	8	A7, IB8, IP2, IP4, N34, T3, TP33	137	CORROSIVE

Sym-bols	Hazardous materials descriptions and proper shipping names	Hazard class or Division	Identification Numbers	PG	Label Codes	Special provisions (§172.102)	ERG Guide No.	Placard Advisory Consult §172.504 & §172.505 *Placard any quantity
(1)	(2)	(3)	(4)	(5)	(6)	(7)		
	Phosphorus pentafluoride	2.3	UN2198		2.3, 8	2, B9, B14	125	POISON GAS*
	Phosphorus pentasulfide, *free from yellow or white phosphorus*	4.3	UN1340	II	4.3, 4.1	A20, B59, IB4, T3, TP33	139	DANGEROUS WHEN WET*
	Phosphorus pentoxide	8	UN1807	II	8	A7, IB8, IP2, IP4, N34, T3, TP33	137	CORROSIVE
	Phosphorus sesquisulfide, *free from yellow or white phosphorus*	4.1	UN1341	II	4.1	A20, IB4, N34, T3, TP33	139	FLAMMABLE SOLID
	Phosphorus tribromide	8	UN1808	II	8	A3, A6, A7, B2, B25, IB2, N34, N43, T7, TP2	137	CORROSIVE
	Phosphorus trichloride	6.1	UN1809	I	6.1, 8	2, B9, B14, B15, B32, B74, B77, N34, T20, TP2, TP13, TP38, TP45	137	POISON INHALAZTION HAZARD*
	Phosphorus trioxide	8	UN2578	III	8	IB8, IP3, T1, TP33	157	CORROSIVE
	Phosphorus trisulfide, *free from yellow or white phosphorus*	4.1	UN1343	II	4.1	A20, IB4, N34, T3, TP33	139	FLAMMABLE SOLID
	Phosphorus, white dry *or* **Phosphorus, white, under water** *or* **Phosphorus white, in solution** *or* **Phosphorus, yellow dry** *or* **Phosphorus, yellow, under water** *or* **Phosphorus, yellow, in solution**	4.2	UN1381	I	4.2, 6.1	B9, B26, N34, T9, TP3, TP31	136	SPONTANEOUSLY COMBUSTIBLE
	Phosphorus white, molten	4.2	UN2447	I	4.2, 6.1	B9, B26, N34, T21, TP3, TP7, TP26	136	SPONTANEOUSLY COMBUSTIBLE

Sym-bols	Hazardous materials descriptions and proper shipping names	Hazard class or Division	Identification Numbers	PG	Label Codes	Special provisions (§172.102)	ERG Guide No.	Placard Advisory Consult §172.504 & §172.505 *Placard any quantity
(1)	(2)	(3)	(4)	(5)	(6)	(7)		
	Phosphorus (white or red) and a chlorate, mixtures of	Forbidden						
	Phosphoryl chloride, see **Phosphorus oxychloride**							
	Phthalic anhydride *with more than .05 percent maleic anhydride*	8	UN2214	III	8	IB8, IP3, T1, TP33	156	CORROSIVE
	Picolines	3	UN2313	III	3	B1, IB3, T4, TP1	129	FLAMMABLE
	Picric acid, *see* **Trinitrophenol,** *etc.*							
	Picrite, *see* **Nitroguanidine,** *etc.*							
	Picryl chloride, *see* **Trinitrochlorobenzene**							
	Pine oil	3	UN1272	III	3	B1, IB3, T2, TP1	129	FLAMMABLE
	alpha-Pinene	3	UN2368	III	3	B1, IB3, T2, TP1	128	FLAMMABLE
	Piperazine	8	UN2579	III	8	IB8, IP3, T1, TP33	153	CORROSIVE
	Piperidine	8	UN2401	I	8, 3	A10, T10, TP2	132	CORROSIVE
	Pivaloyl chloride, see **Trimethylacetyl chloride**							
	Plastic molding compound *in dough, sheet or extruded rope form evolving flammable vapor*	9	UN3314	III	9	32, IB8, IP3, IP7	171	CLASS 9
	Plastic solvent, n.o.s., see **Flammable liquids, n.o.s.**							

Symbols	Hazardous materials descriptions and proper shipping names	Hazard class or Division	Identification Numbers	PG	Label Codes	Special provisions (§172.102)	ERG Guide No.	Placard Advisory Consult §172.504 & §172.505 *Placard any quantity
(1)	(2)	(3)	(4)	(5)	(6)	(7)		
	Plastics, nitrocellulose-based, self-heating, n.o.s.	4.2	UN2006	III	4.2		135	SPONTANEOUSLY COMBUSTIBLE
	Poisonous gases, n.o.s., see **Compressed** *or* **liquefied gases, flammable** *or* **toxic, n.o.s.**							
	Polyalkylamines, n.o.s., see **Amines,** *etc.*							
	Polychlorinated biphenyls, liquid	9	UN2315	II	9	9, 81, 140, IB3, T4, TP1	171	CLASS 9
	Polychlorinated biphenyls, solid	9	UN3432	II	9	9, 81, 140, IB8, T3, TP33	171	CLASS 9
	Polyester resin kit	3	UN3269		3	40, 149	128	FLAMMABLE
	Polyhalogenated biphenyls, liquid *or* **Polyhalogenated terphenyls liquid**	9	UN3151	II	9	IB2	171	CLASS 9
	Polyhalogenated biphenyls, solid *or* **Polyhalogenated terphenyls, solid**	9	UN3152	II	9	IB8, IP2, IP4, T3, TP33	171	CLASS 9
	Polymeric beads, expandable, *evolving flammable vapor*	9	UN2211	III	9	32, IB8, IP3, IP7, T1, TP33	133	CLASS 9
	Potassium	4.3	UN2257	I	4.3	A7, A19, A20, B27, IB4, IP1, N6, N34, T9, TP7, TP33	138	DANGEROUS WHEN WET*
	Potassium arsenate	6.1	UN1677	II	6.1	IB8, IP2, IP4, T3, TP33	151	POISON

Symbols	Hazardous materials descriptions and proper shipping names	Hazard class or Division	Identification Numbers	PG	Label Codes	Special provisions (§172.102)	ERG Guide No.	Placard Advisory Consult §172.504 & §172.505 *Placard any quantity
(1)	(2)	(3)	(4)	(5)	(6)	(7)		
	Potassium arsenite	6.1	UN1678	II	6.1	IB8, IP2, IP4, T3, TP33	154	POISON
	Potassium bisulfite solution, see **Bisulfites, aqueous solutions, n.o.s.**							
	Potassium borohydride	4.3	UN1870	I	4.3	A19, N40	138	DANGEROUS WHEN WET*
	Potassium bromate	5.1	UN1484	II	5.1	IB8, IP4, T3, TP33	140	OXIDIZER
	Potassium carbonyl	Forbidden						
	Potassium chlorate	5.1	UN1485	II	5.1	A9, IB8, IP4, N34, T3, TP33	140	OXIDIZER
	Potassium chlorate, aqueous solution	5.1	UN2427	II	5.1	A2, IB2, T4, TP1	140	OXIDIZER
				III	5.1	A2, IB2, T4, TP1	140	OXIDIZER
	Potassium chlorate mixed with mineral oil, see **Explosive, blasting, type C**							
	Potassium cuprocyanide	6.1	UN1679	II	6.1	IB8, IP2, IP4, T3, TP33	157	POISON
	Potassium cyanide, solid	6.1	UN1680	I	6.1	B69, B77, IB7, IP1, N74, N75, T6, TP33	157	POISON
	Potassium cyanide solution	6.1	UN3413	I	6.1	B69, B77, N74, N75, T14, TP2, TP13	157	POISON

Symbols	Hazardous materials descriptions and proper shipping names	Hazard class or Division	Identification Numbers	PG	Label Codes	Special provisions (§172.102)	ERG Guide No.	Placard Advisory Consult §172.504 & §172.505 *Placard any quantity
(1)	(2)	(3)	(4)	(5)	(6)	(7)		
				II	6.1	B69, B77, IB2, N74, N75, T11, TP2, TP13, TP27	157	POISON
				III	6.1	B69, B77, IB3, N74, N75, T7, TP2, TP13, TP28	157	POISON
	Potassium dichloro isocyanurate or Potassium dichloro-s-triazinetrione, see **Dichloroisocyanuric acid, dry** *or* **Dichloroisocyanuric acid salts** *etc.*							
	Potassium dithionite *or* **Potassium hydrosulfite**	4.2	UN1929	II	4.2	A8, A19, A20, IB6, IP2, T3, TP33	135	SPONTANEOUSLY COMBUSTIBLE
	Potassium fluoride, solid	6.1	UN1812	III	6.1	IB8, IP3, T1, TP33	154	POISON
	Potassium fluoride solution	6.1	UN3422	III	6.1	IB3, T4, TP1	154	POISON
	Potassium fluoroacetate	6.1	UN2628	I	6.1	IB7, IP1, T6, TP33	151	POISON
	Potassium fluorosilicate	6.1	UN2655	III	6.1	IB8, IP3, T1, TP33	151	POISON
	Potassium hydrate, see **Potassium hydroxide, solid**							
	Potassium hydrogen fluoride, see **Potassium hydrogen difluoride**							
	Potassium hydrogen fluoride solution, see **Corrosive liquid, n.o.s.**							
	Potassium hydrogen sulfate	8	UN2509	II	8	A7, IB8, IP2, IP4, N34, T3, TP33	154	CORROSIVE

Symbols	Hazardous materials descriptions and proper shipping names	Hazard class or Division	Identification Numbers	PG	Label Codes	Special provisions (§172.102)	ERG Guide No.	Placard Advisory Consult §172.504 & §172.505 *Placard any quantity
(1)	(2)	(3)	(4)	(5)	(6)	(7)		
	Potassium hydrogendifluoride solid	8	UN1811	II	8, 6.1	IB8, IP2, IP4, N3, N34, T3, TP33	154	CORROSIVE
	Potassium hydrogendifluoride solution	8	UN3421	II	8, 6.1	IB2, N3, N34, T7, TP2	154	CORROSIVE
				III	8, 6.1	IB3, N3, N34, T4, TP1	154	CORROSIVE
	Potassium hydrosulfite, *see* **Potassium dithionite**							
	Potassium hydroxide, liquid, see **Potassium hydroxide solution**							
	Potassium hydroxide, solid	8	UN1813	II	8	IB8, IP2, IP4, T3, TP33	154	CORROSIVE
	Potassium hydroxide, solution	8	UN1814	II	8	B2, IB2, T7, TP2	154	CORROSIVE
				III	8	IB3, T4, TP1	154	CORROSIVE
	Potassium hypochlorite, solution, see **Hypochlorite solutions,** *etc.*							
	Potassium, metal alloys, liquid	4.3	UN1420	I	4.3	A7, A19, A20, B27	138	DANGEROUS WHEN WET*
	Potassium, metal alloys, solid	4.3	UN3403	I	4.3	A19, A20, B27, IB4, IP1, T9, TP7, TP33	138	DANGEROUS WHEN WET*
	Potassium metavanadate	6.1	UN2864	II	6.1	IB8, IP2, IP4, T3, TP33	151	POISON
	Potassium monoxide	8	UN2033	II	8	IB8, IP2, IP4, T3, TP33	154	CORROSIVE

Sym-bols	Hazardous materials descriptions and proper shipping names	Hazard class or Division	Identifica-tion Numbers	PG	Label Codes	Special provisions (§172.102)	ERG Guide No.	Placard Advisory Consult §172.504 & §172.505 *Placard any quantity
(1)	(2)	(3)	(4)	(5)	(6)	(7)		
	Potassium nitrate	5.1	UN1486	III	5.1	A1, A29, IB8, IP3, T1, TP33	140	OXIDIZER
	Potassium nitrate and sodium nitrite mixtures	5.1	UN1487	II	5.1	B78, IB8, IP4, T3, TP33	140	OXIDIZER
	Potassium nitrite	5.1	UN1488	II	5.1	IB8, IP4, T3, TP33	140	OXIDIZER
	Potassium perchlorate	5.1	UN1489	II	5.1	IB6, IP2, T3, TP33	140	OXIDIZER
	Potassium permanganate	5.1	UN1490	II	5.1	IB8, IP4, T3, TP33	140	OXIDIZER
	Potassium peroxide	5.1	UN1491	I	5.1	A20, IB6, IP1, N34	144	OXIDIZER
	Potassium persulfate	5.1	UN1492	III	5.1	A1, A29, IB8, IP3, T1, TP33	140	OXIDIZER
	Potassium phosphide	4.3	UN2012	I	4.3, 6.1	A19, N40	139	DANGEROUS WHEN WET*
	Potassium selenate, see **Selenates** *or* **Selenites**							
	Potassium selenite, see **Selenates** *or* **Selenites**							
	Potassium sodium alloys, liquid	4.3	UN1422	I	4.3	A7, A19, B27, N34, N40, T9, TP3, TP7, TP31	138	DANGEROUS WHEN WET*

Sym-bols	Hazardous materials descriptions and proper shipping names	Hazard class or Division	Identifica-tion Numbers	PG	Label Codes	Special provisions (§172.102)	ERG Guide No.	Placard Advisory Consult §172.504 & §172.505 *Placard any quantity
(1)	(2)	(3)	(4)	(5)	(6)	(7)		
	Potassium sodium alloys, solid	4.3	UN3404	I	4.3	A19, B27, N34, N40, T9, TP7, TP33	138	DANGEROUS WHEN WET*
	Potassium sulfide, anhydrous *or* **Potassium sulfide** *with less than 30 percent water of crystallization*	4.2	UN1382	II	4.2	A19, A20, B16, IB6, IP2, N34, T3, TP33	135	SPONTANEOUSLY COMBUSTIBLE
	Potassium sulfide, hydrated *with not less than 30 percent water of crystallization*	8	UN1847	II	8	IB8, IP2, IP4, T3, TP33	153	CORROSIVE
	Potassium superoxide	5.1	UN2466	I	5.1	A20, IB6, IP1	143	OXIDIZER
	Powder cake, wetted *or* **Powder paste, wetted** *with not less than 17 percent alcohol by mass*	1.1C	UN0433	II	1.1C		112	EXPLOSIVES 1.1*
	Powder cake, wetted *or* **Powder paste, wetted** *with not less than 25 percent water, by mass*	1.3C	UN0159	II	1.3C		112	EXPLOSIVES 1.3*
	Powder paste, *see* **Powder cake,** *etc.*							
	Powder, smokeless	1.1C	UN0160	II	1.1C		112	EXPLOSIVES 1.1*
	Powder, smokeless	1.3C	UN0161	II	1.3C		112	EXPLOSIVES 1.3*
	Power device, explosive, see **Cartridges, power device**							
	Primers, cap type	1.4S	UN0044	II	None		114	NONE
	Primers, cap type	1.1B	UN0377	II	1.1B		112	EXPLOSIVES 1.1*

Sym-bols	Hazardous materials descriptions and proper shipping names	Hazard class or Division	Identifica-tion Numbers	PG	Label Codes	Special provisions (§172.102)	ERG Guide No.	Placard Advisory Consult §172.504 & §172.505 *Placard any quantity
(1)	(2)	(3)	(4)	(5)	(6)	(7)		
	Primers, cap type	1.4B	UN0378	II	1.4B		114	EXPLOSIVES 1.4
	Primers, small arms, see **Primers, cap type**							
	Primers, tubular	1.3G	UN0319	II	1.3G		112	EXPLOSIVES 1.3*
	Primers, tubular	1.4G	UN0320	II	1.4G		114	EXPLOSIVES 1.4
	Primers, tubular	1.4S	UN0376	II	None		114	NONE
	Printing ink, *flammable or* **Printing ink related material** *(including printing ink thinning or reducing compound), flammable*	3	UN1210	I	3	T11, TP1,TP8	129	FLAMMABLE
				II	3	149, IB2, T4, TP1, TP8	129	FLAMMABLE
				III	3	B1, IB3, T2, TP1	129	FLAMMABLE
	Projectiles, illuminating, see **Ammunition, illuminating,** *etc.*							
	Projectiles, *inert with tracer*	1.4S	UN0345	II	1.4S		114	EXPLOSIVES 1.4
	Projectiles, *inert, with tracer*	1.3G	UN0424	II	1.3G		112	EXPLOSIVES 1.3*
	Projectiles, *inert, with tracer*	1.4G	UN0425	II	1.4G		114	EXPLOSIVES 1.4
	Projectiles, *with burster or expelling charge*	1.2D	UN0346	II	1.2D		112	EXPLOSIVES 1.2*
	Projectiles, *with burster or expelling charge*	1.4D	UN0347	II	1.4D		114	EXPLOSIVES 1.4

Sym-bols	Hazardous materials descriptions and proper shipping names	Hazard class or Division	Identifica-tion Numbers	PG	Label Codes	Special provisions (§172.102)	ERG Guide No.	Placard Advisory Consult §172.504 & §172.505 *Placard any quantity
(1)	(2)	(3)	(4)	(5)	(6)	(7)		
	Projectiles, *with burster or expelling charge*	1.2F	UN0426	II	1.2F		112	EXPLOSIVES 1.2*
	Projectiles, *with burster or expelling charge*	1.4F	UN0427	II	1.4F		114	EXPLOSIVES 1.4
	Projectiles, *with burster or expelling charge*	1.2G	UN0434	II	1.2G		112	EXPLOSIVES 1.2*
	Projectiles, *with burster or expelling charge*	1.4G	UN0435	II	1.4G		114	EXPLOSIVES 1.4
	Projectiles, *with bursting charge*	1.1F	UN0167	II	1.1F		112	EXPLOSIVES 1.1*
	Projectiles, *with bursting charge*	1.1D	UN0168	II	1.1D		112	EXPLOSIVES 1.1*
	Projectiles, *with bursting charge*	1.2D	UN0169	II	1.2D		112	EXPLOSIVES 1.2*
	Projectiles, *with bursting charge*	1.2F	UN0324	II	1.2F		112	EXPLOSIVES 1.2*
	Projectiles, *with bursting charge*	1.4D	UN0344	II	1.4D		114	EXPLOSIVES 1.4
	Propadiene, stabilized	2.1	UN2200		2.1		116P	FLAMMABLE GAS
	Propadiene mixed with methyl acetylene, see **Methyl acetylene and propadiene mixtures, stabilized**							
	Propane *see also* **Petroleum gases, liquefied**	2.1	UN1978		2.1	19, T50	115	FLAMMABLE GAS
	Propanethiols	3	UN2402	II	3	A6, IB2, T4, TP1, TP13	130	FLAMMABLE
	n-Propanol *or* **Propyl alcohol, normal**	3	UN1274	II	3	B1, IB2, T4, TP1	129	FLAMMABLE

Sym-bols	Hazardous materials descriptions and proper shipping names	Hazard class or Division	Identifica-tion Numbers	PG	Label Codes	Special provisions (§172.102)	ERG Guide No.	Placard Advisory Consult §172.504 & §172.505 *Placard any quantity
(1)	(2)	(3)	(4)	(5)	(6)	(7)		
				III	3	B1, IB3, T2, TP1	129	FLAMMABLE
	Propellant, liquid	1.3C	UN0495	II	1.3C	37	112	EXPLOSIVES 1.3*
	Propellant, liquid	1.1C	UN0497	II	1.1C	37	112	EXPLOSIVES 1.1*
	Propellant, solid	1.1C	UN0498	II	1.1C		112	EXPLOSIVES 1.1*
	Propellant, solid	1.3C	UN0499	II	1.3C		112	EXPLOSIVES 1.3*
	Propellant, soild	1.4C	UN0501		1.4C		114	EXPLOSIVES 1.4
	Propionaldehyde	3	UN1275	II	3	IB2, T7, TP1	129	FLAMMABLE
	Propionic acid	8	UN1848	III	8	IB3, T4, TP1	132	CORROSIVE
	Propionic anhydride	8	UN2496	III	8	IB3, T4, TP1	156	CORROSIVE
	Propionitrile	3	UN2404	II	3, 6.1	IB2, T7, TP1, TP13	131	FLAMMABLE
	Propionyl chloride	3	UN1815	II	3, 8	IB1, T7, TP1	132	FLAMMABLE
	n-Propyl acetate	3	UN1276	II	3	IB2, T4, TP1	129	FLAMMABLE
	Propyl alcohol, *see* **Propanol**							
	n-Propyl benzene	3	UN2364	III	3	B1, IB3, T2, TP1	128	FLAMMABLE
	Propyl chloride see **1-Chloropropane**							
	n-Propyl chloroformate	6.1	UN2740	I	6.1, 3, 8	2, B9, B14, B32, B74, B77, N34, T20, TP2, TP13, TP38, TP44	155	POISON INHALATION HAZARD*
	Propyl formates	3	UN1281	II	3	IB2, T4, TP1	129	FLAMMABLE

Symbols	Hazardous materials descriptions and proper shipping names	Hazard class or Division	Identification Numbers	PG	Label Codes	Special provisions (§172.102)	ERG Guide No.	Placard Advisory Consult §172.504 & §172.505 *Placard any quantity
(1)	(2)	(3)	(4)	(5)	(6)	(7)		
	n-Propyl isocyanate	6.1	UN2482	I	6.1, 3	1, B9, B14, B30, B72, T22, TP2, TP13, TP38, TP44	155	POISON INHALATION HAZARD*
	Propyl mercaptan, see **Propanethiols**							
	n-Propyl nitrate	3	UN1865	II	3	IB9	131	FLAMMABLE
	Propylamine	3	UN1277	II	3, 8	A7, IB2, N34, T7, TP1	132	FLAMMABLE
	Propylene *see also* **Petroleum gases, liquefied**	2.1	UN1077		2.1	19, T50	115	FLAMMABLE GAS
	Propylene chlorohydrin	6.1	UN2611	II	6.1, 3	IB2, T7, TP2, TP13	131	POISON
	Propylene oxide	3	UN1280	I	3	A3, N34, T11, TP2, TP7	127P	FLAMMABLE
	Propylene tetramer	3	UN2850	III	3	B1, IB3, T2, TP1	128	FLAMMABLE
	1,2-Propylenediamine	8	UN2258	II	8, 3	A3, A6, IB2, N34, T7, TP2	132	CORROSIVE
	Propyleneimine, stabilized	3	UN1921	I	3, 6.1	A3, N34, T14, TP2, TP13	131P	FLAMMABLE
	Propyltrichlorosilane	8	UN1816	II	8, 3	A7, B2, B6, IB2, N34, T7, TP2, TP13	155	CORROSIVE
	Prussic acid, see **Hydrogen cyanide**							

Symbols	Hazardous materials descriptions and proper shipping names	Hazard class or Division	Identification Numbers	PG	Label Codes	Special provisions (§172.102)	ERG Guide No.	Placard Advisory Consult §172.504 & §172.505 *Placard any quantity
(1)	(2)	(3)	(4)	(5)	(6)	(7)		
	Pyrethroid pesticide, liquid, flammable, toxic, *flash point less than 23 degrees C*	3	UN3350	I	3, 6.1	T14, TP2, TP13, TP27	131	FLAMMABLE
				II	3, 6.1	IB2, T11, TP2, TP13, TP27	131	FLAMMABLE
	Pyrethroid pesticide, liquid toxic	6.1	UN3352	I	6.1	T14, TP2, TP13, TP27	151	POISON
				II	6.1	IB2, T11, TP2, TP27	151	POISON
				III	6.1	IB3, T7, TP2, TP28	151	POISON
	Pyrethroid pesticide, liquid, toxic, flammable, *flash point not less than 23 degrees C*	6.1	UN3351	I	6.1, 3	T14, TP2, TP13, TP27	131	POISON
				II	6.1, 3	IB2, T11, TP2, TP13, TP27	131	POISON
				III	6.1, 3	IB3, T7, TP2, TP28	131	POISON
	Pyrethroid pesticide, solid, toxic	6.1	UN3349	I	6.1	IB7, IP1, T6, TP33	151	POISON
				II	6.1	IB8, IP2, IP4, T3, TP33	151	POISON
				III	6.1	IB8, IP3, T1, TP33	151	POISON
	Pyridine	3	UN1282	II	3	IB2, T4, TP2	129	FLAMMABLE
	Pyridine perchlorate	Forbidden						

Symbols	Hazardous materials descriptions and proper shipping names	Hazard class or Division	Identification Numbers	PG	Label Codes	Special provisions (§172.102)	ERG Guide No.	Placard Advisory Consult §172.504 & §172.505 *Placard any quantity
(1)	(2)	(3)	(4)	(5)	(6)	(7)		
G	**Pyrophoric liquid, inorganic, n.o.s.**	4.2	UN3194	I	4.2		135	SPONTANEOUSLY COMBUSTIBLE
G	**Pyrophoric liquids, organic, n.o.s.**	4.2	UN2845	I	4.2	B11, T22, TP2, TP7	135	SPONTANEOUSLY COMBUSTIBLE
G	**Pyrophoric metals, n.o.s.,** *or* **Pyrophoric alloys, n.o.s.**	4.2	UN1383	I	4.2	B11, T21, TP7, TP33	135	SPONTANEOUSLY COMBUSTIBLE
G	**Pyrophoric solid, inorganic, n.o.s.**	4.2	UN3200	I	4.2	T21, TP7, TP33	135	SPONTANEOUSLY COMBUSTIBLE
G	**Pyrophoric solids, organic, n.o.s.**	4.2	UN2846	I	4.2		135	SPONTANEOUSLY COMBUSTIBLE
	Pyrosulfuryl chloride	8	UN1817	II	8	B2, IB2, T8, TP2, TP12	137	CORROSIVE
	Pyroxylin solution or solvent, see **Nitrocellulose**							
	Pyrrolidine	3	UN1922	II	3, 8	IB2, T7, TP1	132	FLAMMABLE
	Quebrachitol pentanitrate	Forbidden						
	Quicklime, see **Calcium oxide**							
	Quinoline	6.1	UN2656	III	6.1	IB3, T4, TP1	154	POISON
	R 12, see **Dichlorodifluoromethane**							
	R 12B1, see **Chlorodifluorobromomethane**							
	R 13, see **Chlorotrifluoromethane**							

Sym-bols	Hazardous materials descriptions and proper shipping names	Hazard class or Division	Identifica-tion Numbers	PG	Label Codes	Special provisions (§172.102)	ERG Guide No.	Placard Advisory Consult §172.504 & §172.505 *Placard any quantity
(1)	(2)	(3)	(4)	(5)	(6)	(7)		
	R 13B1, see **Bromotrifluoromethane**							
	R 14, see **Tetrafluoromethane**							
	R 21, see **Dichlorofluoromethane**							
	R 22, see **Chlorodifluoromethane**							
	R 114, see **Dichlorotetrafluoroethane**							
	R 115, see **Chloropentafluoroethane**							
	R 116, see **Hexafluoroethane**							
	R 124, see **Chlorotetrafluoroethane**							
	R 133a, see **Chlorotrifluoroethane**							
	R 152a, see **Difluoroethane**							
	R 500, see **Dichlorodifluoromethane and difluorethane**, *etc.*							
	R 502, see **Chlorodifluoromethane and chloropentafluoroethane mixture**, *etc.*							
	R 503, see **Chlorotrifluoromethane and trifluoromethane**, *etc.*							
	Radioactive material, excepted package-articles manufactured from natural uranium *or* **natural thorium**	7	UN2909		None		161	
	Radioactive material, excepted package-empty packaging	7	UN2908		Empty		161	NONE

Symbols	Hazardous materials descriptions and proper shipping names	Hazard class or Division	Identification Numbers	PG	Label Codes	Special provisions (§172.102)	ERG Guide No.	Placard Advisory Consult §172.504 & §172.505 *Placard any quantity
(1)	(2)	(3)	(4)	(5)	(6)	(7)		
	Radioactive material, **excepted** package-instruments *or* articles	7	UN2911		None		161	NONE
	Radioactive material, excepted package-limited quantity of material	7	UN2910		None		161	NONE
	Radioactive material, low specific activity **(LSA-I)** *non fissile or fissile-excepted*	7	UN2912		7	A56, T5, TP4, W7	162	RADIOACTIVE* (YELLOW III LABEL OR EXCLUSIVE USE SHIPMENTS)
	Radioactive material, low specific activity **(LSA-II)** *non fissile or fissile-excepted*	7	UN3321		7	A56, T5, TP4, W7	162	RADIOACTIVE* (YELLOW III LABEL OR EXCLUSIVE USE SHIPMENTS)
	Radioactive material, low specific activity **(LSA-III)** *non fissile or fissile excepted*	7	UN3322		7	A56, T5, TP4, W7	162	RADIOACTIVE* (YELLOW III LABEL OR EXCLUSIVE USE SHIPMENTS)
	Radioactive material, surface contaminated objects (SCO-I *or* SCO-II) *non fissile or fissile-excepted*	7	UN2913		7	A56	162	RADIOACTIVE* (YELLOW III LABEL OR EXCLUSIVE USE SHIPMENTS)
	Radioactive material, transported under special arrangement, *non fissile or fissile excepted*	7	UN2919		7	A56, 139	163	RADIOACTIVE* (YELLOW III LABEL OR EXCLUSIVE USE SHIPMENTS)

Symbols	Hazardous materials descriptions and proper shipping names	Hazard class or Division	Identification Numbers	PG	Label Codes	Special provisions (§172.102)	ERG Guide No.	Placard Advisory Consult §172.504 & §172.505 *Placard any quantity
(1)	(2)	(3)	(4)	(5)	(6)	(7)		
	Radioactive material, transported under special arrangement, fissile	7	UN3331		7	A56, 139	165	RADIOACTIVE* (YELLOW III LABEL OR EXCLUSIVE USE SHIPMENTS)
	Radioactive material, Type A package, fissile *non-special form*	7	UN3327		7	A56, W7, W8	165	RADIOACTIVE* (YELLOW III LABEL OR EXCLUSIVE USE SHIPMENTS)
	Radioactive material, Type A package, *non-special form, non fissile or fissile-excepted*	7	UN2915		7	A56, W7, W8	163	RADIOACTIVE* (YELLOW III LABEL OR EXCLUSIVE USE SHIPMENTS)
	Radioactive material, Type A package, special form *non fissile or fissile-excepted*	7	UN3332		7	A56, W7, W8	164	RADIOACTIVE* (YELLOW III LABEL OR EXCLUSIVE USE SHIPMENTS)
	Radioactive material, Type A package, special form, fissile	7	UN3333		7	A56, W7, W8	165	RADIOACTIVE* (YELLOW III LABEL OR EXCLUSIVE USE SHIPMENTS)
	Radioactive material, Type B(M) package, fissile	7	UN3329		7	A56	165	RADIOACTIVE* (YELLOW III LABEL OR EXCLUSIVE USE SHIPMENTS)

Sym-bols	Hazardous materials descriptions and proper shipping names	Hazard class or Division	Identifica-tion Numbers	PG	Label Codes	Special provisions (§172.102)	ERG Guide No.	Placard Advisory Consult §172.504 & §172.505 *Placard any quantity
(1)	(2)	(3)	(4)	(5)	(6)	(7)		
	Radioactive material, Type B(M) package *non fissile or fissile-excepted*	7	UN2917		7	A56	163	RADIOACTIVE* (YELLOW III LABEL OR EXCLUSIVE USE SHIPMENTS)
	Radioactive material, Type B(U) package, fissile	7	UN3328		7	A56	165	RADIOACTIVE* (YELLOW III LABEL OR EXCLUSIVE USE SHIPMENTS)
	Radioactive material, Type B(U) package *non fissile or fissile-excepted*	7	UN2916		7	A56	163	RADIOACTIVE* (YELLOW III LABEL OR EXCLUSIVE USE SHIPMENTS)
	Radioactive material, uranium hexafluoride *non fissile or fissile-excepted*	7	UN2978		7, 8		166	RADIOACTIVE* (YELLOW III LABEL OR EXCLUSIVE USE SHIPMENTS)
I	**Radioactive material, uranium hexafluoride, fissile**	7	UN2977		7, 8		166	RADIOACTIVE* (YELLOW III LABEL OR EXCLUSIVE USE SHIPMENTS)
A W	**Rags, oily**	4.2	UN1856	III	4.2		133	SPONTANEOUSLY COMBUSTIBLE
	Railway torpedo, see **Signals, railway track, explosive**							
	Rare gases and nitrogen mixtures, compressed	2.2	UN1981		2.2		121	NONFLAMMABLE GAS

Symbols	Hazardous materials descriptions and proper shipping names	Hazard class or Division	Identification Numbers	PG	Label Codes	Special provisions (§172.102)	ERG Guide No.	Placard Advisory Consult §172.504 & §172.505 *Placard any quantity
(1)	(2)	(3)	(4)	(5)	(6)	(7)		
	Rare gases and oxygen mixtures, compressed	2.2	UN1980		2.2	79	121	NONFLAMMABLE GAS
	Rare gases mixtures, compressed	2.2	UN1979		2.2		121	NONFLAMMABLE GAS
	RC 318, see **Octafluorocyclobutane**							
	RDX and cyclotetramethylenetetranitramine, wetted *or* **desensitized** *see* **RDX and HMX mixtures, wetted** *or* **desensitized**							
	RDX and HMX mixtures, wetted *with not less than 15 percent water by mass or* **RDX and HMX mixtures, desensitized** *with not less than 10 percent phlegmatizer by mass*	1.1D	UN0391	II	1.1D		112	EXPLOSIVES 1.1*
	RDX and Octogen mixtures, wetted *or* **desensitized** *see* **RDX and HMX mixtures, wetted** *or* **desensitized** *etc.*							
	RDX, see **Cyclotrimethylene trinitramine,** *etc.*							
	Receptacles, small, containing gas (gas cartridges) *flammable, without release device, not refillable and not exceeding 1 L capacity*	2.1	UN2037		2.1		115	FLAMMABLE GAS

Symbols	Hazardous materials descriptions and proper shipping names	Hazard class or Division	Identification Numbers	PG	Label Codes	Special provisions (§172.102)	ERG Guide No.	Placard Advisory Consult §172.504 & §172.505 *Placard any quantity
(1)	(2)	(3)	(4)	(5)	(6)	(7)		
	Receptacles, small, containing gas (gas cartridges) *non-flammable, without release device, not refillable and not exceeding 1 L capacity*	2.2	UN2037		2.2		115	NONFLAMMABLE GAS
	Red phosphorus, see **Phosphorus, amorphous**							
	Refrigerant gas R 404A	2.2	UN3337		2.2	T50	126	NONFLAMMABLE GAS
	Refrigerant gas R 407A	2.2	UN3338		2.2	T50	126	NONFLAMMABLE GAS
	Refrigerant gas R 407B	2.2	UN3339		2.2	T50	126	NONFLAMMABLE GAS
	Refrigerant gas R 407C	2.2	UN3340		2.2	T50	126	NONFLAMMABLE GAS
G	**Refrigerant gases, n.o.s.**	2.2	UN1078		2.2	T50	126	NONFLAMMABLE GAS
D	**Refrigerant gases, n.o.s.** *or* **Dispersant gases, n.o.s.**	2.1	NA1954		2.1	T50	115	FLAMMABLE GAS
	Refrigerating machines, *containing flammable, non-toxic, liquefied gas*	2.1	UN3358		2.1		115	FLAMMABLE GAS
	Refrigerating machines, *containing non-flammable, non-toxic gases, or ammonia solutions (UN2672)*	2.2	UN2857		2.2	A53	126	NONFLAMMABLE GAS
	Regulated medical waste	6.2	UN3291	II	6.2	A13	158	NONE

Symbols	Hazardous materials descriptions and proper shipping names	Hazard class or Division	Identification Numbers	PG	Label Codes	Special provisions (§172.102)	ERG Guide No.	Placard Advisory Consult §172.504 & §172.505 *Placard any quantity
(1)	(2)	(3)	(4)	(5)	(6)	(7)		
	Release devices, explosive	1.4S	UN0173	II	1.4S		114	EXPLOSIVES 1.4
	Resin solution, *flammable*	3	UN1866	I	3	B52, T11, TP1, TP8, TP28	127	FLAMMABLE
				II	3	149, B52, IB2, T4, TP1, TP8	127	FLAMMABLE
				III	3	B1, B52, IB3, T2, TP1	127	FLAMMABLE
	Resorcinol	6.1	UN2876	III	6.1	IB8, IP3, T1, TP33	153	POISON
	Rifle grenade, see **Grenades,** *hand or rifle, etc.*							
	Rifle powder, see **Powder, smokeless (UN 0160)**							
	Rivets, explosive	1.4S	UN0174	II	1.4S		114	EXPLOSIVES 1.4
	Road asphalt or tar liquid, see **Tars, liquid,** *etc.*							
	Rocket motors	1.3C	UN0186	II	1.3C	109	112	EXPLOSIVES 1.3*
	Rocket motors	1.1C	UN0280	II	1.1C	109	112	EXPLOSIVES 1.1*
	Rocket motors	1.2C	UN0281	II	1.2C	109	112	EXPLOSIVES 1.2*
	Rocket motors, liquid fueled	1.2J	UN0395	II	1.2J	109	112	EXPLOSIVES 1.2*
	Rocket motors, liquid fueled	1.3J	UN0396	II	1.3J	109	112	EXPLOSIVES 1.3*
	Rocket motors with hypergolic liquids *with or without an expelling charge*	1.3L	UN0250	II	1.3L	109	112	EXPLOSIVES 1.3*

Symbols	Hazardous materials descriptions and proper shipping names	Hazard class or Division	Identification Numbers	PG	Label Codes	Special provisions (§172.102)	ERG Guide No.	Placard Advisory Consult §172.504 & §172.505 *Placard any quantity
(1)	(2)	(3)	(4)	(5)	(6)	(7)		
	Rocket motors with hypergolic liquids *with or without an expelling charge*	1.2L	UN0322	II	1.2L	109	112	EXPLOSIVES 1.2*
	Rockets, line-throwing	1.2G	UN0238	II	1.2G		112	EXPLOSIVES 1.2*
	Rockets, line-throwing	1.3G	UN0240	II	1.3G		112	EXPLOSIVES 1.3*
	Rockets, line-throwing	1.4G	UN0453	II	1.4G		114	EXPLOSIVES 1.4
	Rockets, liquid fueled *with bursting charge*	1.1J	UN0397	II	1.1J		112	EXPLOSIVES 1.1*
	Rockets, liquid fueled *with bursting charge*	1.2J	UN0398	II	1.2J		112	EXPLOSIVES 1.2*
	Rockets, *with bursting charge*	1.1F	UN0180	II	1.1F		112	EXPLOSIVES 1.1*
	Rockets, *with bursting charge*	1.1E	UN0181	II	1.1E		112	EXPLOSIVES 1.1*
	Rockets, *with bursting charge*	1.2E	UN0182	II	1.2E		112	EXPLOSIVES 1.2*
	Rockets, *with bursting charge*	1.2F	UN0295	II	1.2F		112	EXPLOSIVES 1.2*
	Rockets, *with expelling charge*	1.2C	UN0436	II	1.2C		112	EXPLOSIVES 1.2*
	Rockets, *with expelling charge*	1.3C	UN0437	II	1.3C		112	EXPLOSIVES 1.3*
	Rockets, *with expelling charge*	1.4C	UN0438	II	1.4C		114	EXPLOSIVES 1.4
	Rockets, *with inert head*	1.3C	UN0183	II	1.3C		112	EXPLOSIVES 1.3*
	Rockets, *with inert head*	1.2C	UN0502		1.2C		112	EXPLOSIVES 1.2*
	Rosin oil	3	UN1286	II	3	IB2, T4, TP1	127	FLAMMABLE
				III	3	B1, IB3, T2, TP1	127	FLAMMABLE

Symbols	Hazardous materials descriptions and proper shipping names	Hazard class or Division	Identification Numbers	PG	Label Codes	Special provisions (§172.102)	ERG Guide No.	Placard Advisory Consult §172.504 & §172.505 *Placard any quantity
(1)	(2)	(3)	(4)	(5)	(6)	(7)		
	Rubber scrap *or* **shoddy** *powdered or granulated, not exceeding 840 microns and rubber content exceeding 45%*	4.1	UN1345	II	4.1	IB8, IP2, IP4, T3, TP33	133	FLAMMABLE SOLID
	Rubber solution	3	UN1287	II	3	149, IB2, T4, TP1, TP8	127	FLAMMABLE
				III	3	B1, IB3, T2, TP1	127	FLAMMABLE
	Rubidium	4.3	UN1423	I	4.3	22, A7, A19, IB4, IP1, N34, N40, N45	138	DANGEROUS WHEN WET*
	Rubidium hydroxide	8	UN2678	II	8	IB8, IP2, IP4, T3, TP33	154	CORROSIVE
	Rubidium hydroxide solution	8	UN2677	II	8	B2, IB2, T7, TP2	154	CORROSIVE
				III	8	IB3, T4, TP1	154	CORROSIVE
	Safety fuse, see **Fuse, safety**							
G	**Samples, explosive,** *other than initiating explosives*		UN0190	II		113	—	—
	Sand acid, see **Fluorosilicic acid**							
	Seed cake, *containing vegetable oil solvent extractions and expelled seeds, with not more than 10 percent of oil and when the amount of moisture is higher than 11 percent, with not more than 20 percent of oil and moisture combined.*	4.2	UN1386	III	None	IB8, IP3, IP6, N7	135	SPONTANEOUSLY COMBUSTIBLE

Sym-bols	Hazardous materials descriptions and proper shipping names	Hazard class or Division	Identifica-tion Numbers	PG	Label Codes	Special provisions (§172.102)	ERG Guide No.	Placard Advisory Consult §172.504 & §172.505 *Placard any quantity
(1)	(2)	(3)	(4)	(5)	(6)	(7)		
I	**Seed cake** *with more than 1.5 percent oil and not more than 11 percent moisture*	4.2	UN1386	III	None	IB8, IP3, IP6, N7	135	SPONTANEOUSLY COMBUSTIBLE
I	**Seed cake** *with not more than 1.5 percent oil and not more than 11 percent moisture*	4.2	UN2217	III	None	IB8, IP3, IP6, N7	135	SPONTANEOUSLY COMBUSTIBLE
	Selenates *or* **Selenites**	6.1	UN2630	I	6.1	IB7, IP1, T6, TP33	151	POISON
	Selenic acid	8	UN1905	I	8	IB7, IP1, N34, T6, TP33	154	CORROSIVE
	Selenium compound, solid, n.o.s.	6.1	UN3283	I	6.1	IB7, IP1, T6, TP33	151	POISON
				II	6.1	IB8, IP2, IP4, T3, TP33	151	POISON
				III	6.1	IB8, IP3, T1, TP33	151	POISON
	Selenium compound, liquid, n.o.s.	6.1	UN3440	I	6.1	T14, TP2, TP27	151	POISON
				II	6.1	IB2, T11, TP2, TP27	151	POISON
				III	6.1	IB3, T7, TP1, TP28	151	POISON
	Selenium disulfide	6.1	UN2657	II	6.1	IB8, IP2, IP4, T3, TP33	153	POISON
	Selenium hexafluoride	2.3	UN2194		2.3, 8	1	125	POISON GAS*
	Selenium nitride	Forbidden						

Sym-bols	Hazardous materials descriptions and proper shipping names	Hazard class or Division	Identifica-tion Numbers	PG	Label Codes	Special provisions (§172.102)	ERG Guide No.	Placard Advisory Consult §172.504 & §172.505 *Placard any quantity
(1)	(2)	(3)	(4)	(5)	(6)	(7)		
	Selenium oxychloride	8	UN2879	I	8, 6.1	A3, A6, A7, N34, T10, TP2, TP12, TP13	157	CORROSIVE
	Self-defense spray, aerosol, see **Aerosols**, *etc.*							
+ A D	**Self-defense spray, non-pressurized**	9	NA3334	III	9	A37	171	CLASS 9
G	**Self-heating liquid, corrosive, inorganic, n.o.s.**	4.2	UN3188	II	4.2, 8	IB2	136	SPONTANEOUSLY COMBUSTIBLE
				III	4.2, 8	IB2	136	SPONTANEOUSLY COMBUSTIBLE
G	**Self-heating liquid, corrosive, organic, n.o.s.**	4.2	UN3185	II	4.2, 8	IB2	136	SPONTANEOUSLY COMBUSTIBLE
				III	4.2, 8	IB2	136	SPONTANEOUSLY COMBUSTIBLE
G	**Self-heating liquid, inorganic, n.o.s.**	4.2	UN3186	II	4.2	IB2	135	SPONTANEOUSLY COMBUSTIBLE
				III	4.2	IB2	135	SPONTANEOUSLY COMBUSTIBLE
G	**Self-heating liquid, organic, n.o.s.**	4.2	UN3183	II	4.2	IB2	135	SPONTANEOUSLY COMBUSTIBLE
				III	4.2	IB2	135	SPONTANEOUSLY COMBUSTIBLE
G	**Self-heating liquid, toxic, inorganic, n.o.s.**	4.2	UN3187	II	4.2, 6.1	IB2	136	SPONTANEOUSLY COMBUSTIBLE

Symbols	Hazardous materials descriptions and proper shipping names	Hazard class or Division	Identification Numbers	PG	Label Codes	Special provisions (§172.102)	ERG Guide No.	Placard Advisory Consult §172.504 & §172.505 *Placard any quantity
(1)	(2)	(3)	(4)	(5)	(6)	(7)		
				III	4.2, 6.1	IB2	136	SPONTANEOUSLY COMBUSTIBLE
G	**Self-heating liquid, toxic, organic, n.o.s.**	4.2	UN3184	II	4.2, 6.1	IB2	136	SPONTANEOUSLY COMBUSTIBLE
				III	4.2, 6.1	IB2	136	SPONTANEOUSLY COMBUSTIBLE
G	**Self-heating solid, corrosive, inorganic, n.o.s.**	4.2	UN3192	II	4.2, 8	IB5, IP2, T3, TP33	136	SPONTANEOUSLY COMBUSTIBLE
				III	4.2, 8	IB8, IP3, T1, TP33	136	SPONTANEOUSLY COMBUSTIBLE
G	**Self-heating, solid, corrosive, organic, n.o.s.**	4.2	UN3126	II	4.2, 8	IB5, IP2, T3, TP33	136	SPONTANEOUSLY COMBUSTIBLE
				III	4.2, 8	IB8, IP3, T1, TP33	136	SPONTANEOUSLY COMBUSTIBLE
G	**Self-heating solid, inorganic, n.o.s.**	4.2	UN3190	II	4.2	IB6, IP2, T3, TP33	135	SPONTANEOUSLY COMBUSTIBLE
				III	4.2	IB8, IP3, T1, TP33	135	SPONTANEOUSLY COMBUSTIBLE
G	**Self-heating, solid, organic, n.o.s.**	4.2	UN3088	II	4.2	IB6, IP2, T3, TP33	135	SPONTANEOUSLY COMBUSTIBLE
				III	4.2	IB8, IP3, T1, TP33	135	SPONTANEOUSLY COMBUSTIBLE
G	**Self-heating, solid, oxidizing, n.o.s.**	4.2	UN3127		4.2, 5.1		135	SPONTANEOUSLY COMBUSTIBLE

Sym-bols	Hazardous materials descriptions and proper shipping names	Hazard class or Division	Identifica-tion Numbers	PG	Label Codes	Special provisions (§172.102)	ERG Guide No.	Placard Advisory Consult §172.504 & §172.505 *Placard any quantity
(1)	(2)	(3)	(4)	(5)	(6)	(7)		
G	**Self-heating solid, toxic, inorganic, n.o.s.**	4.2	UN3191	II	4.2, 6.1	IB5, IP2, T3, TP33	136	SPONTANEOUSLY COMBUSTIBLE
				III	4.2, 6.1	IB8, IP3, T1, TP33	136	SPONTANEOUSLY COMBUSTIBLE
G	**Self-heating, solid, toxic, organic, n.o.s.**	4.2	UN3128	II	4.2, 6.1	IB5, IP2, T3, TP33	136	SPONTANEOUSLY COMBUSTIBLE
				III	4.2, 6.1	IB8, IP3, T1, TP33	136	SPONTANEOUSLY COMBUSTIBLE
	Self-propelled vehicle, see **Engines** *or* **Batteries** *etc.*							
G	**Self-reactive liquid type B**	4.1	UN3221	II	4.1	53	149	FLAMMABLE SOLID
G	**Self-reactive liquid type B, temperature controlled**	4.1	UN3231	II	4.1	53	150	FLAMMABLE SOLID
G	**Self-reactive liquid type C**	4.1	UN3223	II	4.1		149	FLAMMABLE SOLID
G	**Self-reactive liquid type C, temperature controlled**	4.1	UN3233	II	4.1		150	FLAMMABLE SOLID
G	**Self-reactive liquid type D**	4.1	UN3225	II	4.1		149	FLAMMABLE SOLID
G	**Self-reactive liquid type D, temperature controlled**	4.1	UN3235	II	4.1		150	FLAMMABLE SOLID
G	**Self-reactive liquid type E**	4.1	UN3227	II	4.1		149	FLAMMABLE SOLID

Sym-bols	Hazardous materials descriptions and proper shipping names	Hazard class or Division	Identifica-tion Numbers	PG	Label Codes	Special provisions (§172.102)	ERG Guide No.	Placard Advisory Consult §172.504 & §172.505 *Placard any quantity
(1)	(2)	(3)	(4)	(5)	(6)	(7)		
G	**Self-reactive liquid type E, temperature controlled**	4.1	UN3237	II	4.1		150	FLAMMABLE SOLID
G	**Self-reactive liquid type F**	4.1	UN3229	II	4.1		149	FLAMMABLE SOLID
G	**Self-reactive liquid type F, temperature controlled**	4.1	UN3239	II	4.1		150	FLAMMABLE SOLID
G	**Self-reactive solid type B**	4.1	UN3222	II	4.1	53	149	FLAMMABLE SOLID
G	**Self-reactive solid type B, temperature controlled**	4.1	UN3232	II	4.1	53	150	FLAMMABLE SOLID
G	**Self-reactive solid type C**	4.1	UN3224	II	4.1		149	FLAMMABLE SOLID
G	**Self-reactive solid type C, temperature controlled**	4.1	UN3234	II	4.1		150	FLAMMABLE SOLID
G	**Self-reactive solid type D**	4.1	UN3226	II	4.1		149	FLAMMABLE SOLID
G	**Self-reactive solid type D, temperature controlled**	4.1	UN3236	II	4.1		150	FLAMMABLE SOLID
G	**Self-reactive solid type E**	4.1	UN3228	II	4.1		149	FLAMMABLE SOLID
G	**Self-reactive solid type E, temperature controlled**	4.1	UN3238	II	4.1		150	FLAMMABLE SOLID
G	**Self-reactive solid type F**	4.1	UN3230	II	4.1		149	FLAMMABLE SOLID

Symbols	Hazardous materials descriptions and proper shipping names	Hazard class or Division	Identification Numbers	PG	Label Codes	Special provisions (§172.102)	ERG Guide No.	Placard Advisory Consult §172.504 & §172.505 *Placard any quantity
(1)	(2)	(3)	(4)	(5)	(6)	(7)		
G	**Self-reactive solid type F, temperature controlled**	4.1	UN3240	II	4.1		150	FLAMMABLE SOLID
	Shale oil	3	UN1288	I	3	T11, TP1, TP8, TP27	128	FLAMMABLE
				II	3	IB2, T4, TP1, TP8	128	FLAMMABLE
				III	3	B1, IB3, T2, TP1	128	FLAMMABLE
	Shaped charges, see **Charges, shaped,** *etc.*							
	Signal devices, hand	1.4G	UN0191	II	1.4G		114	EXPLOSIVES 1.4
	Signal devices, hand	1.4S	UN0373	II	1.4S		114	EXPLOSIVES 1.4
	Signals, distress, *ship*	1.1G	UN0194	II	1.1G		112	EXPLOSIVES 1.1*
	Signals, distress, *ship*	1.3G	UN0195	II	1.3G		112	EXPLOSIVES 1.3*
	Signals, highway, see **Signal devices, hand**							
	Signals, railway track, explosive	1.1G	UN0192	II	1.1G		112	EXPLOSIVES 1.1*
	Signals, railway track, explosive	1.4S	UN0193	II	1.4S		114	EXPLOSIVES 1.4
	Signals, railway track, explosive	1.3G	UN0492		1.3G		112	EXPLOSIVES 1.3*
	Signals, railway track, explosive	1.4G	UN0493		1.4G		114	EXPLOSIVES 1.4
	Signals, ship distress, water-activated, see **Contrivances, water-activated,** *etc.*							
	Signals, smoke	1.1G	UN0196	II	1.1G		112	EXPLOSIVES 1.1*

Symbols	Hazardous materials descriptions and proper shipping names	Hazard class or Division	Identification Numbers	PG	Label Codes	Special provisions (§172.102)	ERG Guide No.	Placard Advisory Consult §172.504 & §172.505 *Placard any quantity
(1)	(2)	(3)	(4)	(5)	(6)	(7)		
	Signals, smoke	1.4G	UN0197	II	1.4G		114	EXPLOSIVES 1.4
	Signals, smoke	1.2G	UN0313	II	1.2G		112	EXPLOSIVES 1.2*
	Signals, smoke	1.3G	UN0487	II	1.3G		112	EXPLOSIVES 1.3*
	Silane	2.1	UN2203		2.1		116	FLAMMABLE GAS
	Silicofluoric acid, see **Fluorosilicic acid**							
	Silicon chloride, see **Silicon tetrachloride**							
	Silicon powder, amorphous	4.1	UN1346	III	4.1	A1, IB8, IP3, T1, TP33	170	FLAMMABLE SOLID
	Silicon tetrachloride	8	UN1818	II	8	A3, A6, B2, B6, IB2, T7, TP2, TP7	157	CORROSIVE
	Silicon tetrafluoride	2.3	UN1859		2.3, 8	2	125	POISON GAS*
	Silver acetylide (dry)	Forbidden						
	Silver arsenite	6.1	UN1683	II	6.1	IB8, IP2, IP4, T3, TP33	151	POISON
	Silver azide (dry)	Forbidden						
	Silver chlorite (dry)	Forbidden						
	Silver cyanide	6.1	UN1684	II	6.1	IB8, IP2, IP4, T3, TP33	151	POISON
	Silver fulminate (dry)	Forbidden						
	Silver nitrate	5.1	UN1493	II	5.1	IB8, IP4, T3, TP33	140	OXIDIZER

Symbols	Hazardous materials descriptions and proper shipping names	Hazard class or Division	Identification Numbers	PG	Label Codes	Special provisions (§172.102)	ERG Guide No.	Placard Advisory Consult §172.504 & §172.505 *Placard any quantity
(1)	(2)	(3)	(4)	(5)	(6)	(7)		
	Silver oxalate (dry)	Forbidden						
	Silver picrate (dry)	Forbidden						
	Silver picrate, wetted *with not less than 30 percent water, by mass*	4.1	UN1347	I	4.1	23	113	FLAMMABLE SOLID
	Sludge, acid	8	UN1906	II	8	A3, A7, B2, IB2, N34, T8, TP2, TP12, TP28	153	CORROSIVE
D	**Smokeless powder for small arms** *(100 pounds or less)*	4.1	NA3178	I	4.1	16	133	FLAMMABLE SOLID
	Soda lime *with more than 4 percent sodium hydroxide*	8	UN1907	III	8	IB8, IP3, T1, TP33	154	CORROSIVE
	Sodium	4.3	UN1428	I	4.3	A7, A8, A19, A20, B9, B48, B68, IB4, IP1, N34, T9, TP7, TP33, TP46	138	DANGEROUS WHEN WET*
	Sodium aluminate, solid	8	UN2812	III	8	IB8, IP3, T1, TP33	154	CORROSIVE
	Sodium aluminate, solution	8	UN1819	II	8	B2, IB2, T7, TP2	154	CORROSIVE
				III	8	IB3, T4, TP1	154	CORROSIVE
	Sodium aluminum hydride	4.3	UN2835	II	4.3	A8, A19, A20, IB4, T3, TP33	138	DANGEROUS WHEN WET*
	Sodium ammonium vanadate	6.1	UN2863	II	6.1	IB8, IP2, IP4, T3, TP33	154	POISON
	Sodium arsanilate	6.1	UN2473	III	6.1	IB8, IP3, T1, TP33	154	POISON

Sym-bols	Hazardous materials descriptions and proper shipping names	Hazard class or Division	Identifica-tion Numbers	PG	Label Codes	Special provisions (§172.102)	ERG Guide No.	Placard Advisory Consult §172.504 & §172.505 *Placard any quantity
(1)	(2)	(3)	(4)	(5)	(6)	(7)		
	Sodium arsenate	6.1	UN1685	II	6.1	IB8, IP2, IP4, T3, TP33	151	POISON
	Sodium arsenite, aqueous solutions	6.1	UN1686	II	6.1	IB2, T7, TP2	154	POISON
				III	6.1	IB3, T4, TP2	154	POISON
	Sodium arsenite, solid	6.1	UN2027	II	6.1	IB8, IP2, IP4, T3, TP33	151	POISON
	Sodium azide	6.1	UN1687	II	6.1	IB8, IP2, IP4	153	POISON
	Sodium bifluoride, see **Sodium hydrogendifluoride**							
	Sodium bisulfite, solution, see **Bisulfites, aqueous solutions, n.o.s.**							
	Sodium borohydride	4.3	UN1426	I	4.3	N40	138	DANGEROUS WHEN WET*
	Sodium borohydride and sodium hydroxide solution, *with not more than 12 percent sodium borohydride and not more than 40 percent sodium hydroxide by mass*	8	UN3320	II	8	B2, IB2, N34, T7, TP2	157	CORROSIVE
				III	8	B2, IB3, N34, T4, TP2	157	CORROSIVE
	Sodium bromate	5.1	UN1494	II	5.1	IB8, IP4, T3, TP33	141	OXIDIZER
	Sodium cacodylate	6.1	UN1688	II	6.1	IB8, IP2, IP4, T3, TP33	152	POISON

Sym-bols	Hazardous materials descriptions and proper shipping names	Hazard class or Division	Identifica-tion Numbers	PG	Label Codes	Special provisions (§172.102)	ERG Guide No.	Placard Advisory Consult §172.504 & §172.505 *Placard any quantity
(1)	(2)	(3)	(4)	(5)	(6)	(7)		
	Sodium carbonate peroxyhydrate	5.1	UN3378	II	5.1	IB8, IP2, IP4, T3, TP33	140	OXIDIZER
				III	5.1	IB8, IP3, T1, TP33	140	OXIDIZER
	Sodium chlorate	5.1	UN1495	II	5.1	A9, IB8, IP4, N34, T3, TP33	140	OXIDIZER
	Sodium chlorate, aqueous solution	5.1	UN2428	II	5.1	A2, IB2, T4, TP1	140	OXIDIZER
				III	5.1	A2, IB2, T4, TP1	140	OXIDIZER
	Sodium chlorate mixed with dinitrotoluene, see **Explosive blasting, type C**							
	Sodium chlorite	5.1	UN1496	II	5.1	A9, IB8, IP2, IP4, N34, T3, TP33	143	OXIDIZER
	Sodium chloroacetate	6.1	UN2659	III	6.1	IB8, IP3, T1, TP33	151	POISON
	Sodium cuprocyanide, solid	6.1	UN2316	I	6.1	IB7, IP1, T6, TP33	157	POISON
	Sodium cuprocyanide, solution	6.1	UN2317	I	6.1	T14, TP2, TP13	157	POISON
	Sodium cyanide, solid	6.1	UN1689	I	6.1	B69, B77, IB7, N74, N75, T6, TP33	157	POISON
	Sodium cyanide solution	6.1	UN3414	I	6.1	B69, B77, N74, N75, T14, TP2, TP13	157	POISON
				II	6.1	B69, B77, IB2, N74, N75, T11, TP2, TP13, TP27	157	POISON

Symbols	Hazardous materials descriptions and proper shipping names	Hazard class or Division	Identification Numbers	PG	Label Codes	Special provisions (§172.102)	ERG Guide No.	Placard Advisory Consult §172.504 & §172.505 *Placard any quantity
(1)	(2)	(3)	(4)	(5)	(6)	(7)		
				III	6.1	B69, B77, IB3, N74, N75, T7, TP2, TP13, TP28	157	POISON
	Sodium dichloroisocyanurate or Sodium dichloro-s-triazinetrione, see **Dichloroisocyanuric acid** *etc.*							
	Sodium dinitro-o-cresolate, *dry or wetted with less than 15 percent water, by mass*	1.3C	UN0234	II	1.3C		112	EXPLOSIVES 1.3*
	Sodium dinitro-o-cresolate, wetted, *with not less than 10% waters, by mass*	4.1	UN3369	I	4.1	162, A8, A19, N41, N84	113	FLAMMABLE SOLID
	Sodium dinitro-o-cresolate, wetted *with not less than 15 percent water, by mass*	4.1	UN1348	I	4.1, 6.1	23, A8, A19, A20, N41	113	FLAMMABLE SOLID
	Sodium dithionite *or* **Sodium hdrosulfite**	4.2	UN1384	II	4.2	A19, A20, IB6, IP2, T3, TP33	135	SPONTANEOUSLY COMBUSTIBLE
	Sodium fluoride, solid	6.1	UN1690	III	6.1	IB8, IP3, T1, TP33	154	POISON
	Sodium fluoride solution	6.1	UN3415	III	6.1	IB3, T4, TP1	154	POISON
	Sodium fluoroacetate	6.1	UN2629	I	6.1	IB7, IP1, T6, TP33	151	POISON
	Sodium fluorosilicate	6.1	UN2674	III	6.1	IB8, IP3, T1, TP33	154	POISON
	Sodium hydrate, see **Sodium hydroxide, solid**							

Symbols	Hazardous materials descriptions and proper shipping names	Hazard class or Division	Identification Numbers	PG	Label Codes	Special provisions (§172.102)	ERG Guide No.	Placard Advisory Consult §172.504 & §172.505 *Placard any quantity
(1)	(2)	(3)	(4)	(5)	(6)	(7)		
	Sodium hydride	4.3	UN1427	I	4.3	A19, N40	138	DANGEROUS WHEN WET*
	Sodium hydrogendifluoride	8	UN2439	II	8	IB8, IP2, IP4, N3, N34, T3, TP33	154	CORROSIVE
	Sodium hydrosulfide, *with less than 25 percent water of crystallization*	4.2	UN2318	II	4.2	A7, A19, A20, IB6, IP2, T3, TP33	135	SPONTANEOUSLY COMBUSTIBLE
	Sodium hydrosulfide *with not less than 25 percent water of crystallization*	8	UN2949	II	8	A7, IB8, IP2, IP4, T7, TP2	154	CORROSIVE
	Sodium hydrosulfite, *see* **Sodium dithionite**							
	Sodium hydroxide, solid	8	UN1823	II	8	IB8, IP2, IP4, T3, TP33	154	CORROSIVE
	Sodium hydroxide solution	8	UN1824	II	8	B2, IB2, N34, T7, TP2	154	CORROSIVE
				III	8	IB3, N34, T4, TP1	154	CORROSIVE
	Sodium hypochlorite, solution, see **Hypochlorite solutions** *etc.*							
	Sodium metal, liquid alloy, see **Alkali metal alloys, liquid, n.o.s.**							
	Sodium methylate	4.2	UN1431	II	4.2, 8	A7, A19, IB5, IP2, T3, TP33	138	SPONTANEOUSLY COMBUSTIBLE
	Sodium methylate solutions *in alcohol*	3	UN1289	II	3, 8	IB2, T7, TP1, TP8	132	FLAMMABLE

Symbols	Hazardous materials descriptions and proper shipping names	Hazard class or Division	Identification Numbers	PG	Label Codes	Special provisions (§172.102)	ERG Guide No.	Placard Advisory Consult §172.504 & §172.505 *Placard any quantity
(1)	(2)	(3)	(4)	(5)	(6)	(7)		
				III	3, 8	B1, IB3, T4, TP1	132	FLAMMABLE
	Sodium monoxide	8	UN1825	II	8	IB8, IP2, IP4, T3, TP33	157	CORROSIVE
	Sodium nitrate	5.1	UN1498	III	5.1	A1, A29, IB8, IP3, T1, TP33	140	OXIDIZER
	Sodium nitrate and potassium nitrate mixtures	5.1	UN1499	III	5.1	A1, A29, IB8, IP3, T1, TP33	140	OXIDIZER
	Sodium nitrite	5.1	UN1500	III	5.1, 6.1	A1, A29, IB8, IP3, T1, TP33	140	OXIDIZER
	Sodium pentachlorophenate	6.1	UN2567	II	6.1	IB8, IP2, IP4, T3, TP33	154	POISON
	Sodium perborate monohydrate	5.1	UN3377	III	5.1	IB8, IP3, T1, TP33	140	OXIDIZER
	Sodium perchlorate	5.1	UN1502	II	5.1	IB6, IP2, T3, TP33	140	OXIDIZER
	Sodium permanganate	5.1	UN1503	II	5.1	IB6, IP2, T3, TP33	140	OXIDIZER
	Sodium peroxide	5.1	UN1504	I	5.1	A20, IB5, IP1, N34	144	OXIDIZER
	Sodium peroxoborate, anhydrous	5.1	UN3247	II	5.1	IB8, IP4, T3, TP33	140	OXIDIZER
	Sodium persulfate	5.1	UN1505	III	5.1	A1, IB8, IP3, T1, TP33	140	OXIDIZER
	Sodium phosphide	4.3	UN1432	I	4.3, 6.1	A19, N40	139	DANGEROUS WHEN WET*
	Sodium picramate, *dry or wetted with less than 20 percent water, by mass*	1.3C	UN0235	II	1.3C		112	EXPLOSIVES 1.3*

Symbols	Hazardous materials descriptions and proper shipping names	Hazard class or Division	Identification Numbers	PG	Label Codes	Special provisions (§172.102)	ERG Guide No.	Placard Advisory Consult §172.504 & §172.505 *Placard any quantity
(1)	(2)	(3)	(4)	(5)	(6)	(7)		
	Sodium picramate, wetted *with not less than 20 percent water, by mass*	4.1	UN1349	I	4.1	23, A8, A19, N41	113	FLAMMABLE SOLID
	Sodium picryl peroxide	Forbidden						
	Sodium potassium alloys, see **Potassium sodium alloys**							
	Sodium selenate, see **Selenates** *or* **Selenites**							
	Sodium sulfide, anhydrous *or* **Sodium sulfide** *with less than 30 percent water of crystallization*	4.2	UN1385	II	4.2	A19, A20, IB6, IP2, N34, T3, TP33	135	SPONTANEOUSLY COMBUSTIBLE
	Sodium sulfide, hydrated *with not less than 30 percent water*	8	UN1849	II	8	IB8, IP2, IP4, T3, TP33	153	CORROSIVE
	Sodium superoxide	5.1	UN2547	I	5.1	A20, IB6, IP1, N34	143	OXIDIZER
	Sodium tetranitride	Forbidden						
G	**Solids containing corrosive liquid, n.o.s.**	8	UN3244	II	8	49, IB5, T3, TP33	154	CORROSIVE
G	**Solids containing flammable liquid, n.o.s.**	4.1	UN3175	II	4.1	47, IB6, IP2, T3, TP33	133	FLAMMABLE SOLID
G	**Solids containing toxic liquid, n.o.s.**	6.1	UN3243	II	6.1	48, IB2, T2, TP33	151	POISON
	Sounding devices, explosive	1.2F	UN0204	II	1.2F		112	EXPLOSIVES 1.2*
	Sounding devices, explosive	1.1F	UN0296	II	1.1F		112	EXPLOSIVES 1.1*
	Sounding devices, explosive	1.1D	UN0374	II	1.1D		112	EXPLOSIVES 1.1*

Sym-bols	Hazardous materials descriptions and proper shipping names	Hazard class or Division	Identification Numbers	PG	Label Codes	Special provisions (§172.102)	ERG Guide No.	Placard Advisory Consult §172.504 & §172.505 *Placard any quantity
(1)	(2)	(3)	(4)	(5)	(6)	(7)		
	Sounding devices, explosive	1.2D	UN0375	II	1.2D		112	EXPLOSIVES 1.2*
	Spirits of salt, see **Hydrochloric acid**							
	Squibs, see **Igniters** *etc.*							
	Stannic chloride, anhydrous	8	UN1827	II	8	B2, IB2, T7, TP2	137	CORROSIVE
	Stannic chloride pentahydrate	8	UN2440	III	8	IB8, IP3, T1, TP33	154	CORROSIVE
	Stannic phosphide	4.3	UN1433	I	4.3, 6.1	A19, N40	139	DANGEROUS WHEN WET*
	Steel swarf, see **Ferrous metal borings,** *etc.*							
	Stibine	2.3	UN2676		2.3, 2.1	1	119	POISON GAS*
	Storage batteries, wet, see **Batteries,** *wet etc.*							
	Strontium arsenite	6.1	UN1691	II	6.1	IB8, IP2, IP4, T3, TP33	151	POISON
	Strontium chlorate	5.1	UN1506	II	5.1	A1, A9, IB8, IP2, IP4, N34, T3, TP33	143	OXIDIZER
	Strontium nitrate	5.1	UN1507	III	5.1	A1, A29, IB8, IP3, T1, TP33	140	OXIDIZER
	Strontium perchlorate	5.1	UN1508	II	5.1	IB6, IP2, T3, TP33	140	OXIDIZER
	Strontium peroxide	5.1	UN1509	II	5.1	IB6, IP2, T3, TP33	143	OXIDIZER

Symbols	Hazardous materials descriptions and proper shipping names	Hazard class or Division	Identification Numbers	PG	Label Codes	Special provisions (§172.102)	ERG Guide No.	Placard Advisory Consult §172.504 & §172.505 *Placard any quantity
(1)	(2)	(3)	(4)	(5)	(6)	(7)		
	Strontium phosphide	4.3	UN2013	I	4.3, 6.1	A19, N40	139	DANGEROUS WHEN WET*
	Strychnine *or* **Strychnine salts**	6.1	UN1692	I	6.1	IB7, IP1, T6, TP33	151	POISON
	Styphnic acid, *see* **Trinitroresorcinol,** *etc.*							
	Styrene monomer, stabilized	3	UN2055	III	3	B1, IB3, T2, TP1	128P	FLAMMABLE
G	**Substances, explosive, n.o.s.**	1.1L	UN0357	II	1.1L	101	112	EXPLOSIVE 1.1*
G	**Substances, explosive, n.o.s.**	1.2L	UN0358	II	1.2L	101	112	EXPLOSIVES 1.2*
G	**Substances, explosive, n.o.s.**	1.3L	UN0359	II	1.3L	101	112	EXPLOSIVES 1.3*
G	**Substances, explosive, n.o.s.**	1.1A	UN0473	II	1.1A	101, 111	112	EXPLOSIVES 1.1*
G	**Substances, explosive, n.o.s.**	1.1C	UN0474	II	1.1C	101	112	EXPLOSIVES 1.1*
G	**Substances, explosive, n.o.s.**	1.1D	UN0475	II	1.1D	101	112	EXPLOSIVES 1.1*
G	**Substances, explosive, n.o.s.**	1.1G	UN0476	II	1.1G	101	112	EXPLOSIVES 1.1*
G	**Substances, explosive, n.o.s.**	1.3C	UN0477	II	1.3C	101	112	EXPLOSIVES 1.3*
G	**Substances, explosive, n.o.s.**	1.3G	UN0478	II	1.3G	101	112	EXPLOSIVES 1.3*
G	**Substances, explosive, n.o.s.**	1.4C	UN0479	II	1.4C	101	114	EXPLOSIVES 1.4
G	**Substances, explosive, n.o.s.**	1.4D	UN0480	II	1.4D	101	114	EXPLOSIVES 1.4
G	**Substances, explosive, n.o.s.**	1.4S	UN0481	II	1.4S	101	114	EXPLOSIVES 1.4
G	**Substances, explosive, n.o.s.**	1.4G	UN0485	II	1.4G	101	114	EXPLOSIVES 1.4

Symbols	Hazardous materials descriptions and proper shipping names	Hazard class or Division	Identification Numbers	PG	Label Codes	Special provisions (§172.102)	ERG Guide No.	Placard Advisory Consult §172.504 & §172.505 *Placard any quantity
(1)	(2)	(3)	(4)	(5)	(6)	(7)		
G	**Substances, explosive, very insensitive, n.o.s.,** *or* **Substances, EVI, n.o.s.**	1.5D	UN0482	II	1.5D	101	112	EXPLOSIVES 1.5
	Substituted nitrophenol pesticides, liquid, flammable, toxic, *flash point less than 23 degrees C*	3	UN2780	I	3, 6.1	T14, TP2, TP13, TP27	131	FLAMMABLE
				II	3, 6.1	IB2, T11, TP2, TP13, TP27	131	FLAMMABLE
	Substituted nitrophenol pesticides, liquid, toxic	6.1	UN3014	I	6.1	T14, TP2, TP13, TP27	153	POISON
				II	6.1	IB2, T11, TP2, TP13, TP27	153	POISON
				III	6.1	IB3, T7, TP2, TP28	153	POISON
	Substituted nitrophenol pesticides, liquid, toxic, flammable *flash point not less than 23 degrees C*	6.1	UN3013	I	6.1, 3	T14, TP2, TP13, TP27	131	POISON
				II	6.1, 3	IB2, T11, TP2, TP13, TP27	131	POISON
				III	6.1, 3	B1, IB3, T7, TP2, TP28	131	POISON
	Substituted nitrophenol pesticides, solid, toxic	6.1	UN2779	I	6.1	IB7, IP1, T6, TP33	153	POISON
				II	6.1	IB8, IP2, IP4, T3, TP33	153	POISON

Sym-bols	Hazardous materials descriptions and proper shipping names	Hazard class or Division	Identifica-tion Numbers	PG	Label Codes	Special provisions (§172.102)	ERG Guide No.	Placard Advisory Consult §172.504 & §172.505 *Placard any quantity
(1)	(2)	(3)	(4)	(5)	(6)	(7)		
				III	6.1	IB8, IP3, T1, TP33	153	POISON
	Sucrose octanitrate (dry)	Forbidden						
	Sulfamic acid	8	UN2967	III	8	IB8, IP3, T1, TP33	154	CORROSIVE
D	**Sulfur**	9	NA1350	III	9	30, IB8, IP2	133	CLASS 9
I	**Sulfur**	4.1	UN1350	III	4.1	30, IB8, IP3, T1, TP33	133	FLAMMABLE SOLID
	Sulfur and chlorate, loose mixtures of	Forbidden						
	Sulfur chlorides	8	UN1828	I	8	5, A3, A7, A10, B10, B77, N34, T20, TP2, TP12	137	CORROSIVE
	Sulfur dichloride, see **Sulfur chlorides**							
	Sulfur dioxide	2.3	UN1079		2.3, 8	3, B14, T50, TP19	125	POISON GAS*
	Sulfur dioxide solution, see **Sulfurous acid**							
	Sulfur hexafluoride	2.2	UN1080		2.2		126	NONFLAMMABLE GAS
D	**Sulfur, molten**	9	NA2448	III	9	30, IB3, T1, TP3	133	CLASS 9
I	**Sulfur, molten**	4.1	UN2448	III	4.1	30, IB1, T1, TP3	133	FLAMMABLE SOLID
	Sulfur tetrafluoride	2.3	UN2418		2.3, 8	1	125	POISON GAS*

Symbols	Hazardous materials descriptions and proper shipping names	Hazard class or Division	Identification Numbers	PG	Label Codes	Special provisions (§172.102)	ERG Guide No.	Placard Advisory Consult §172.504 & §172.505 *Placard any quantity
(1)	(2)	(3)	(4)	(5)	(6)	(7)		
+	**Sulfur trioxide, stabilized**	8	UN1829	I	8, 6.1	2, B9, B14, B32, B49, B74, B77, N34, T20, TP4, TP12, TP13, TP25, TP26, TP38, TP45	137	CORROSIVE, POISON INHALATION HAZARD*
	Sulfuretted hydrogen, see **Hydrogen sulfide**							
	Sulfuric acid, fuming *with less than 30 percent free sulfur trioxide*	8	UN1831	I	8	A3, A7, B84, N34, T20, TP2, TP12, TP13	137	CORROSIVE
+	**Sulfuric acid, fuming** *with 30 percent or more free sulfur trioxide*	8	UN1831	I	8, 6.1	2, B9, B14, B32, B74, B77, B84, N34, T20, TP2, TP12, TP13	137	CORROSIVE, POISON INHALATION HAZARD*
	Sulfuric acid, spent	8	UN1832	II	8	A3, A7, B2, B83, B84, IB2, N34, T8, TP2, TP12	137	CORROSIVE
	Sulfuric acid *with more than 51 percent acid*	8	UN1830	II	8	A3, A7, B3, B83, B84, IB2, N34, T8, TP2, TP12	137	CORROSIVE
	Sulfuric acid *with not more than 51% acid*	8	UN2796	II	8	A3, A7, B2, B15, IB2, N6, N34, T8, TP2, TP12	157	CORROSIVE
	Sulfuric and hydrofluoric acid mixtures, *see* **Hydrofluoric and sulfuric acid mixtures**							

Symbols	Hazardous materials descriptions and proper shipping names	Hazard class or Division	Identification Numbers	PG	Label Codes	Special provisions (§172.102)	ERG Guide No.	Placard Advisory Consult §172.504 & §172.505 *Placard any quantity
(1)	(2)	(3)	(4)	(5)	(6)	(7)		
	Sulfuric anhydride, see **Sulfur trioxide, stabilized**							
	Sulfurous acid	8	UN1833	II	8	B3, IB2, T7, TP2	154	CORROSIVE
+	**Sulfuryl chloride**	8	UN1834	I	8, 6.1	1, B6, B9, B10, B14, B30, B74, B77, N34, T22, TP2, TP12, TP38, TP44	137	CORROSIVE, POISON INHALATION HAZARD*
	Sulfuryl fluoride	2.3	UN2191		2.3	4	123	POISON GAS*
	Tars, liquid *including road asphalt and oils, bitumen and cut backs*	3	UN1999	II	3	149, B13, IB2, T3, TP3, TP29	130	FLAMMABLE
				III	3	B1, B13, IB3, T1, TP3	130	FLAMMABLE
	Tear gas candles	6.1	UN1700	II	6.1, 4.1		159	POISON
	Tear gas cartridges, see **Ammunition, tear-producing,** *etc.*							
D	**Tear gas devices** *with more than 2 percent tear gas substances, by mass*	6.1	NA1693	I	6.1		159	POISON
				II	6.1		159	POISON
	Tear gas devices, with not more than 2 percent tear gas substances, by mass, see **Aerosols,** *etc.*							

Sym-bols	Hazardous materials descriptions and proper shipping names	Hazard class or Division	Identifica-tion Numbers	PG	Label Codes	Special provisions (§172.102)	ERG Guide No.	Placard Advisory Consult §172.504 & §172.505 *Placard any quantity
(1)	(2)	(3)	(4)	(5)	(6)	(7)		
	Tear gas grenades, see **Tear gas candles**							
G	**Tear gas substances, liquid, n.o.s.**	6.1	UN1693	I	6.1		159	POISON
				II	6.1	IB2	159	POISON
G	**Tear gas substance, solid, n.o.s.**	6.1	UN3448	I	6.1	T6, TP33	159	POISON
				II	6.1	IB8, IP2, IP4, T3, TP33	159	POISON
	Tellurium compound, n.o.s.	6.1	UN3284	I	6.1	IB7, IP1, T6, TP33	151	POISON
				II	6.1	IB8, IP2, IP4, T3, TP33	151	POISON
				III	6.1	IB8, IP3, T1, TP33	151	POISON
	Tellurium hexafluoride	2.3	UN2195		2.3, 8	1	125	POISON GAS*
	Terpene hydrocarbons, n.o.s.	3	UN2319	III	3	B1, IB3, T4, TP1, TP29	128	FLAMMABLE
	Terpinolene	3	UN2541	III	3	B1, IB3, T2, TP1	128	FLAMMABLE
	Tetraazido benzene quinone	Forbidden						
	Tetrabromoethane	6.1	UN2504	III	6.1	IB3, T4, TP1	159	POISON
	1,1,2,2-Tetrachloroethane	6.1	UN1702	II	6.1	IB2, N36, T7, TP2	151	POISON
	Tetrachloroethylene	6.1	UN1897	III	6.1	IB3, N36, T4, TP1	160	POISON
	Tetraethyl dithiopyrophosphate	6.1	UN1704	II	6.1	IB2, T7, TP2	153	POISON
	Tetraethyl silicate	3	UN1292	III	3	B1, IB3, T2, TP1	129	FLAMMABLE

Sym-bols	Hazardous materials descriptions and proper shipping names	Hazard class or Division	Identifica-tion Numbers	PG	Label Codes	Special provisions (§172.102)	ERG Guide No.	Placard Advisory Consult §172.504 & §172.505 *Placard any quantity
(1)	(2)	(3)	(4)	(5)	(6)	(7)		
	Tetraethylammonium perchlorate (dry)	Forbidden						
	Tetraethylenepentamine	8	UN2320	III	8	IB3, T4, TP1	153	CORROSIVE
	1,1,1,2-Tetrafluoroethane *or* **Refrigerant gas R 134a**	2.2	UN3159		2.2	T50	126	NONFLAMMABLE GAS
	Tetrafluoroethylene, stabilized	2.1	UN1081		2.1		116P	FLAMMABLE GAS
	Tetrafluoromethane, *or* **Refrigerant gas R 14**	2.2	UN1982		2.2		126	NONFLAMMABLE GAS
	1,2,3,6-Tetrahydrobenzaldehyde	3	UN2498	III	3	B1, IB3, T2, TP1	129	FLAMMABLE
	Tetrahydrofuran	3	UN2056	II	3	IB2, T4, TP1	127	FLAMMABLE
	Tetrahydrofurfurylamine	3	UN2943	III	3	B1, IB3, T2, TP1	129	FLAMMABLE
	Tetrahydrophthalic anhydrides *with more than 0.05 percent of maleic anhydride*	8	UN2698	III	8	IB8, IP3, T1, TP33	156	CORROSIVE
	1,2,3,6-Tetrahydropyridine	3	UN2410	II	3	IB2, T4, TP1	129	FLAMMABLE
	Tetrahydrothiophene	3	UN2412	II	3	IB2, T4, TP1	130	FLAMMABLE
	Tetramethylammonium hydroxide, solid	8	UN3423	II	8	B2, IB8, IP2, IP4, T3, TP33	153	CORROSIVE
	Tetramethylammonium hydroxide solution	8	UN1835	II	8	B2, IB2, T7, TP2	153	CORROSIVE
				III	8	B2, IB3, T7, TP2	153	CORROSIVE
	Tetramethylene diperoxide dicarbamide	Forbidden						
	Tetramethylsilane	3	UN2749	I	3	A7, T14, TP2	130	FLAMMABLE

Sym-bols	Hazardous materials descriptions and proper shipping names	Hazard class or Division	Identifica-tion Numbers	PG	Label Codes	Special provisions (§172.102)	ERG Guide No.	Placard Advisory Consult §172.504 & §172.505 *Placard any quantity
(1)	(2)	(3)	(4)	(5)	(6)	(7)		
	Tetranitro diglycerin	Forbidden						
	Tetranitroaniline	1.1D	UN0207	II	1.1D		112	EXPLOSIVES 1.1*
+	**Tetranitromethane**	5.1	UN1510	I	5.1, 6.1	2, B9, B14, B32, B74, T20, TP2, TP13, TP38, TP44	143	OXIDIZDER, POISON INHALATION HAZARD*
	2,3,4,6-Tetranitrophenol	Forbidden						
	2,3,4,6-Tetranitrophenyl methyl nitramine	Forbidden						
	2,3,4,6-Tetranitrophenylnitramine	Forbidden						
	Tetranitroresorcinol (dry)	Forbidden						
	2,3,5,6-Tetranitroso-1,4-dinitrobenzene	Forbidden						
	2,3,5,6-Tetranitroso nitrobenzene (dry)	Forbidden						
	Tetrapropylorthotitanate	3	UN2413	III	3	B1, IB3, T4, TP1	128	FLAMMABLE
	Tetrazene, *see* **Guanyl nitrosaminoguanyltetrazene**							
	Tetrazine (dry)	Forbidden						
	Tetrazol-1-acetic acid	1.4C	UN0407	II	1.4C		114	EXPLOSIVES 1.4
	1H-Tetrazole	1.1D	UN0504		1.1D		112	EXPLOSIVES 1.1*
	Tetrazolyl azide (dry)	Forbidden						
	Tetryl, *see* **Trinitrophenylmethylnitramine**							

Symbols	Hazardous materials descriptions and proper shipping names	Hazard class or Division	Identification Numbers	PG	Label Codes	Special provisions (§172.102)	ERG Guide No.	Placard Advisory Consult §172.504 & §172.505 *Placard any quantity
(1)	(2)	(3)	(4)	(5)	(6)	(7)		
A I W	**Textile waste, wet**	4.2	UN1857	III	4.2		133	SPONTANEOUSLY COMBUSTIBLE
	Thallium chlorate	5.1	UN2573	II	5.1, 6.1	IB6, IP2, T3, TP33	141	OXIDIZER
	Thallium compounds, n.o.s.	6.1	UN1707	II	6.1	IB8, IP2, IP4, T3, TP33	151	POISON
	Thallium nitrate	6.1	UN2727	II	6.1, 5.1	IB6, IP2, T3, TP33	141	POISON
	4-Thiapentanal	6.1	UN2785	III	6.1	IB3, T4, TP1	152	POISON
	Thioacetic acid	3	UN2436	II	3	IB2, T4, TP1	129	FLAMMABLE
	Thiocarbamate pesticide, liquid, flammable, toxic, *flash point less than 23 degrees C*	3	UN2772	I	3, 6.1	T14, TP2, TP13, TP27	131	FLAMMABLE
				II	3, 6.1	IB2, T11, TP13, TP27	131	FLAMMABLE
	Thiocarbamate pesticide, liquid, toxic, flammable, *flash point not less than 23 degrees C*	6.1	UN3005	I	6.1, 3	T14, TP2, TP13	131	POISON
				II	6.1, 3	IB2, T11, TP2, TP13, TP27	131	POISON
				III	6.1, 3	IB3, T7, TP2, TP28	131	POISON
	Thiocarbamate pesticide, liquid, toxic	6.1	UN3006	I	6, 1	T14, TP2, TP13	151	POISON

Sym-bols	Hazardous materials descriptions and proper shipping names	Hazard class or Division	Identifica-tion Numbers	PG	Label Codes	Special provisions (§172.102)	ERG Guide No.	Placard Advisory Consult §172.504 & §172.505 *Placard any quantity
(1)	(2)	(3)	(4)	(5)	(6)	(7)		
				II	6.1	IB2, T11, TP2, TP13, TP27	151	POISON
				III	6.1	IB3, T7, TP2, TP28	151	POISON
	Thiocarbamate pesticides, solid, toxic	6.1	UN2771	I	6.1	IB7, IP1, T6, TP33	151	POISON
				II	6.1	IB8, IP2, IP4, T3, TP33	151	POISON
				III	6.1	IB8, IP3, T1, TP33	151	POISON
	Thiocarbonylchloride, see **Thiophosgene**							
	Thioglycol	6.1	UN2966	II	6.1	IB2, T7, TP2	153	POISON
	Thioglycolic acid	8	UN1940	II	8	A7, B2, IB2, N34, T7, TP2	153	CORROSIVE
	Thiolactic acid	6.1	UN2936	II	6.1	IB2, T7, TP2	153	POISON
	Thionyl chloride	8	UN1836	I	8	B6, B10, N34, T10, TP2, TP12, TP13	137	CORROSIVE
	Thiophene	3	UN2414	II	3	IB2, T4, TP1	130	FLAMMABLE
+	**Thiophosgene**	6.1	UN2474	II	6.1	2, B9, B14, B32, B74, N33, N34, T20, TP2, TP38, TP45	157	POISON INHALATION HAZARD*

Sym-bols	Hazardous materials descriptions and proper shipping names	Hazard class or Division	Identification Numbers	PG	Label Codes	Special provisions (§172.102)	ERG Guide No.	Placard Advisory Consult §172.504 & §172.505 *Placard any quantity
(1)	(2)	(3)	(4)	(5)	(6)	(7)		
	Thiophosphoryl chloride	8	UN1837	II	8	A3, A7, B2, B8, B25, IB2, N34, T7, TP2	157	CORROSIVE
	Thiourea dioxide	4.2	UN3341	II	4.2	IB6, IP2, T3, TP33	135	SPONTANEOUSLY COMBUSTIBLE
				III	4.2	IB8, IP3, T1, TP33	135	SPONTANEOUSLY COMBUSTIBLE
	Tin chloride, fuming, see **Stannic chloride, anhydrous**							
	Tin perchloride or Tin tetrachloride, see **Stannic chloride, anhydrous**							
	Tinctures, medicinal	3	UN1293	II	3	IB2, T4, TP1, TP8	127	FLAMMABLE
				III	3	B1, IB3, T2, TP1	127	FLAMMABLE
	Tinning flux, see **Zinc chloride**							
	Titanium disulphide	4.2	UN3174	III	4.2	IB8, IP3, T1, TP33	135	SPONTANEOUSLY COMBUSTIBLE
	Titanium hydride	4.1	UN1871	II	4.1	A19, A20, IB4, N34, T3, TP33	170	FLAMMABLE SOLID
	Titanium powder, dry	4.2	UN2546	I	4.2		135	SPONTANEOUSLY COMBUSTIBLE
				II	4.2	A19, A20, IB6, IP2, N5, N34, T3, TP33	135	SPONTANEOUSLY COMBUSTIBLE

Sym-bols	Hazardous materials descriptions and proper shipping names	Hazard class or Division	Identifica-tion Numbers	PG	Label Codes	Special provisions (§172.102)	ERG Guide No.	Placard Advisory Consult §172.504 & §172.505 *Placard any quantity
(1)	(2)	(3)	(4)	(5)	(6)	(7)		
				III	4.2	IB8, IP3, T1, TP33	135	SPONTANEOUSLY COMBUSTIBLE
	Titanium powder, wetted *with not less than 25 percent water (a visible excess of water must be present) (a) mechanically produced, particle size less than 53 microns; (b) chemically produced, particle size less than 840 microns*	4.1	UN1352	II	4.1	A19, A20, IB6, IP2, N34, T3, TP33	170	FLAMMABLE SOLID
	Titanium sponge granules *or* **Titanium sponge powders**	4.1	UN2878	III	4.1	A1, IB8, IP3, T1, TP33	170	FLAMMABLE SOLID
+	**Titanium tetrachloride**	8	UN1838	II	8, 6.1	2, B7, B9, B14, B32, B74, B77, T20, TP2, TP13, TP38, TP45	137	CORROSIVE, POISON INHALATION HAZARD*
	Titanium trichloride mixtures	8	UN2869	II	8	A7, IB8, IP2, IP4, N34, T3, TP33	157	CORROSIVE
				III	8	A7, IB8, IP3, N34, T1, TP33	157	CORROSIVE
	Titanium trichloride, pyrophoric *or* **Titanium trichloride mixtures, pyrophoric**	4.2	UN2441	I	4.2, 8	N34	135	SPONTANEOUSLY COMBUSTIBLE
	TNT mixed with aluminum, see **Tritonal**							
	TNT, *see* **Trinitrotoluene,** *etc.*							
	Toluene	3	UN1294	II	3	IB2, T4, TP1	130	FLAMMABLE

Sym-bols	Hazardous materials descriptions and proper shipping names	Hazard class or Division	Identification Numbers	PG	Label Codes	Special provisions (§172.102)	ERG Guide No.	Placard Advisory Consult §172.504 & §172.505 *Placard any quantity
(1)	(2)	(3)	(4)	(5)	(6)	(7)		
+	**Toluene diisocyanate**	6.1	UN2078	II	6.1	IB2, T7, TP2, TP13	156	POISON
	Toluene sulfonic acid, see **Alkyl,** *or* **Aryl sulfonic acid** *etc.*							
+	**Toluidines, liquid**	6.1	UN1708	II	6.1	IB2, T7, TP2	153	POISON
+	**Toluidines, solid**	6.1	UN3451	II	6.1	IB8, IP2, IP4, T3, TP33	153	POISON
	2,4-Toluylenediamine, solid *or* **2, 4-Toluenediamine, solid**	6.1	UN1709	III	6.1	IB8, IP3, T1, TP33	151	POISON
	2,4-Toluylenediamine solution *or* **2,4-Toluenediamine solution**	6.1	UN3418	III	6.1	IB3, T4, TP1	151	POISON
	Torpedoes, liquid fueled, *with inert head*	1.3J	UN0450	II	1.3J		112	EXPLOSIVES 1.3*
	Torpedoes, liquid fueled, *with or without bursting charge*	1.1J	UN0449	II	1.1J		112	EXPLOSIVES 1.1*
	Torpedoes *with bursting charge*	1.1E	UN0329	II	1.1E		112	EXPLOSIVES 1.1*
	Torpedoes *with bursting charge*	1.1F	UN0330	II	1.1F		112	EXPLOSIVES 1.1*
	Torpedoes *with bursting charge*	1.1D	UN0451	II	1.1D		112	EXPLOSIVES 1.1*
G	**Toxic by inhalation liquid, n.o.s.** *with an inhalation toxicity lower than or equal to 200 ml/m3 and saturated vapor concentration greater than or equal to 500 LC50.*	6.1	UN3381	I	6.1	1,B9, B14, B30, B72, T22, TP2, TP13, TP27, TP38, TP44	151	POISON INHALATION HAZARD*

Sym-bols	Hazardous materials descriptions and proper shipping names	Hazard class or Division	Identifica-tion Numbers	PG	Label Codes	Special provisions (§172.102)	ERG Guide No.	Placard Advisory Consult §172.504 & §172.505 *Placard any quantity
(1)	(2)	(3)	(4)	(5)	(6)	(7)		
G	**Toxic by inhalation liquid, n.o.s.** *with an inhalation toxicity lower than or equal to 1000 ml/m3 and saturated vapor concentration greater than or equal to 10 LC50.*	6.1	UN3382	I	6.1	2, B9, B14, B32, B74, T20, TP2, TP13, TP27, TP38, TP45	151	POISON INHALATION HAZARD*
G	**Toxic by inhalation liquid, flammable, n.o.s.** *with an inhalation toxicity lower than or equal to 200 ml/m3 and saturated vapor concentration greater than or equal to 500 LC50.*	6.1	UN3383	I	6.1, 3	1,B9, B14, B30, B72, T22, TP2, TP13, TP27, TP38, TP44	131	POISON INHALATION HAZARD*
G	**Toxic by inhalation liquid, flammable, n.o.s.** *with an inhalation toxicity lower than or equal to 1000 ml/m3 and saturated vapor concentration greater than or equal to 10 LC50.*	6.1	UN3384	I	6.1, 3	2,B9, B14, B32, B74, T20, TP2, TP13, TP27, TP38, TP45	131	POISON INHALATION HAZARD*
G	**Toxic by inhalation liquid, water-reactive, n.o.s.** *with an inhalation toxicity lower than or equal to 200 ml/m3 and saturated vapor concentration greater than or equal to 500 LC50.*	6.1	UN3385	I	6.1, 4.3	1,B9, B14, B30, B72, T22, TP2, TP13, TP38, TP44	139	POISON INHALATION HAZARD*
G	**Toxic by inhalation liquid, water-reactive, n.o.s.** *with an inhalation toxicity lower than or equal to 1000 ml/m3 and saturated vapor concentration greater than or equal to 10 LC50.*	6.1	UN3386	I	6.1, 4.3	2, B9, B14, B32, B74, T20, TP2, TP13, TP38, TP44	139	POISON INHALATION HAZARD*

Sym-bols	Hazardous materials descriptions and proper shipping names	Hazard class or Division	Identifica-tion Numbers	PG	Label Codes	Special provisions (§172.102)	ERG Guide No.	Placard Advisory Consult §172.504 & §172.505 *Placard any quantity
(1)	(2)	(3)	(4)	(5)	(6)	(7)		
G	**Toxic by inhalation liquid, oxidizing, n.o.s.** *with an inhalation toxicity lower than or equal to 200 ml/m3 and saturated vapor concentration greater than or equal to 500 LC50.*	6.1	UN3387	I	6.1, 5.1	1,B9, B14, B30, B72, T22, TP2, TP13, TP38, TP44	142	POISON INHALATION HAZARD*
G	**Toxic by inhalation liquid, oxidizing, n.o.s.** *with an inhalation toxicity lower than or equal to 1000 ml/m3 and saturated vapor concentration greater than or equal to 10 LC50.*	6.1	UN3388	I	6.1, 5.1	2, B9, B14, B32, T20, TP2, TP13, TP38, TP44	142	POISON INHALATION HAZARD*
G	**Toxic by inhalation liquid, corrosive, n.o.s.** *with an inhalation toxicity lower than or equal to 200 ml/m3 and saturated vapor concentration greater than or equal to 500 LC50.*	6.1	UN3389	I	6.1, 8	1,B9, B14, B30, B72, T22, TP2, TP13, TP27, TP38, TP44	154	POISON INHALATION HAZARD*
G	**Toxic by inhalation liquid, corrosive, n.o.s.** *with an inhalation toxicity lower than or equal to 1000 ml/m3 and saturated vapor concentration greater than or equal to 10 LC50.*	6.1	UN3390	I	6.1, 8	2, B9, B14, B32, B74, T20, TP2, TP13, TP27, TP38, TP45	154	POISON INHALATION HAZARD*
G	**Toxic liquid, corrosive, inorganic, n.o.s.**	6.1	UN3289	I	6.1, 8	T14, TP2, TP13, TP27	154	POISON
				II	6.1, 8	IB2, T11, TP2, TP27	154	POISON
G	**Toxic liquid, inorganic, n.o.s.**	6.1	UN3287	I	6.1	T14, TP2, TP13, TP27	151	POISON

Symbols	Hazardous materials descriptions and proper shipping names	Hazard class or Division	Identification Numbers	PG	Label Codes	Special provisions (§172.102)	ERG Guide No.	Placard Advisory Consult §172.504 & §172.505 *Placard any quantity
(1)	(2)	(3)	(4)	(5)	(6)	(7)		
				II	6.1	IB2, T11, TP2, TP27	151	POISON
				III	6.1	IB3, T7, TP1,TP28	151	POISON
G	**Toxic liquids, corrosive, organic, n.o.s.**	6.1	UN2927	I	6.1, 8	T14, TP2, TP13, TP27	154	POISON
				II	6.1, 8	IB2, T11, TP2, TP27	154	POISON
G	**Toxic liquids, flammable, organic, n.o.s.**	6.1	UN2929	I	6.1, 3	T14, TP2, TP13,TP27	131	POISON
				II	6.1, 3	IB2, T11, TP2, TP13, TP27	131	POISON
G	**Toxic, liquids, organic, n.o.s.**	6.1	UN2810	I	6.1	T14, TP2, TP13, TP27	153	POISON
				II	6.1	IB2, T11, TP2, TP13, TP27	153	POISON
				III	6.1	IB3, T7, TP1, TP28	153	POISON
G	**Toxic liquids, oxidizing, n.o.s.**	6.1	UN3122	I	6.1, 5.1	A4	142	POISON
				II	6.1, 5.1	IB2	142	POISON
G	**Toxic liquids, water-reactive, n.o.s.**	6.1	UN3123	I	6.1, 4.3	A4	139	POISON, DANGEROUS WHEN WET*

Sym-bols	Hazardous materials descriptions and proper shipping names	Hazard class or Division	Identification Numbers	PG	Label Codes	Special provisions (§172.102)	ERG Guide No.	Placard Advisory Consult §172.504 & §172.505 *Placard any quantity
(1)	(2)	(3)	(4)	(5)	(6)	(7)		
				II	6.1, 4.3	IB2	139	POISON, DANGEROUS WHEN WET*
G	**Toxic solid, corrosive, inorganic, n.o.s.**	6.1	UN3290	I	6.1, 8	IB7, T6, TP33	154	POISON
				II	6.1, 8	IB6, IP2, T3, TP33	154	POISON
G	**Toxic solid, inorganic, n.o.s.**	6.1	UN3288	I	6.1	IB7, T6, TP33	151	POISON
				II	6.1	IB8, IP2, IP4, T3, TP33	151	POISON
				III	6.1	IB8, IP3, T1, TP33	151	POISON
G	**Toxic solids, corrosive, organic, n.o.s.**	6.1	UN2928	I	6.1, 8	IB7, T6, TP33	154	POISON
				II	6.1, 8	IB6, IP2, T3, TP33	154	POISON
G	**Toxic solids, flammable, organic, n.o.s.**	6.1	UN2930	I	6.1, 4.1	IB6, T6, TP33	134	POISON
				II	6.1, 4.1	IB8, IP2, IP4, T3, TP33	134	POISON
G	**Toxic solids, organic, n.o.s.**	6.1	UN2811	I	6.1	IB7, T6, TP33	154	POISON
				II	6.1	IB8, IP2, IP4, T3, TP33	154	POISON
				III	6.1	IB8, IP3, T1, TP33	154	POISON
G	**Toxic solids, oxidizing, n.o.s.**	6.1	UN3086	I	6.1, 5.1	T6, TP33	141	POISON

Symbols	Hazardous materials descriptions and proper shipping names	Hazard class or Division	Identification Numbers	PG	Label Codes	Special provisions (§172.102)	ERG Guide No.	Placard Advisory Consult §172.504 & §172.505 *Placard any quantity
(1)	(2)	(3)	(4)	(5)	(6)	(7)		
				II	6.1, 5.1	IB6, IP2, T3, TP33	141	POISON
G	**Toxic solids, self-heating, n.o.s.**	6.1	UN3124	I	6.1, 4.2	A5, T6, TP33	136	POISON
				II	6.1, 4.2	IB6, IP2, T3, TP33	136	POISON
G	**Toxic solids, water-reactive, n.o.s.**	6.1	UN3125	I	6.1, 4.3	A5, T6, TP33	139	POISON, DANGEROUS WHEN WET*
				II	6.1, 4.3	IB6, IP2, T3, TP33	139	POISON, DANGEROUS WHEN WET*
G	**Toxins, extracted from living sources, liquid, n.o.s.**	6.1	UN3172	I	6.1	141	153	POISON
				II	6.1	141, IB2	153	POISON
				III	6.1	141, IB3	153	POISON
G	**Toxins, extracted from living sources, solid, n.o.s.**	6.1	UN3462	I	6.1	141, IB7, IP1, T6, TP33	153	POISON
				II	6.1	141, IB8, IP2, IP4, T3, TP33	153	POISON
				III	6.1	141, IB8, IP3, T1, TP33	153	POISON
D	**Toy Caps**	1.4S	NA0337	II	1.4S		114	EXPLOSIVES 1.4

Sym-bols	Hazardous materials descriptions and proper shipping names	Hazard class or Division	Identifica-tion Numbers	PG	Label Codes	Special provisions (§172.102)	ERG Guide No.	Placard Advisory Consult §172.504 & §172.505 *Placard any quantity
(1)	(2)	(3)	(4)	(5)	(6)	(7)		
	Tracers for ammunition	1.3G	UN0212	II	1.3G		112	EXPLOSIVES 1.3*
	Tracers for ammunition	1.4G	UN0306	II	1.4G		114	EXPLOSIVES 1.4
	Tractors, see **Vehicle,** *etc.*							
	Tri-(b-nitroxyethyl) ammonium nitrate	Forbidden						
	Triallyl borate	6.1	UN2609	III	6.1	IB3	156	POISON
	Triallylamine	3	UN2610	III	3, 8	B1, IB3, T4, TP1	132	FLAMMABLE
	Triazine pesticides, liquid, flammable, toxic, *flash point less than 23 degrees C*	3	UN2764	I	3, 6.1	T14, TP2, TP13, TP27	131	FLAMMABLE
				II	3, 6.1	IB2, T11, TP2, TP13, TP27	131	FLAMMABLE
	Triazine pesticides, liquid, toxic	6.1	UN2998	I	6.1	T14, TP2, TP13, TP27	151	POISON
				II	6.1	IB2, T11, TP2, TP13, TP27	151	POISON
				III	6.1	IB3, T7, TP2, TP28	151	POISON
	Triazine pesticides, liquid, toxic, flammable, *flash point not less than 23 degrees C*	6.1	UN2997	I	6.1, 3	T14, TP2, TP13, TP27	131	POISON
				II	6.1, 3	IB2, T11, TP2, TP13, TP27	131	POISON
				III	6.1, 3	IB3, T7, TP2, TP28	131	POISON

Symbols	Hazardous materials descriptions and proper shipping names	Hazard class or Division	Identification Numbers	PG	Label Codes	Special provisions (§172.102)	ERG Guide No.	Placard Advisory Consult §172.504 & §172.505 *Placard any quantity
(1)	(2)	(3)	(4)	(5)	(6)	(7)		
	Triazine pesticides, solid, toxic	6.1	UN2763	I	6.1	IB7, IP1, T6, TP33	151	POISON
				II	6.1	IB8, IP2, IP4, T3, TP33	151	POISON
				III	6.1	IB8, IP3, T1, TP33	151	POISON
	Tributylamine	6.1	UN2542	II	6.1	IB2, T7, TP2	153	POISON
	Tributylphosphane	4.2	UN3254	I	4.2	T21, TP7, TP33	135	SPONTANEOUSLY COMBUSTIBLE
	Trichloro-s-triazinetrione dry, with more than 39 percent available chlorine, see **Trichloroisocyanuric acid, dry**							
	Trichloroacetic acid	8	UN1839	II	8	A7, IB8, IP2, IP4, N34, T3, TP33	153	CORROSIVE
	Trichloroacetic acid, solution	8	UN2564	II	8	A3, A6, A7, B2, IB2, N34, T7, TP2	153	CORROSIVE
				III	8	A3, A6, A7, IB3, N34, T4, TP1	153	CORROSIVE
+	**Trichloroacetyl chloride**	8	UN2442	II	8, 6.1	2, B9, B14, B32, B74, N34, T20, TP2, TP38, TP45	156	CORROSIVE, POISON INHALATION HAZARD*
	Trichlorobenzenes, liquid	6.1	UN2321	III	6.1	IB3, T4, TP1	153	POISON
	Trichlorobutene	6.1	UN2322	II	6.1	IB2, T7, TP2	152	POISON
	1,1,1-Trichloroethane	6.1	UN2831	III	6.1	IB3, N36, T4, TP1	160	POISON

Symbols	Hazardous materials descriptions and proper shipping names	Hazard class or Division	Identification Numbers	PG	Label Codes	Special provisions (§172.102)	ERG Guide No.	Placard Advisory Consult §172.504 & §172.505 *Placard any quantity
(1)	(2)	(3)	(4)	(5)	(6)	(7)		
	Trichloroethylene	6.1	UN1710	III	6.1	IB3, N36, T4, TP1	160	POISON
	Trichloroisocyanuric acid, dry	5.1	UN2468	II	5.1	IB8, IP4, T3, TP33	140	OXIDIZER
	Trichloromethyl perchlorate	Forbidden						
	Trichlorosilane	4.3	UN1295	I	4.3, 3, 8	N34, T14, TP2, TP7, TP13	139	DANGEROUS WHEN WET*
	Tricresyl phosphate *with more than 3 percent ortho isomer*	6.1	UN2574	II	6.1	A3, IB2, N33, N34, T7, TP2	151	POISON
	Triethyl phosphite	3	UN2323	III	3	B1, IB3, T2, TP1	130	FLAMMABLE
	Triethylamine	3	UN1296	II	3, 8	IB2, T7, TP1	132	FLAMMABLE
	Triethylenetetramine	8	UN2259	II	8	B2, IB2, T7, TP2	153	CORROSIVE
	Trifluoroacetic acid	8	UN2699	I	8	A3, A6, A7, B4, N3, N34, N36, T10, TP2, TP12	154	CORROSIVE
	Trifluoroacetyl chloride	2.3	UN3057		2.3, 8	2, B7, B9, B14, T50, TP21	125	POISON GAS*
	Trifluorochloroethylene, stabilized	2.3	UN1082		2.3, 2.1	3, B14, T50	119P	POISON GAS*
	1,1,1-Trifluoroethane *or* **Refrigerant gas, R 143a**	2.1	UN2035		2.1	T50	115	FLAMMABLE GAS
	Trifluoromethane *or* **Refrigerant gas R 23**	2.2	UN1984		2.2		126	NONFLAMMABLE GAS
	Trifluoromethane, refrigerated liquid	2.2	UN3136		2.2	T75, TP5	120	NONFLAMMABLE GAS

Symbols	Hazardous materials descriptions and proper shipping names	Hazard class or Division	Identification Numbers	PG	Label Codes	Special provisions (§172.102)	ERG Guide No.	Placard Advisory Consult §172.504 & §172.505 *Placard any quantity
(1)	(2)	(3)	(4)	(5)	(6)	(7)		
	2-Trifluoromethylaniline	6.1	UN2942	III	6.1	IB3	153	POISON
	3-Trifluoromethylaniline	6.1	UN2948	II	6.1	IB2, T7, TP2	153	POISON
	Triformoxime trinitrate	Forbidden						
	Triisobutylene	3	UN2324	III	3	B1, IB3, T4, TP1	128	FLAMMABLE
	Triisopropyl borate	3	UN2616	II	3	IB2, T4, TP1	129	FLAMMABLE
				III	3	B1, IB3, T2, TP1	129	FLAMMABLE
D	**Trimethoxysilane**	6.1	NA9269	I	6.1, 3	2, B9, B14, B32, B74, T20, TP4, TP12, TP13, TP38, TP45	132	POISON INHALATION HAZARD*
	Trimethyl borate	3	UN2416	II	3	IB2, T7, TP1	129	FLAMMABLE
	Trimethyl phosphite	3	UN2329	III	3	B1, IB3, T2, TP1	130	FLAMMABLE
	1,3,5-Trimethyl-2,4,6-trinitrobenzene	Forbidden						
	Trimethylacetyl chloride	6.1	UN2438	I	6.1, 8, 3	2, B3, B9, B14, B32, B74, N34, T20, TP2, TP13, TP38, TP45,	132	POISON INHALATION HAZARD*
	Trimethylamine, anhydrous	2.1	UN1083		2.1	T50	118	FLAMMABLE GAS
	Trimethylamine, aqueous solutions *with not more than 50 percent trimethylamine by mass*	3	UN1297	I	3, 8	T11, TP1	132	FLAMMABLE
				II	3, 8	B1, IB2, T7, TP1	132	FLAMMABLE

Symbols	Hazardous materials descriptions and proper shipping names	Hazard class or Division	Identification Numbers	PG	Label Codes	Special provisions (§172.102)	ERG Guide No.	Placard Advisory Consult §172.504 & §172.505 *Placard any quantity
(1)	(2)	(3)	(4)	(5)	(6)	(7)		
				III	3, 8	B1, IB3, T7, TP1	132	FLAMMABLE
	1,3,5-Trimethylbenzene	3	UN2325	III	3	B1, IB3, T2, TP1	129	FLAMMABLE
	Trimethylchlorosilane	3	UN1298	II	3, 8	A3, A7, B77, IB2, N34, T7, TP2, TP13	155	FLAMMABLE
	Trimethylcyclohexylamine	8	UN2326	III	8	IB3, T4, TP1	153	CORROSIVE
	Trimethylene glycol diperchlorate	Forbidden						
	Trimethylhexamethylene diisocyanate	6.1	UN2328	III	6.1	IB3, T4, TP2, TP13	156	POISON
	Trimethylhexamethylenediamines	8	UN2327	III	8	IB3, T4, TP1	153	CORROSIVE
	Trimethylol nitromethane trinitrate	Forbidden						
	Trinitro-meta-cresol	1.1D	UN0216	II	1.1D		112	EXPLOSIVES 1.1*
	2,4,6-Trinitro-1,3-diazobenzene	Forbidden						
	2,4,6-Trinitro-1,3,5-triazido benzene (dry)	Forbidden						
	Trinitroacetic acid	Forbidden						
	Trinitroacetonitrile	Forbidden						
	Trinitroamine cobalt	Forbidden						
	Trinitroaniline *or* **Picramide**	1.1D	UN0153	II	1.1D		112	EXPLOSIVES 1.1*
	Trinitroanisole	1.1D	UN0213	II	1.1D		112	EXPLOSIVES 1.1*

Sym-bols	Hazardous materials descriptions and proper shipping names	Hazard class or Division	Identification Numbers	PG	Label Codes	Special provisions (§172.102)	ERG Guide No.	Placard Advisory Consult §172.504 & §172.505 *Placard any quantity
(1)	(2)	(3)	(4)	(5)	(6)	(7)		
	Trinitrobenzene, *dry or wetted with less than 30 percent water, by mass*	1.1D	UN0214	II	1.1D		112	EXPLOSIVES 1.1*
	Trinitrobenzene, wetted, *with not less than 10% by mass*	4.1	UN3367	I	4.1	162, A8, A19, N41, N84	113	FLAMMABLE SOLID
	Trinitrobenzene, wetted *with not less than 30 percent water, by mass*	4.1	UN1354	I	4.1	23, A2, A8, A19, N41	113	FLAMMABLE SOLID
	Trinitrobenzenesulfonic acid	1.1D	UN0386	II	1.1D		112	EXPLOSIVES 1.1*
	Trinitrobenzoic acid, *dry or wetted with less than 30 percent water, by mass*	1.1D	UN0215	II	1.1D		112	EXPLOSIVES 1.1*
	Trinitrobenzoic acid, wetted, *with not less than 10% water by mass*	4.1	UN3368	I	4.1	162, A8, A19, N41, N84	113	FLAMMABLE SOLID
	Trinitrobenzoic acid, wetted *with not less than 30 percent water, by mass*	4.1	UN1355	I	4.1	23, A2, A8, A19, N41	113	FLAMMABLE SOLID
	Trinitrochlorobenzene *or* **Picryl chloride**	1.1D	UN0155	II	1.1D		112	EXPLOSIVES 1.1*
	Trinitrochlorobenzene (picryl chloride), wetted, *with not less than 10% water by mass*	4.1	UN3365	I	4.1	162, A8, A19, N41, N84	113	FLAMMABLE SOLID
	Trinitroethanol	Forbidden						
	Trinitroethylnitrate	Forbidden						
	Trinitrofluorenone	1.1D	UN0387	II	1.1D		112	EXPLOSIVES 1.1*
	Trinitromethane	Forbidden						
	1,3,5-Trinitronaphthalene	Forbidden						

Sym-bols	Hazardous materials descriptions and proper shipping names	Hazard class or Division	Identifica-tion Numbers	PG	Label Codes	Special provisions (§172.102)	ERG Guide No.	Placard Advisory Consult §172.504 & §172.505 *Placard any quantity
(1)	(2)	(3)	(4)	(5)	(6)	(7)		
	Trinitronaphthalene	1.1D	UN0217	II	1.1D		112	EXPLOSIVES 1.1*
	Trinitrophenetole	1.1D	UN0218	II	1.1D		112	EXPLOSIVES 1.1*
	Trinitrophenol *or* **Picric acid,** *dry or wetted with less than 30 percent water, by mass*	1.1D	UN0154	II	1.1D		112	EXPLOSIVES 1.1*
	Trinitrophenol (picric acid), wetted, *with not less than 10 percent water by mass*	4.1	UN3364	I	4.1	162, A8, A19, N41, N84	113	FLAMMABLE SOLID
	Trinitrophenol, wetted *with not less than 30 percent water, by mass*	4.1	UN1344	I	4.1	23, A8, A19, N41	113	FLAMMABLE SOLID
	2,4,6-Trinitrophenyl guanidine (dry)	Forbidden						
	2,4,6-Trinitrophenyl nitramine	Forbidden						
	2,4,6-Trinitrophenyl trimethylol methyl nitramine trinitrate (dry)	Forbidden						
	Trinitrophenylmethylnitramine *or* **Tetryl**	1.1D	UN0208	II	1.1D		112	EXPLOSIVES 1.1*
	Trinitroresorcinol *or* **Styphnic acid,** *dry or wetted with less than 20 percent water, or mixture of alcohol and water, by mass*	1.1D	UN0219	II	1.1D		112	EXPLOSIVES 1.1*
	Trinitroresorcinol, wetted *or* **Styphnic acid, wetted** *with not less than 20 percent water, or mixture of alcohol and water by mass*	1.1D	UN0394	II	1.1D		112	EXPLOSIVES 1.1*

Symbols	Hazardous materials descriptions and proper shipping names	Hazard class or Division	Identification Numbers	PG	Label Codes	Special provisions (§172.102)	ERG Guide No.	Placard Advisory Consult §172.504 & §172.505 *Placard any quantity
(1)	(2)	(3)	(4)	(5)	(6)	(7)		
	2,4,6-Trinitroso-3-methyl nitraminoanisole	Forbidden						
	Trinitrotetramine cobalt nitrate	Forbidden						
	Trinitrotoluene and Trinitrobenzene mixtures *or* **TNT and trinitrobenzene mixtures** *or* **TNT and hexanitrostilbene mixtures** *or* **Trinitrotoluene and hexanitrostilnene mixtures**	1.1D	UN0388	II	1.1D		112	EXPLOSIVES 1.1*
	Trinitrotoluene mixtures containing Trinitrobenzene and Hexanitrostilbene *or* **TNT mixtures containing trinitrobenzene and hexanitrostilbene**	1.1D	UN0389	II	1.1D		112	EXPLOSIVES 1.1*
	Trinitrotoluene *or* **TNT,** *dry or wetted with less than 30 percent water, by mass*	1.1D	UN0209	II	1.1D		112	EXPLOSIVES 1.1*
	Trinitrotoluene (TNT), wetted, *with not less than 10 percent water by mass*	4.1	UN3366	I	4.1	162, A8, A19, N41, N84	113	FLAMMABLE SOLID
	Trinitrotoluene, wetted *with not less than 30 percent water, by mass*	4.1	UN1356	I	4.1	23, A2, A8, A19, N41	113	FLAMMABLE SOLID
	Tripropylamine	3	UN2260	III	3, 8	B1, IB3, T4, TP1	132	FLAMMABLE
	Tripropylene	3	UN2057	II	3	IB2, T4, TP1	128	FLAMMABLE
				III	3	B1, IB3, T2, TP1	128	FLAMMABLE

Sym-bols	Hazardous materials descriptions and proper shipping names	Hazard class or Division	Identifica-tion Numbers	PG	Label Codes	Special provisions (§172.102)	ERG Guide No.	Placard Advisory Consult §172.504 & §172.505 *Placard any quantity
(1)	(2)	(3)	(4)	(5)	(6)	(7)		
	Tris-(1-aziridinyl)phosphine oxide, solution	6.1	UN2501	II	6.1	IB2, T7, TP2	152	POISON
				III	6.1	IB3, T4, TP1	152	POISON
	Tris, bis-bifluoroamino diethoxy propane (TVOPA)	Forbidden						
	Tritonal	1.1D	UN0390	II	1.1D		112	EXPLOSIVES 1.1*
	Tungsten hexafluoride	2.3	UN2196		2.3, 8	2	125	POISON GAS*
	Turpentine	3	UN1299	III	3	B1, IB3, T2, TP1	128	FLAMMABLE
	Turpentine substitute	3	UN1300	I	3	T11, TP1, TP8, TP27	128	FLAMMABLE
				II	3	IB2, T4, TP1	128	FLAMMABLE
				III	3	B1, IB3, T2, TP1	128	FLAMMABLE
	Undecane	3	UN2330	III	3	B1, IB3, T2, TP1	128	FLAMMABLE
	Urea hydrogen peroxide	5.1	UN1511	III	5.1, 8	A1, A7, A29, IB8, IP3, T1, TP33	140	OXIDIZER
	Urea nitrate, *dry or wetted with less than 20 percent water, by mass*	1.1D	UN0220	II	1.1D	119	112	EXPLOSIVES 1.1*
	Urea nitrate, wetted, *with not less than 10 percent water by mass*	4.1	UN3370	I	4.1	162, A8, A19, N41, N83	113	FLAMMABLE SOLID
	Urea nitrate, wetted *with not less than 20 percent water, by mass*	4.1	UN1357	I	4.1	23, 39, A8, A19, N41	113	FLAMMABLE SOLID

Sym-bols	Hazardous materials descriptions and proper shipping names	Hazard class or Division	Identifica-tion Numbers	PG	Label Codes	Special provisions (§172.102)	ERG Guide No.	Placard Advisory Consult §172.504 & §172.505 *Placard any quantity
(1)	(2)	(3)	(4)	(5)	(6)	(7)		
	Urea peroxide, see **Urea hydrogen peroxide**							
	Valeraldehyde	3	UN2058	II	3	IB2, T4, TP1	129	FLAMMABLE
	Valeric acid, see **Corrosive liquids, n.o.s.**							
	Valeryl chloride	8	UN2502	II	8, 3	A3, A6, A7, B2, IB2, N34, T7, TP2	132	CORROSIVE
	Vanadium compound, n.o.s.	6.1	UN3285	I	6.1	IB7, IP1, T6, TP33	151	POISON
				II	6.1	IB8, IP2, IP4, T3, TP33	151	POISON
				III	6.1	IB8, IP3, T1, TP33	151	POISON
	Vanadium oxytrichloride	8	UN2443	II	8	A3, A6, A7, B2, B16, IB2, N34, T7, TP2	137	CORROSIVE
	Vanadium pentoxide, *non-fused form*	6.1	UN2862	III	6.1	IB8, IP3, T1, TP33	151	POISON
	Vanadium tetrachloride	8	UN2444	I	8	A3, A6, A7, B4, N34, T10, TP2	137	CORROSIVE
	Vanadium trichloride	8	UN2475	III	8	IB8, IP3, T1, TP33	157	CORROSIVE
	Vanadyl sulfate	6.1	UN2931	II	6.1	IB8, IP2, IP4, T3, TP33	151	POISON
	Vehicle, flammable gas powered	9	UN3166		9	135, 157	128	CLASS 9
	Vehicle, flammable liquid powered	9	UN3166		9	135, 157	128	CLASS 9

Symbols	Hazardous materials descriptions and proper shipping names	Hazard class or Division	Identification Numbers	PG	Label Codes	Special provisions (§172.102)	ERG Guide No.	Placard Advisory Consult §172.504 & §172.505 *Placard any quantity
(1)	(2)	(3)	(4)	(5)	(6)	(7)		
	Very signal cartridge, see **Cartridges, signal**							
	Vinyl acetate, stabilized	3	UN1301	II	3	IB2, T4, TP1	129P	FLAMMABLE
	Vinyl bromide, stabilized	2.1	UN1085		2.1	T50	116P	FLAMMABLE GAS
	Vinyl butyrate, stabilized	3	UN2838	II	3	IB2, T4, TP1	129P	FLAMMABLE
	Vinyl chloride, stabilized	2.1	UN1086		2.1	21, B44, T50	116P	FLAMMABLE GAS
	Vinyl chloroacetate	6.1	UN2589	II	6.1, 3	IB2, T7, TP2	155	POISON
	Vinyl ethyl ether, stabilized	3	UN1302	I	3	A3, T11, TP2	127P	FLAMMABLE
	Vinyl fluoride, stabilized	2.1	UN1860		2.1		116P	FLAMMABLE GAS
	Vinyl isobutyl ether, stabilized	3	UN1304	II	3	IB2, T4, TP1	127P	FLAMMABLE
	Vinyl methyl ether, stabilized	2.1	UN1087		2.1	B44, T50	116P	FLAMMABLE GAS
	Vinyl nitrate polymer	Forbidden						
	Vinylidene chloride, stabilized	3	UN1303	I	3	T12, TP2, TP7	130P	FLAMMABLE
	Vinylpyridines, stabilized	6.1	UN3073	II	6.1, 3, 8	IB1, T7, TP2, TP13	131P	POISON
	Vinyltoluenes, stabilized	3	UN2618	III	3	B1, IB3, T2, TP1	130P	FLAMMABLE
	Vinyltrichlorosilane, stabilized	3	UN1305	I	3, 8	A3, A7, B6, N34, T11, TP2, TP13	155P	FLAMMABLE
	Warheads, rocket *with burster or expelling charge*	1.4D	UN0370	II	1.4D		114	EXPLOSIVES 1.4

Symbols	Hazardous materials descriptions and proper shipping names	Hazard class or Division	Identification Numbers	PG	Label Codes	Special provisions (§172.102)	ERG Guide No.	Placard Advisory Consult §172.504 & §172.505 *Placard any quantity
(1)	(2)	(3)	(4)	(5)	(6)	(7)		
	Warheads, rocket *with burster or expelling charge*	1.4F	UN0371	II	1.4F		114	EXPLOSIVES 1.4
	Warheads, rocket *with bursting charge*	1.1D	UN0286	II	1.1D		112	EXPLOSIVES 1.1*
	Warheads, rocket *with bursting charge*	1.2D	UN0287	II	1.2D		112	EXPLOSIVES 1.2*
	Warheads, rocket *with bursting charge*	1.1F	UN0369	II	1.1F		112	EXPLOSIVES 1.1*
	Warheads, torpedo *with bursting charge*	1.1D	UN0221	II	1.1D		112	EXPLOSIVES 1.1*
G	**Water-reactive liquid, corrosive, n.o.s.**	4.3	UN3129	I	4.3, 8		138	DANGEROUS WHEN WET*
				II	4.3, 8	IB1	138	DANGEROUS WHEN WET*
				III	4.3, 8	IB2	138	DANGEROUS WHEN WET*
G	**Water-reactive liquid, n.o.s.**	4.3	UN3148	I	4.3		138	DANGEROUS WHEN WET*
				II	4.3	IB1	138	DANGEROUS WHEN WET*
				III	4.3	IB2	138	DANGEROUS WHEN WET*
G	**Water-reactive liquid, toxic, n.o.s.**	4.3	UN3130	I	4.3, 6.1	A4	139	DANGEROUS WHEN WET*
				II	4.3, 6.1	IB1	139	DANGEROUS WHEN WET*

Symbols	Hazardous materials descriptions and proper shipping names	Hazard class or Division	Identification Numbers	PG	Label Codes	Special provisions (§172.102)	ERG Guide No.	Placard Advisory Consult §172.504 & §172.505 *Placard any quantity
(1)	(2)	(3)	(4)	(5)	(6)	(7)		
				III	4.3, 6.1	IB2	139	DANGEROUS WHEN WET*
G	**Water-reactive solid, corrosive, n.o.s.**	4.3	UN3131	I	4.3, 8	IB4, IP1, N40	138	DANGEROUS WHEN WET*
				II	4.3, 8	IB6, IP2, T3, TP33	138	DANGEROUS WHEN WET*
				III	4.3, 8	IB8, IP4, T1, TP33	138	DANGEROUS WHEN WET*
G	**Water-reactive solid, flammable, n.o.s.**	4.3	UN3132	I	4.3, 4.1	IB4, N40	138	DANGEROUS WHEN WET*
				II	4.3, 4.1	IB4, T3, TP33	138	DANGEROUS WHEN WET*
				III	4.3, 4.1	IB6, T1, TP33	138	DANGEROUS WHEN WET*
G	**Water-reactive solid, n.o.s.**	4.3	UN2813	I	4.3	IB4, N40	138	DANGEROUS WHEN WET*
				II	4.3	IB7, IP2, T3, TP33	138	DANGEROUS WHEN WET*
				III	4.3	IB8, IP4, T1, TP33	138	DANGEROUS WHEN WET*
G	**Water-reactive solid, oxidizing, n.o.s.**	4.3	UN3133	II	4.3, 5.1		138	DANGEROUS WHEN WET*
				III	4.3, 5.1		138	DANGEROUS WHEN WET*

Sym-bols	Hazardous materials descriptions and proper shipping names	Hazard class or Division	Identifica-tion Numbers	PG	Label Codes	Special provisions (§172.102)	ERG Guide No.	Placard Advisory Consult §172.504 & §172.505 *Placard any quantity
(1)	(2)	(3)	(4)	(5)	(6)	(7)		
G	**Water-reactive solid, self-heating, n.o.s.**	4.3	UN3135	I	4.3, 4.2	N40	138	DANGEROUS WHEN WET*
				II	4.3, 4.2	IB5, IP2, T3, TP33	138	DANGEROUS WHEN WET*
				III	4.3, 4.2	IB8, IP4, T1, TP33	138	DANGEROUS WHEN WET*
G	**Water-reactive solid, toxic, n.o.s.**	4.3	UN3134	I	4.3, 6.1	A8, IB4, IP1, N40	139	DANGEROUS WHEN WET*
				II	4.3, 6.1	IB5, IP2, T3, TP33	139	DANGEROUS WHEN WET*
				III	4.3, 6.1	IB8, IP4, T1, TP33	139	DANGEROUS WHEN WET*
	Wheel chair, electric, see **Battery powered vehicle** *or* **Battery powered equipment**							
	White acid, see **Hydrofluoric acid**							
I	**White asbestos** *(chrysotile, actinolite, anthophyllite, tremolite)*	9	UN2590	III	9	156, IB8, IP2, IP3, T1, TP33	171	CLASS 9
	Wood preservatives, liquid	3	UN1306	II	3	149, IB2, T4, TP1, TP8	129	FLAMMABLE
				III	3	B1, IB3, T2, TP1	129	FLAMMABLE
A I W	**Wool waste, wet**	4.2	UN1387	III	4.2		133	SPONTANEOUSLY COMBUSTIBLE

Symbols	Hazardous materials descriptions and proper shipping names	Hazard class or Division	Identification Numbers	PG	Label Codes	Special provisions (§172.102)	ERG Guide No.	Placard Advisory Consult §172.504 & §172.505 *Placard any quantity
(1)	(2)	(3)	(4)	(5)	(6)	(7)		
	Xanthates	4.2	UN3342	II	4.2	IB6, IP2, T3, TP33	135	SPONTANEOUSLY COMBUSTIBLE
				III	4.2	IB8, IP3, T1, TP33	135	SPONTANEOUSLY COMBUSTIBLE
	Xenon	2.2	UN2036		2.2		121	NONFLAMMABLE GAS
	Xenon, refrigerated liquid *(cryogenic liquids)*	2.2	UN2591		2.2	T75, TP5	120	NONFLAMMABLE GAS
	Xylenes	3	UN1307	II	3	IB2, T4, TP1	130	FLAMMABLE
				III	3	B1, IB3, T2, TP1	130	FLAMMABLE
	Xylenols, solid	6.1	UN2261	II	6.1	IB8, IP2, IP4, T3, TP33	153	POISON
	Xylenols, liquid	6.1	UN3430	II	6.1	IB2, T7, TP2	153	POISON
	Xylidines, liquid	6.1	UN1711	II	6.1	IB2, T7, TP2	153	POISON
	Xylidines, solid	6.1	UN3452	II	6.1	IB8, IP2, IP4, T3, TP33	153	POISON
	Xylyl bromide, liquid	6.1	UN1701	II	6.1	A3, A6, A7, IB2, N33, T7, TP2, TP13	152	POISON
	Xylyl bromide, solid	6.1	UN3417	II	6.1	A3, A6, A7, IB8, IP2, IP4, N33, T3, TP33	152	POISON
	p-Xylyl diazide	Forbidden						

Symbols (1)	Hazardous materials descriptions and proper shipping names (2)	Hazard class or Division (3)	Identification Numbers (4)	PG (5)	Label Codes (6)	Special provisions (§172.102) (7)	ERG Guide No.	Placard Advisory Consult §172.504 & §172.505 *Placard any quantity
	Zinc ammonium nitrite	5.1	UN1512	II	5.1	IB8, IP4, T3, TP33	140	OXIDIZER
	Zinc arsenate *or* **Zinc arsenite** *or* **Zinc arsenate and zinc arsenite mixtures.**	6.1	UN1712	II	6.1	IB8, IP2, IP4, T3, TP33	151	POISON
	Zinc ashes	4.3	UN1435	III	4.3	A1, A19, IB8, IP4, T1, TP33	138	DANGEROUS WHEN WET*
	Zinc bisulfite solution, see **Bisulfites, aqueous solutions, n.o.s.**							
	Zinc bromate	5.1	UN2469	III	5.1	A1, A29, IB8, IP3, T1, TP33	140	OXIDIZER
	Zinc chlorate	5.1	UN1513	II	5.1	A9, IB8, IP2, IP4, N34, T3, TP33	140	OXIDIZER
	Zinc chloride, anhydrous	8	UN2331	III	8	IB8, IP3, T1, TP33	154	CORROSIVE
	Zinc chloride, solution	8	UN1840	III	8	IB3, T4, TP1	154	CORROSIVE
	Zinc cyanide	6.1	UN1713	I	6.1	IB7, IP1, T6, TP33	151	POISON
	Zinc dithionite *or* **Zinc hydrosulfite**	9	UN1931	III	None	IB8, IP3, T1, TP33	171	CLASS 9
	Zinc ethyl, see **Diethylzinc**							
	Zinc fluorosilicate	6.1	UN2855	III	6.1	IB8, IP3, T1, TP33	151	POISON
	Zinc hydrosulfite, *see* **Zinc dithionite**							
	Zinc muriate solution, see **Zinc chloride, solution**							
	Zinc nitrate	5.1	UN1514	II	5.1	IB8, IP4, T3, TP33	140	OXIDIZER

Symbols	Hazardous materials descriptions and proper shipping names	Hazard class or Division	Identification Numbers	PG	Label Codes	Special provisions (§172.102)	ERG Guide No.	Placard Advisory Consult §172.504 & §172.505 *Placard any quantity
(1)	(2)	(3)	(4)	(5)	(6)	(7)		
	Zinc permanganate	5.1	UN1515	II	5.1	IB6, IP2, T3, TP33	140	OXIDIZER
	Zinc peroxide	5.1	UN1516	II	5.1	IB6, IP2, T3, TP33	143	OXIDIZER
	Zinc phosphide	4.3	UN1714	I	4.3, 6.1	A19, N40	139	DANGEROUS WHEN WET*
	Zinc powder *or* **Zinc dust**	4.3	UN1436	I	4.3, 4.2	A19, IB4, IP1, N40	138	DANGEROUS WHEN WET*
				II	4.3, 4.2	A19, IB7, IP2, T3, TP33	138	DANGEROUS WHEN WET*
				III	4.3, 4.2	IB8, IP4, T1, TP33	138	DANGEROUS WHEN WET*
	Zinc resinate	4.1	UN2714	III	4.1	A1, IB6, T1, TP33	133	FLAMMABLE SOLID
	Zinc selenate, see **Selenates** *or* **Selenites**							
	Zinc selenite, see **Selenates** *or* **Selenites**							
	Zinc silicofluoride, see **Zinc fluorosilicate**							
	Zirconium, dry, *coiled wire, finished metal sheets, strip (thinner than 254 microns but not thinner than 18 microns)*	4.1	UN2858	III	4.1	A1	170	FLAMMABLE SOLID
	Zirconium, dry, *finished sheets, strip or coiled wire*	4.2	UN2009	III	4.2	A1, A19	135	SPONTANEOUSLY COMBUSTIBLE

Sym-bols	Hazardous materials descriptions and proper shipping names	Hazard class or Division	Identifica-tion Numbers	PG	Label Codes	Special provisions (§172.102)	ERG Guide No.	Placard Advisory Consult §172.504 & §172.505 *Placard any quantity
(1)	(2)	(3)	(4)	(5)	(6)	(7)		
	Zirconium hydride	4.1	UN1437	II	4.1	A19, A20, IB4, N34, T3, TP33	138	FLAMMABLE SOLID
	Zirconium nitrate	5.1	UN2728	III	5.1	A1, A29, IB8, IP3, T1, TP33	140	OXIDIZER
	Zirconium picramate, *dry or wetted with less than 20 percent water, by mass*	1.3C	UN0236	II	1.3C		112	EXPLOSIVES 1.3*
	Zirconium picramate, wetted *with not less than 20 percent water, by mass*	4.1	UN1517	I	4.1	23, N41	113	FLAMMABLE SOLID
	Zirconium powder, dry	4.2	UN2008	I	4.2	T21, TP7, TP33	135	SPONTANEOUSLY COMBUSTIBLE
				II	4.2	A19, A20, IB6, IP2, N5, N34, T3, TP33	135	SPONTANEOUSLY COMBUSTIBLE
				III	4.2	IB8, IP3, T1, TP33	135	SPONTANEOUSLY COMBUSTIBLE
	Zirconium powder, wetted *with not less than 25 percent water (a visible excess of water must be present) (a) mechanically produced, particle size less than 53 microns; (b) chemically produced, particle size less than 840 microns*	4.1	UN1358	II	4.1	A19, A20, IB6, IP2, N34, T3, TP33	170	FLAMMABLE SOLID
	Zirconium scrap	4.2	UN1932	III	4.2	IB8, IP3, N34, T1, TP33	135	SPONTANEOUSLY COMBUSTIBLE
	Zirconium suspended in a liquid	3	UN1308	I	3		170	FLAMMABLE

Symbols	Hazardous materials descriptions and proper shipping names	Hazard class or Division	Identification Numbers	PG	Label Codes	Special provisions (§172.102)	ERG Guide No.	Placard Advisory Consult §172.504 & §172.505 *Placard any quantity
(1)	(2)	(3)	(4)	(5)	(6)	(7)		
				II	3	IB2	170	FLAMMABLE
				III	3	B1, IB2	170	FLAMMABLE
	Zirconium tetrachloride	8	UN2503	III	8	IB8, IP3, T1, TP33	137	CORROSIVE

Appendix A to §172.101 – List of Hazardous Substances and Reportable Quantities

1. This Appendix lists materials and their corresponding reportable quantities (RQs) that are listed or designated as "hazardous substances" under section 101(14) of the Comprehensive Environmental Response, Compensation, and Liability Act, 42 U.S.C. 9601(14) (CERCLA; 42 U.S.C. 9601 *et seq*). This listing fulfills the requirement of CERCLA, 42 U.S.C. 9656 (a), that all "hazardous substances," as defined in 42 U.S.C. 9601 (14), be listed and regulated as hazardous materials under 49 U.S.C. 5101-5127. That definition includes substances listed under sections 311(b)(2)(A) and 307(a) of the Federal Water Pollution Control Act, 33 U.S.C. 1321(b)(2)(A) and 1317(a), section 3001 of the Solid Waste Disposal Act, 42 U.S.C. 6921, and Section 112 of the Clean Air Act, 42 U.S.C. 7412. In addition, this list contains materials that the Administrator of the Environmental Protection Agency has determined to be hazardous substances in accordance with section 102 of CERCLA, 42 U.S.C. 9602. It should be noted that 42 U.S.C. 9656(b) provides that common and contract carriers may be held liable under laws other than CERCLA for the release of a hazardous substance as defined in that Act, during transportation that commenced before the effective date of the listing and regulating of that substance as a hazardous material under 49 U.S.C. 5101-5127.

2. This Appendix is divided into two TABLES which are entitled "TABLE 1—HAZARDOUS SUBSTANCES OTHER THAN RADIONUCLIDES" and "TABLE 2—RADIONUCLIDES." A material listed in this Appendix is regulated as a hazardous material and a hazardous substance under this subchapter if it meets the definition of a hazardous substance in §171.8 of this subchapter.

3. The procedure for selecting a proper shipping name for a hazardous substance is set forth in §172.101(c).

4. Column 1 of TABLE 1, entitled *"Hazardous substance"*, contains the names of those elements and compounds that are hazardous substances. Following the listing of elements and compounds is a listing of waste streams. These waste streams appear on the list in numerical sequence and are referenced by

the appropriate "D", "F", or "K" numbers. Column 2 of TABLE 1, entitled *"Reportable quantity (RQ)"*, contains the reportable quantity (RQ), in pounds and kilograms, for each hazardous substance listed in Column 1 of TABLE 1.

5. A series of notes is used throughout TABLE 1 and TABLE 2 to provide additional information concerning certain hazardous substances. These notes are explained at the end of each TABLE.

6. TABLE 2 lists radionuclides that are hazardous substances and their corresponding RQ's. The RQ's in TABLE 2 for radionuclides are expressed in units of curies and terabecquerels, whereas those in TABLE 1 are expressed in units of pounds and kilograms. If a material is listed in both TABLE 1 and TABLE 2, the lower RQ shall apply. Radionuclides are listed in alphabetical order. The RQs for radionuclides are given in the radiological unit of measure of curie, abbreviated "Ci", followed, in parentheses, by an equivalent unit measured in terabecquerels, abbreviated "TBq".

7. For mixtures of radionuclides, the following requirements shall be used in determining if a package contains an RQ of a hazardous substance: (i) if the identity and quantity (in curies or terabecquerels) of each radionuclide in a mixture or solution is known, the ratio between the quantity per package (in curies or terabecquerels) and the RQ for the radionuclide must be determined for each radionuclide. A package contains an RQ of a hazardous substance when the sum of the ratios for the radionuclides in the mixture or solution is equal to or greater than one; (ii) if the identity of each radionuclide in a mixture or solution is known but the quantity per package (in curies or terabecquerels) of one or more of the radionuclides is unknown, an RQ of a hazardous substance is present in a package when the total quantity (in curies or terabecquerels) of the mixture or solution is equal to or greater than the lowest RQ of any individual radionuclide in the mixture or solution; and (iii) if the identity of one or more radionuclides in a mixture or solution is unknown (or if the identity of a radionuclide by itself is unknown), an RQ of a hazardous substance is present when the total quantity (in curies or terabecquerels) in a package is equal to or greater than either one curie or the lowest RQ of any known individual radionuclide in the mixture or solution, whichever is lower.

Hazardous Substances	RQ: lbs (kg)
Acenaphthene	100 (45.4)
Acenaphthylene	5000 (2270)
Acetaldehyde	1000 (454)
Acetaldehyde, chloro-	1000 (454)
Acetaldehyde, trichloro-	5000 (2270)
Acetamide	100 (45.4)
Acetamide, N-(aminothioxomethyl)-	1000 (454)
Acetamide, N-(4-ethoxyphenyl)-	100 (45.4)
Acetamide, N-fluoren-2-yl-	1 (0.454)
Acetamide, 2-fluoro-	100 (45.4)
Acetic acid	5000 (2270)
Acetic acid (2,4-dichlorophenoxy)-	100 (45.4)
Acetic acid, ethyl ester	5000 (2270)
Acetic acid, fluoro-, sodium salt	10 (4.54)
Acetic acid, lead (2+)salt	10 (4.54)
Acetic acid, thallium(I+) salt	100 (45.4)
Acetic acid, (2,4,5-trichlorophenoxy)	1000 (454)
Acetic anhydride	5000 (2270)
Acetone	5000 (2270)
Acetone cyanohydrin	10 (4.54)
Acetonitrile	5000 (2270)
Acetophenone	5000 (2270)
2-Acetylaminofluorene	1 (0.454)
Acetyl bromide	5000 (2270)
Acetyl chloride	5000 (2270)
1-Acetyl-2-thiourea	1000 (454)
Acrolein	1 (0.454)
Acrylamide	5000 (2270)
Acrylic acid	5000 (2270)
Acrylonitrile	100 (45.4)
Adipic acid	5000 (2270)
Aldicarb	1 (0.454)
Aldrin	1 (0.454)
Allyl alcohol	100 (45.4)
Allyl chloride	1000 (454)
Aluminum phosphide	100 (45.4)
Aluminum sulfate	5000 (2270)
4-Aminobiphenyl	1 (0.454)
5-(Aminomethyl)-3-isoxazolol	1000 (454)
4-Aminopyridine	1000 (454)
Amitrole	10 (4.54)
Ammonia	100 (45.4)
Ammonium acetate	5000 (2270)
Ammonium benzoate	5000 (2270)

Hazardous Substances	RQ: lbs (kg)
Ammonium bicarbonate	5000 (2270)
Ammonium bichromate	10 (4.54)
Ammonium bifluoride	100 (45.4)
Ammonium bisulfite	5000 (2270)
Ammonium carbamate	5000 (2270)
Ammonium carbonate	5000 (2270)
Ammonium chloride	5000 (2270)
Ammonium chromate	10 (4.54)
Ammonium citrate, dibasic	5000 (2270)
Ammonium dichromate @	10 (4.54)
Ammonium fluoborate	5000 (2270)
Ammonium fluoride	100 (45.4)
Ammonium hydroxide	1000 (454)
Ammonium oxalate	5000 (2270)
Ammonium picrate	10 (4.54)
Ammonium silicofluoride	1000 (454)
Ammonium sulfamate	5000 (2270)
Ammonium sulfide	100 (45.4)
Ammonium sulfite	5000 (2270)
Ammonium tartrate	5000 (2270)
Ammonium thiocyanate	5000 (2270)
Ammonium vanadate	1000 (454)
Amyl acetate	5000 (2270)
iso-Amyl acetate	
sec-Amyl acetate	
tert-Amyl acetate	
Aniline	5000 (2270)
o-Anisidine	100 (45.4)
Anthracene	5000 (2270)
Antimony¢	5000 (2270)
Antimony pentachloride	1000 (454)
Antimony potassium tartrate	100 (45.4)
Antimony tribromide	1000 (454)
Antimony trichloride	1000 (454)
Antimony trifluoride	1000 (454)
Antimony trioxide	1000 (454)
Argentate(1-), bis(cyano-C)-, potassium	1 (0.454)
Aroclor 1016	1 (0.454)
Aroclor 1221	1 (0.454)
Aroclor 1232	1 (0.454)
Aroclor 1242	1 (0.454)
Aroclor 1248	1 (0.454)
Aroclor 1254	1 (0.454)
Aroclor 1260	1 (0.454)

Hazardous Substances	RQ: lbs (kg)
Arsenic¢	1 (0.454)
Arsenic acid	1 (0.454)
Arsenic acid H3AsO4	1 (0.454)
Arsenic disulfide	1 (0.454)
Arsenic oxide As2O3	1 (0.454)
Arsenic oxide As2O5	1 (0.454)
Arsenic pentoxide	1 (0.454)
Arsenic trichloride	1 (0.454)
Arsenic trioxide	1 (0.454)
Arsenic trisulfide	1 (0.454)
Arsine, diethyl-	1 (0.454)
Arsinic acid, dimethyl-	1 (0.454)
Arsonous dichloride, phenyl-	1 (0.454)
Asbestos ¢¢	1 (0.454)
Auramine	100 (45.4)
Azaserine	1 (0.454)
Aziridine	1 (0.454)
Aziridine, 2-methyl-	1 (0.454)
Azirino(2',3',3',4)pytrolo(1,2-a)indole-4,7-dione, 6-amino-8-[((aminocarbonyl)oxy)methyl]-1,1a,2,8,8a,8b-hexahydro-8a-methoxy-5-methyl-, [1aS-[aalpha,8beta,8aalpha,8balpha)]-	10 (4.54)
Barium cyanide	10 (4.54)
Benz[j]aceanthrylene, 1,2-dihydro-3-methyl-	10 (4.54)
Benz[c]acridine	100 (45.4)
3,4-Benzacridine	100 (45.4)
Benzal chloride	5000 (2270)
Benzamide,3,5-dichloro-N-(1,1-dimethyl-2-propynyl)	5000 (2270)
Benz[a]anthracene	10 (4.54)
1,2-Benzanthracene	10 (4.54)
Benz[a]anthracene, 7,12-dimethyl-	1 (0.454)
Benzenamine	5000 (2270)
Benzenamine, 4,4'-carbonimidoylbis(N,N-dimethyl-	100 (45.4)
Benzenamine, 4-chloro-	1000 (454)
Benzenamine, 4-chloro-2-methyl-,hydrochloride	100 (45.4)
Benzenamine, N,N-dimethyl-4-(phenylazo)-	10 (4.54)
Benzenamine, 2-methyl-	100 (45.4)
Benzenamine, 4-methyl-	100 (45.4)
Benzenamine, 4,4'-methylenebis(2-chloro-	10 (4.54)
Benzenamine,2-methyl-, hydrochloride	100 (45.4)
Benzenamine,2-methyl-5-nitro-	100 (45.4)
Benzenamine,4-nitro-	5000 (2270)
Benzene	10 (4.54)
Benzene, 1-bromo-4-phenoxy-	100 (45.4)
Benzene, chloro-	100 (45.4)
Benzene, chloromethyl-	100 (45.4)

Hazardous Substances	RQ: lbs (kg)
Benzene,1,2-dichloro-	100 (45.4)
Benzene, 1,3-dichloro-	100 (45.4)
Benzene, 1,4-dichloro-	100 (45.4)
Benzene, 1,1'-(2,2-dichloroethylidene)bis[4-chloro	1 (0.454)
Benzene, dichloromethyl-	5000 (2270)
Benzene, 1,3-diisocyanatomethyl	100 (45.4)
Benzene, dimethyl-	100 (45.4)
Benzene, m-dimethyl-	1000 (454)
Benzene, o-dimethyl-	1000 (454)
Benzene, p-dimethyl-	100 (45.4)
Benzene, hexachloro-	10 (4.54)
Benzene, hexahydro-	1000 (454)
Benzene, hydroxy-	1000 (454)
Benzene, methyl-	1000 (454)
Benzene, 1-methyl-2,4-dinitro-	10 (4.54)
Benzene, 2-methyl-1,3-dinitro-	100 (45.4)
Benzene, 1-methylethyl-	5000 (2270)
Benzene, nitro-	1000 (454)
Benzene, pentachloro-	10 (4.54)
Benzene, pentachloronitro-	100 (45.4)
Benzene, 1,2,4,5-tetrachloro-	5000 (2270)
Benzene, 1,1'-(2,2,2-trichloroethylidene)bis [4-chloro-	1 (0.454)
Benzene, 1,1'-(2,2,2-trichloroethylidene)bis [4-methoxy)-	1 (0.454)
Benzene, (trichloromethyl)	10 (4.54)
Benzene, 1,3,5-trinitro-	10 (4.54)
Benzeneacetic acid, 4-chloro-alpha-(4-chlorophenyl)-alpha-hydroxy-, ethyl ester	10 (4.54)
Benzenebutanoic acid, 4-[bis(2-chloroethyl)amino]-	10 (4.54)
Benzenediamine, ar-methyl-	10 (4.54)
1,2-Benzenedicarboxylic acid,[bis(2-ethylhexyl)] ester	100 (45.4)
1,2-Benzenedicarboxylic acid,dibutyl ester	10 (4.54)
1,2-Benzenedicarboxylic acid, diethyl ester	1000 (454)
1,2-Benzenedicarboxylic acid, dimethyl ester	5000 (2270)
1,2-Benzenedicarboxylic acid, dioctyl ester	5000 (2270)
1,3-Benzenediol	5000 (2270)
1,2-Benzenediol,4-[1- hydroxy-2-(methylamino) ethyl]-	1000 (454)
Benzeneethanamine, alpha,alpha-dimethyl-	5000 (2270)
Benzeneethanamine, alpha,alpha-dimethyl-	5000 (2270)
Benzenesulfonic acid chloride	100 (45.4)
Benzenesulfonyl chloride	100 (45.4)
Benzenethiol	100 (45.4)
Benzidine	1 (0.454)
1,2-Benzisothiazol-3(2H)-one,1,1-dioxide	100 (45.4)
Benzo[a]anthracene	10 (4.54)
1,3-Benzodioxole, 5-(2-propenyl)-	100 (45.4)

Hazardous Substances	RQ: lbs (kg)
1,3-Benzodioxole, 5-(1-propenyl)-	100 (45.4)
1,3-Benzodioxole, 5-propyl-	10 (4.54)
Benzo[b]fluoranthene	1 (0.454)
Benzo[k]fluoranthene	5000 (2270)
Benzo[j,k]fluorene	100 (45.4)
Benzoic acid	5000 (2270)
Benzonitrile	5000 (2270)
Benzo[g,h,i]perylene	5000 (2270)
2H-1-Benzopyran-2-one, 4-hydroxy-3-(3-oxo-1-phenyl-butyl)-, & salts, when present at concentrations greater than 0.3%	100 (45.4)
Benzo[a]pyrene	1 (0.454)
3,4-Benzopyrene	1 (0.454)
p-Benzoquinone	10 (4.54)
Benzo[rst]pentaphene	10 (4.54)
Benzotrichloride	10 (4.54)
Benzoyl chloride	1000 (454)
1,2-Benzphenanthrene	100 (45.4)
Benzyl chloride	100 (45.4)
Beryllium ¢	10 (4.54)
Beryllium chloride	1 (0.454)
Beryllium dust ¢	10 (4.54)
Beryllium fluoride	1 (0.454)
Beryllium nitrate	1 (0.454)
alpha - BHC	10 (4.54)
beta - BHC	1 (0.454)
delta - BHC	1 (0.454)
gamma - BHC	1 (0.454)
2,2'-Bioxirane	10 (4.54)
Biphenyl	100 (45.4)
(1,1'-Biphenyl)-4,4' diamine	1 (0.454)
(1,1'-Biphenyl)-4,4' diamine 3,3'dichloro-	1 (0.454)
(1,1'-Biphenyl)-4,4' diamine 3,3'-dimethoxy-	10 (4.54)
(1,1'-Biphenyl)-4,4' diamine 3,3'-dimethyl-	10 (4.54)
Bis(2-chloroethoxy) methane	1000 (454)
Bis(2-chloroethyl) ether	10 (4.54)
Bis(2-ethylhexyl)phthalate	100 (45.4)
Bromoacetone	1000 (454)
Bromoform	100 (45.4)
4-Bromophenyl phenyl ether	100 (45.4)
Brucine	100 (45.4)
1,3-Butadiene	10 (4.54)
1,3-Butadiene, 1,1,2,3,4,4-hexachloro-	1 (0.454)
1-Butanamine, N-butyl-N-nitroso-	10 (4.54)
1-Butanol	5000 (2270)

Hazardous Substances	RQ: lbs (kg)
2-Butanone	5000 (2270)
2-Butanone, 3,3-dimethyl-1-(methylthio)-,O-[(methy lamino)carbonyl] oxime	100 (45.4)
2-Butanone peroxide	10 (4.54)
2-Butenal	100 (45.4)
2-Butane, 1,4-dichloro-	1 (0.454)
2-Butenoic acid, 2-methyl-,7[[2,3-dihydroxy-2-(1-methoxy-ethyl)-3-methyl-1-oxobutoxy]methyl]-2,3,5,7a-tetrahydro-1H-pyrrolizin-1-ylester,[1S-[1alpha(Z),7(2S*,3R*),7aalpha]]-	10 (4.54)
Butyl acetate	5000 (2270)
iso- Butyl acetate	
sec- Butyl acetate	
tert- Butyl acetate	
n-Butyl alcohol	5000 (2270)
Butylamine	1000 (454)
iso- Butylamine	
sec- Butylamine	
tert- Butylamine	
Butyl benzyl phthalate	100 (45.4)
n-Butyl phthalate	10 (4.54)
Butyric acid	5000 (2270)
iso-Butyric acid	
Cacodylic acid	1 (0.454)
Cadmium ¢	10 (4.54)
Cadmium acetate	10 (4.54)
Cadmium bromide	10 (4.54)
Cadmium chloride	10 (4.54)
Calcium arsenate	1 (0.454)
Calcium arsenite	1 (0.454)
Calcium carbide	10 (4.54)
Calcium chromate	10 (4.54)
Calcium cyanamide	1000 (454)
Calcium cyanide	10 (4.54)
Calcium cyanide Ca(CN)2	10 (4.54)
Calcium dodecylbenzene sulfonate	1000 (454)
Calcium hypochlorite	10 (4.54)
Camphene, octachloro-	1 (0.454)
Captan	10 (4.54)
Carbamic acid, ethyl ester	100 (45.4)
Carbamic acid, methylnitroso-, ethyl ester	1 (0.454)
Carbamic chloride, dimethyl-	1 (0.454)
Carbamide, thio-	10 (4.54)
Carbamimidoselenoic acid	1000 (454)
Carbamothioic acid, bis (1-methylethyl)-, S-(2,3-dichloro-2-) ester	100 (45.4)

Hazardous Substances	RQ: lbs (kg)
Carbaryl	100 (45.4)
Carbofuran	10 (4.54)
Carbon bisulfide	100 (45.4)
Carbon disulfide	100 (45.4)
Carbonic acid, dithallium (I+)	100 (45.4)
Carbonic dichloride	10 (4.54)
Carbonic difluoride	1000 (454)
Carbonochloridic acid, methyl ester	1000 (454)
Carbonyl sulfide	100 (45.4)
Carbon oxyfluoride	1000 (454)
Carbon tetrachloride	10 (4.54)
Catechol	100 (45.4)
Chloral	5000 (2270)
Chloramben	100 (45.4)
Chlorambucil	10 (4.54)
Chlordane	1 (0.454)
Chlordane, alpha & gamma isomers	1 (0.454)
Chlordane, technical	1 (0.454)
Chlorine	10 (4.54)
Chlornaphazine	100 (45.4)
Chloroacetaldehyde	1000 (454)
2-Chloroacetophenone	100 (45.4)
p-Chloroaniline	1000 (454)
Chlorobenzene	100 (45.4)
Chlorobenzilate	10 (4.54)
4-Chloro-m-cresol	5000 (2270)
p-Chloro-m-cresol	5000 (2270)
Chlorodibromomethane	100 (45.4)
Chloroethane	100 (45.4)
2-Chloroethyl vinyl ether	1000 (454)
Chloroform	10 (4.54)
Chloromethane	100 (45.4)
Chloromethyl methyl ether	10 (4.54)
beta-Chloronaphthalene	5000 (2270)
2-Chloronaphthalene	5000 (2270)
2-Chlorophenol	100 (45.4)
o-Chlorophenol	100 (45.4)
4-Chlorophenyl phenyl ether	5000 (2270)
1-(o-Chlorophenyl)thiourea	100 (45.4)
Chloroprene	100 (45.4)
3-Chloropropionitrile	1000 (454)
Chlorosulfonic acid	1000 (454)
4-Chloro-o-toluidine, hydrochloride	100 (45.4)
Chlorpyrifos	1 (0.454)

Hazardous Substances	RQ: lbs (kg)
Chromic acetate	1000 (454)
Chromic acid	10 (4.54)
Chromic acid H2CrO4, calcium salt	10 (4.54)
Chromic sulfate	1000 (454)
Chromium ¢	5000 (2270)
Chromous chloride	1000 (454)
Chrysene	100 (45.4)
Cobaltous bromide	1000 (454)
Cobaltous formate	1000 (454)
Cobaltous sulfamate	1000 (454)
Coke Oven Emissions	1 (0.454)
Copper ¢	5000 (2270)
Copper chloride @	10 (4.54)
Copper cyanide	10 (4.54)
Copper cyanide CuCN	10 (4.54)
Coumaphos	10 (4.54)
Creosote	1 (0.454)
Cresols (isomers and mixture)	100 (45.4)
m-Cresol	100 (45.4)
o-Cresol	100 (45.4)
p-Cresol	100 (45.4)
Cresylic acid (isomers and mixture)	100 (45.4)
m-Cresylic acid	100 (45.4)
o-Cresylic acid	100 (45.4)
p-Cresylic acid	100 (45.4)
Crotonaldehyde	100 (45.4)
Cumene	5000 (2270)
Cupric acetate	100 (45.4)
Cupric acetoarsenite	1 (0.454)
Cupric chloride	10 (4.54)
Cupric nitrate	100 (45.4)
Cupric oxalate	100 (45.4)
Cupric sulfate	10 (4.54)
Cupric sulfate ammoniated	100 (45.4)
Cupric tartrate	100 (45.4)
Cyanides (soluble salts and complexes) not otherwise specified	10 (4.54)
Cyanogen	100 (45.4)
Cyanogen bromide	1000 (454)
Cyanogen bromide (CN)Br	1000 (454)
Cyanogen chloride	10 (4.54)
Cyanogen chloride (CN)Cl	10 (4.54)
2,5-Cyclohexadiene-1,4-dione	10 (4.54)
Cyclohexane	1000 (454)
Chloroacetic acid	100 (45.4)

Hazardous Substances	RQ: lbs (kg)
Cyclohexane, 1,2,3,4,5,6-hexachloro-, (1alpha,2alpha,3beta,4alpha,5al pha,6beta)-	1 (0.454)
Cyclohexanone	5000 (2270)
2-Cyclohexyl-4,6-dinitrophenol	100 (45.4)
1,3-Cyclopentadiene, 1,2,3,4,5,5-hexachloro-	10 (4.54)
Cyclophosphamide	10 (4.54)
2,4-D Acid	100 (45.4)
2,4-D Ester	100 (45.4)
Daunomycin	10 (4.54)
DDD	1 (0.454)
4,4'-DDD	1 (0.454)
DDE.	1 (0.454)
4,4'-DDE	1 (0.454)
DDT.	1 (0.454)
4,4' DDT	1 (0.454)
Dialiate	100 (45.4)
Diamine	1 (0.454)
Diazinon	1 (0.454)
Diazomethane	100 (45.4)
Dibenz[a,h]anthracene	1 (0.454)
1,2:5,6-Dibenzanthracene	1 (0.454)
Dibenzo[a,h]anthracene	1 (0.454)
Dibenzofuran	100 (45.4)
Dibenz[a,i]pyrene	10 (4.54)
1,2-Dibromo-3-chloropropane	1 (0.454)
Dibutyl phthalate	10 (4.54)
Di-n-butylphthalate	10 (4.54)
Dicamba	1000 (454)
Dichlobenil	100 (45.4)
Dichlone	1 (0.454)
Dichlorobenzene	100 (45.4)
1,2-Dichlorobenzene	100 (45.4)
1,3-Dichlorobenzene	100 (45.4)
1,4-Dichlorobenzene	100 (45.4)
m-Dichlorobenzene	100 (45.4)
o-Dichlorobenzene	100 (45.4)
p-Dichlorobenzene	100 (45.4)
3,3'-Dichlorobenzidine	1 (0.454)
Dichlorobromomethane	5000 (2270)
1,4-Dichloro-2-butene	1 (0.454)
Dichlorodifluoromethane	5000 (2270)
1,1-Dichloroethane	1000 (454)
1,2-Dichloroethane	100 (45.4)
1,1-Dichloroethylene	100 (45.4)
1,2-Dichloroethylene	1000 (454)

Hazardous Substances	RQ: lbs (kg)
Dichloroethyl ether	10 (4.54)
Dichloroisopropyl-ether.	1000 (454)
Dichloromethane@.	1000 (454)
Dichloromethoxy ethane.	1000 (454)
Dichloromethyl ether.	10 (4.54)
2,4-Dichlorophenol	100 (45.4)
2,6-Dichlorophenol	100 (45.4)
Dichlorophenylarsine	1 (0.454)
Dichloropropane	1000 (454)
1,1-Dichloropropane	
1,3-Dichloropropane	
1,2-Dichloropropane.	1000 (454)
Dichloropropane - Dichloropropene (mixture)	100 (45.4)
Dichloropropene.	100 (45.4)
2,3-Dichloropropene	
1,3-Dichloropropene.	100 (45.4)
2,2-Dichloropropionic acid	5000 (2270)
Dichlorvos.	10 (4.54)
Dicofol	10 (4.54)
Dieldrin.	1 (0.454)
1,2:3,4-Diepoxybutane	10 (4.54)
Diethanolamine	100 (45.4)
Diethylamine.	1000 (454)
N,N-diethylaniline	1000 (454)
Diethylarsine.	1 (0.454)
1,4-Diethylenedioxide.	100 (45.4)
Diethylhexyl phthalate	100 (45.4)
N,N'-Diethylhydrazine.	10 (4.54)
O,O-Diethyl S-methyl dithiophosphate	5000 (2270)
Diethyl-p-nitrophenyl phosphate.	100 (45.4)
Diethyl phthalate.	1000 (454)
O,O-Diethyl O-pyrazinyl phosphorothioate.	100 (45.4)
Diethyl sulfate.	10 (4.54)
Diethylstilbestrol	1 (0.454)
Dihydrosafrole	10 (4.54)
Diisopropyl fluorophosphate.	100 (45.4)
1,4,5,8-Dimethanonaphthalene,1,2,3,4,10,10-hexachloro-1, 4,4a,5,8,8a-hexahydro,(1alpha,4alpha,4abeta, 5abeta,8beta,8abeta)-	1 (0.454)
1,4,5,8-Dimethanonaphthalene,1,2,3,4,10,10-10-hexa-chloro-1,4,4a,5,8,8a-hexahydro-, (1alpha,4alpha,4abeta, 5alpha,8alpha,8abeta)-	1 (0.454)
2,7:3,6-Dimethanonaphth[2,3-b]oxirene,3,4,5,6,9,9-hexach loro-1a,2,2a,3,6,6a,7,7a-octahydro-, (1aalpha,2beta, 2abeta,3alpha,6alpha,6abeta,7beta,7aal pha)-	1 (0.454)

Hazardous Substances	RQ: lbs (kg)
2,7:3,6-Dimethanonaphth[2,3-b]oxirene, 3,4,5,6,9,9-hexachloro-1a,2,2a,3,6,6a,7,7a-octahydro,(1aalpha,2beta, 2aalpha,3beta, 6beta,6aalpha,7beta,7aalpha)-	1 (0.454)
Dimethoate	10 (4.54)
3,3'-Dimethoxybenzidine	10 (4.54)
Dimethylamine	1000 (454)
p-Dimethylaminoazobenzene	10 (4.54)
N,N-dimethylaniline	100 (45.4)
7,12-Dimethylbenz[a]anthracene	1 (0.454)
3,3'-Dimethylbenzidine	10 (4.54)
alpha,alpha-Dimethylbenzyl-hydroperoxide	10 (4.54)
Dimethylcarbamoyl chloride	1 (0.454)
Dimethylformamide	100 (45.4)
1,1-Dimethylhydrazine	10 (4.54)
1,2-Dimethylhydrazine	1 (0.454)
Dimethylhydrazine,unsymmetrical@	10 (4.54)
alpha,alpha-Dimethylphenethylamine	5000 (2270)
2,4-Dimethylphenol	100 (45.4)
Dimethyl phthalate	5000 (2270)
Dimethyl sulfate	100 (45.4)
Dinitrobenzene (mixed)	100 (45.4)
m- Dinitrobenzene	
o- Dinitrobenzene	
p- Dinitrobenzene	
4,6-Dinitro-o-cresol and salts	10 (4.54)
Dinitrogen tetroxide @	10 (4.54)
Dinitrophenol	10 (4.54)
2,5- Dinitrophenol	
2,4-Dinitrophenol	10 (4.54)
Dinitrotoluene	10 (4.54)
3,4-Dinitrotoluene	
2,4-Dinitrotoluene	10 (4.54)
2,6-Dinitrotoluene	100 (45.4)
Dinoseb	1000 (454)
Di-n-octyl phthalate	5000 (2270)
1,4-Dioxane	100 (45.4)t
1,2-Diphenylhydrazine	10 (4.54)
Diphosphoramide, octamethyl-	100 (45.4)
Diphosphoric acid,tetraethyl ester	10 (4.54)
Dipropylamine	5000 (2270)
Di-n-propylnitrosamine	10 (4.54)
Diquat	1000 (454)
Disulfoton	1 (0.454)
Dithiobiuret	100 (45.4)
Diuron	100 (45.4)

Hazardous Substances	RQ: lbs (kg)
Dodecylbenzenesulfonic acid	1000 (454)
2,4-D, salts and esters	100 (45.4)
Endosulfan	1 (0.454)
alpha - Endosulfan	1 (0.454)
beta - Endosulfan	1 (0.454)
Endosulfan sulfate	1 (0.454)
Endothall	1000 (454)
Endrin	1 (0.454)
Endrin, & metabolites	1 (0.454)
Endrin aldehyde	1 (0.454)
Epichlorohydrin	100 (45.4)
Epinephrine	1000 (454)
1,2-Epoxybutane	100 (45.4)
Ethanal	1000 (454)
Ethanamine, N-ethyl-N-nitroso-	1 (0.454)
Ethane, 1,2-dibromo-	1 (0.454)
Ethane, 1,1-dichloro-	1000 (454)
Ethane, 1,2-dichloro-	100 (45.4)
Ethane, hexachloro-	100 (45.4)
Ethane, 1,1'-[methylenebis(oxy)]bis(2-chloro-	1000 (454)
Ethane, 1,1'-oxybis-	100 (45.4)
Ethane, 1,1'-oxybis(2-chloro-	10 (4.54)
Ethane, pentachloro-	10 (4.54)
Ethane, 1,1,1,2-tetrachloro-	100 (45.4)
Ethane, 1,1,2,2-tetrachloro-	100 (45.4)
Ethane, 1,1,2-trichloro-	100 (45.4)
Ethane, 1,1,1-trichloro-	1000 (454)
1,2-Ethanediamine, N,N-dimethyl-N'-2-pyridinyl-N'-(2-thienyl- methyl)-	5000 (2270)
Ethanedinitrile	100 (45.4)
Ethanenitrile	5000 (2270)
Ethanethiobamide	10 (4.54)
Ethanimidothioic acid, N-[[(methylamino)carbonyl] oxy]-,methyl ester	100 (45.4)
Ethanol, 2-ethoxy-	1000 (454)
Ethanol, 2,2'-(nitrosoimino)bis-	1 (0.454)
Ethanone, 1-phenyl-	5000 (2270)
Ethanoyl chloride	5000 (2270)
Ethene, chloro-	1 (0.454)
Ethene, 2-chloroethoxy-	1000 (454)
Ethene, 1,1-dichloro-	100 (45.4)
Ethene, 1,2-dichloro-(E)	1000 (454)
Ethene, tetrachloro-	100 (45.4)
Ethene, trichloro-	100 (45.4)
Ethion	10 (4.54)

Hazardous Substances	RQ: lbs (kg)
Ethyl acetate	5000 (2270)
Ethyl acrylate	1000 (454)
Ethylbenzene	1000 (454)
Ethyl carbamate (Urethan)	100 (45.4)
Ethyl chloride @	100 (45.4)
Ethyl cyanide	10 (4.54)
Ethylene dibromide	1 (0.454)
Ethylene dichloride	100 (45.4)
Ethylene glycol	5000 (2270)
Ethylene glycol monoethyl ether	1000 (454)
Ethylene oxide	10 (4.54)
Ethylenebisdithiocarbamic acid	5000 (2270)
Ethylenebisdithiocarbamic acid, salts and esters	5000 (2270)
Ethylenediamine	5000 (2270)
Ethylenediamine tetraacetic acid (EDTA)	5000 (2270)
Ethylenethiourea	10 (4.54)
Ethylenimine	1 (0.454)
Ethyl ether	100 (45.4)
Ethylidene dichloride	1000 (454)
Ethyl methacrylate	1000 (454)
Ethyl methanesulfonate	1(0.454)
Ethyl methyl ketone @	5000 (2270)
Famphur	1000 (454)
Ferric ammonium citrate	1000 (454)
Ferric ammonium oxalate	1000 (454)
Ferric chloride	1000 (454)
Ferric fluoride	100 (45.4)
Ferric nitrate	1000 (454)
Ferric sulfate	1000 (454)
Ferrous ammonium sulfate	1000 (454)
Ferrous chloride	100 (45.4)
Ferrous sulfate	1000 (454)
Fluoranthene	100 (45.4)
Fluorene	5000 (2270)
Fluorine	10 (4.54)
Fluoroacetamide	100 (45.4)
Fluoroacetic acid, sodium salt	10 (4.54)
Formaldehyde	100 (45.4)
Formic acid	5000 (2270)
Fulminic acid, mercury(2+)salt	10 (4.54)
Fumaric acid	5000 (2270)
Furan	100 (45.4)
Furan, tetrahydro-	1000 (454)
2-Furancarboxaldehyde	5000 (2270)

Hazardous Substances	RQ: lbs (kg)
2,5-Furandione	5000 (2270)
Furfural	5000 (2270)
Furfuran	100 (45.4)
Glucopyranose, 2-deoxy-2-(3-methyl-3-nitrosoureido)-	1 (0.454)
D-Glucose, 2-deoxy-2-[[(methylnitrosoamino)-carbonyl]amino]-	1 (0.454)
Glycidylaldehyde	10 (4.54)
Guanidine, N-methyl-N'-nitro-N-nitroso-	10 (4.54)
Guthion	1 (0.454)
Heptachlor	1 (0.454)
Heptachlor epoxide	1 (0.454)
Hexachlorobenzene	10 (4.54)
Hexachlorobutadiene	1 (0.454)
Hexachlorocyclohexane (gamma isomer)	1 (0.454)
Hexachlorocyclopentadiene	10 (4.54)
Hexachloroethane	100 (45.4)
1,2,3,4,10-10-Hexachloro-1,4,4a,5,8,8a-hexahydro-1,4:5,8-endo,exo-dimethanonaphthalene	1 (0.454)
Hexachlorophene	100 (45.4)
Hexachloropropene	1000 (454)
Hexaethyl tetraphosphate	100 (45.4)
Hexamethylene-1,6-diisocyanate	100 (45.4)
Hexamethylphosphoramide	1 (0.454)
Hexane	5000 (2270)
Hydrazine	1 (0.454)
Hydrazine, 1,2-diethyl-	10 (4.54)
Hydrazine, 1,1-dimethyl-	10 (4.54)
Hydrazine, 1,2-dimethyl-	1 (0.454)
Hydrazine, 1,2-diphenyl-	10 (4.54)
Hydrazine, methyl-	10 (4.54)
Hydrazinecarbothioamide	100 (45.4)
Hydrochloric acid	5000 (2270)
Hydrocyanic acid	10 (4.54)
Hydrofluoric acid	100 (45.4)
Hydrogen chloride	5000 (2270)
Hydrogen cyanide	10 (4.54)
Hydrogen fluoride	100 (45.4)
Hydrogen phosphide	100 (45.4)
Hydrogen sulfide	100 (45.4)
Hydrogen sulfide H2S	100 (45.4)
Hydroperoxide, 1-methyl-1-phenylethyl-	10 (4.54)
Hydroquinone	100 (45.4)
2-Imidazolidinethione	10 (4.54)
Indeno(1,2,3-cd)pyrene	100 (45.4)
1,3-Isobenzofurandione	5000 (2270)

Hazardous Substances	RQ: lbs (kg)
Isobutyl alcohol	5000 (2270)
Isodrin	1 (0.454)
Isophorone	5000 (2270)
Isoprene	100 (45.4)
Isopropanolamine dodecylbenzene sulfonate	1000 (454)
Isosafrole	100 (45.4)
3(2H)-Isoxazolone, 5-(aminomethyl)-	1000 (454)
Kepone	1 (0.454)
Lasiocarpine	10 (4.54)
Lead ¢	10 (4.54)
Lead acetate	10 (4.54)
Lead arsenate	1 (0.454)
Lead,bis(acetato-O)tetrahydroxytri	10 (4.54)
Lead chloride	10 (4.54)
Lead fluoborate	10 (4.54)
Lead fluoride	10 (4.54)
Lead iodide	10 (4.54)
Lead nitrate	10 (4.54)
Lead phosphate	10 (4.54)
Lead stearate	10 (4.54)
Lead subacetate	10 (4.54)
Lead sulfate	10 (4.54)
Lead sulfide	10 (4.54)
Lead thiocyanate	10 (4.54)
Lindane	1 (0.454)
Lithium chromate	10 (4.54)
Malathion	100 (45.4)
Maleic acid	5000 (2270)
Maleic anhydride	5000 (2270)
Maleic hydrazide	5000 (2270)
Malononitrile	1000 (454)
MDI	5000 (2270)
Melphalan	1 (0.454)
Mercaptodimethur	10 (4.54)
Mercuric cyanide	1 (0.454)
Mercuric nitrate	10 (4.54)
Mercuric sulfate	10 (4.54)
Mercuric thiocyanate	10 (4.54)
Mercurous nitrate	10 (4.54)
Mercury	1 (0.454)
Mercury, (acetato-O)phenyl-	100 (45.4)
Mercury fulminate	10 (4.54)
Methacrylonitrile	1000 (454)
Methanamine, N-methyl-	1000 (454)

Hazardous Substances	RQ: lbs (kg)
Methanamine, N-methyl-N-nitroso	10 (4.54)
Methane, bromo-	1000 (454)
Methane, chloro-	100 (45.4)
Methane, chloromethoxy-	10 (4.54)
Methane, dibromo-	1000 (454)
Methane, dichloro-	1000 (454)
Methane, dichlorodifluoro-	5000 (2270)
Methane, iodo-	100 (45.4)
Methane, isocyanato-	10 (4.54)
Methane, oxybis(chloro-	10 (4.54)
Methane, tetrachloro-	10 (4.54)
Methane, tetranitro-	10 (4.54)
Methane, tribromo-	100 (45.4)
Methane, trichloro-	10 (4.54)
Methane, trichlorofluoro-	5000 (2270)
Methenesulfenyl chloride, trichloro	100 (45.4)
Methanesulfonic acid, ethyl ester	1 (0.454)
Methanethiol	100 (45.4)
6,9-Methano-2,4,3-benzodioxathiepin, 6,7,8,9,10,10-hexachloro-1,5,5a,6,9,9a-hexahydro-, 3-oxide	1 (0.454)
Methanoic acid	5000 (2270)
4,7-Methano-1H-indene, 1,4,5,6,7,8,8-heptachloro-3a, 4,7,7a-tetrahydro-	1 (0.454)
4,7-Methano-1H-indene,1,4,5,6,7,8,8-octachloro-3,3a,4,7,7a-hexahydro-	1 (0.454)
Methanol	5000 (2270)
Methapyrilene	5000 (2270)
1,3,4-Metheno-2H-cyclobutal[cd]-pentalen-2-one, 1,1a,3,3a,4,5,5,5a,5b,6-decachloroctahydro-	1 (0.454)
Methomyl	100 (45.4)
Methoxychlor	1 (0.454)
Methyl alcohol	5000 (2270)
Methylamine @	100 (45.4)
Methyl bromide	1000 (454)
1-Methylbutadiene	100 (45.4)
Methyl chloride	100 (45.4)
Methyl chlorocarbonate	1000 (414)
Methyl chloroform	1000 (454)
Methyl chloroformate	1000 (454)
Methylchloromethyl ether @	1 (0.454)
3-Methylcholanthrene	10 (4.54)
4,4'-Methylenebis(2-chloroaniline)	10 (4.54)
Methylene bromide	1000 (454)
Methylene chloride	1000 (454)
4,4'-Methylenedianiline	10 (4.54)

Hazardous Substances	RQ: lbs (kg)
Methylene diphenyl diisocyanate	5000 (2270)
Methylene oxide	100 (45.4)
Methyl ethyl ketone(MEK)	5000 (2270)
Methyl ethyl ketone peroxide	10 (4.54)
Methyl hydrazine	10 (4.54)
Methyl iodide	100 (45.4)
Methyl isobutyl ketone	5000 (2270)
Methyl isocyanate	10 (4.54)
2-Methyllactonitrile	10 (4.54)
Methyl mercaptan	100 (45.4)
Methyl methacrylate	1000 (454)
Methyl parathion	100 (45.4)
4-Methyl-2-pentanone	5000 (2270)
Methyl tert-butyl ether	1000 (454)
Methylthiouracil	10 (4.54)
Mevinphos	10 (4.54)
Mexacarbate	1000 (454)
Mitomycin C	10 (4.54)
MNNG	10 (4.54)
Monoethylamine	100 (45.4)
Monomethylamine	100 (45.4)
Muscimol	1000 (454)
Naled	10 (4.54)
5,12-Naphthacenedione, 8-acetyl-10-[3-amino-2,3,6-trideoxy-alpha-L-lyxo-hexopyranosyl)oxy]-7,8,9,10-tetrahdro-6,8,11-trihydroxy-1-methoxy-,(8S-cis)-	10 (4.54)
Naphthalenamine,N,N-bis(2-chloroethyl)-	100 (45.4)
Naphthalene	100 (45.4)
Naphthalene, 2-chloro-	5000 (2270)
1,4-Naphthalenedione	5000 (2270)
2,7-Naphthalenedisulfonic acid,3,3'-[(3,3'-dimethyl-(1,1'-biphenyl)-4,4'-diyl)-bis(azo)]bis(5-amino-4-hydroxy)-tetrasodium salt	10 (4.54)
Naphthenic acid	100 (45.4)
1,4-Naphthoquinone	5000 (2270)
alpha-Naphthylamine	100 (45.4)
beta-Naphthylamine	1 (0.454)
1-Naphthylamine	100 (45.4)
2-Naphthylamine	1 (0.454)
alpha-Naphthylthiourea	100 (45.4)
Nickel ¢	100 (45.4)
Nickel ammonium sulfate	100 (45.4)
Nickel carbonyl	10 (4.54)
Nickel carbonyl Ni(CO)4,(T-4)-	10 (4.54)
Nickel chloride	100 (45.4)

Hazardous Substances	RQ: lbs (kg)
Nickel cyanide	10 (4.54)
Nickel cyanide Ni(CN)2	10 (4.54)
Nickel hydroxide	10 (4.54)
Nickel nitrate	100 (45.4)
Nickel sulfate	100 (45.4)
Nicotine and salts	100 (45.4)
Nitric acid	1000 (454)
Nitric acid, thallium(1+)salt	100 (45.4)
Nitric oxide	10 (4.54)
p-Nitroaniline	5000 (2270)
Nitrobenzene	1000 (454)
4-nitrobiphenyl	10 (4.54)
Nitrogen dioxide	10 (4.54)
Nitrogen oxide NO	10 (4.54)
Nitrogen oxide NO2	10 (4.54)
Nitroglycerine	10 (4.54)
Nitrophenol (mixed)	100 (45.4)
m-	
o-	
p-	
o-Nitrophenol	100 (45.4)
p-Nitrophenol	100 (45.4)
2-Nitrophenol	100 (45.4)
4-Nitrophenol	100 (45.4)
2-Nitropropane	10 (4.54)
N-Nitrosodi-n-butylamine	10 (4.54)
N-Nitrosodiethanolamine	1 (0.454)
N-Nitrosodiethylamine	1 (0.454)
N-Nitrosodimethylamine	10 (4.54)
N-Nitrosodiphenylamine	100 (45.4)
N-Nitroso-N-ethylurea	1 (0.454)
N-Nitroso-N-methylurea	1 (0.454)
N-Nitroso-N-methylurethane	1 (0.454)
N-Nitrosomethylvinylamine	10 (4.54)
n-Nitrosomorpholine	1 (0.454)
N-Nitrosopiperidine	10 (4.54)
N-Nitrosopyrrolidine	1 (0.454)
Nitrotoluene	1000 (454)
m-Nitrotoluene	
o-Nitrotoluene	
p-Nitrotoluene	
5-Nitro-o-toluidine	100 (45.4)
Octamethylpyrophosphoramide	100 (45.4)
Osmium oxide OsO4 (T-4)-	1000 (454)

Hazardous Substances	RQ: lbs (kg)
Osmium tetroxide	1000 (454)
7-Oxabicyclo[2.2.1]heptane-2,3-dicarboxylic acid	1000 (454)
1,2-Oxathiolane, 2,2-dioxide	10 (4.54)
2H-1,3,2-Oxazaphosphorin-2-amine, N,N-bis (2-chloroethyl)tetrahydro-,2-oxide	10 (4.54)
Oxirane	10 (4.54)
Oxiranecarboxyaldehyde	10 (4.54)
Oxirane, (chloromethyl)-	100 (45.4)
Paraformaldehyde	1000 (454)
Paraldehyde	1000 (454)
Parathion	10 (4.54)
Pentachlorobenzene	10 (4.54)
Pentachloroethane	10 (4.54)
Pentachloronitrobenzene (PCNB)	100 (45.4)
Pentachlorophenol	10 (4.54)
1,3-Pentadiene	100 (45.4)
Perchloroethylene	100 (45.4)
Perchloromethyl mercaptan @	100 (45.4)
Phenacetin	100 (45.4)
Phenanthrene	5000 (2270)
Phenol	1000 (454)
Phenol, 2-chloro-	100 (45.4)
Phenol, 4-chloro-3-methyl-	5000 (2270)
Phenol, 2-cyclohexyl-4,6-dinitro-	100 (45.4)
Phenol, 2,4-dichloro-	100 (45.4)
Phenol, 2,6-dichloro-	100 (45.4)
Phenol, 4,4'-(1,2-diethyl-1,2-ethenediyl)bis-, (E)	1 (0.454)
Phenol, 2,4-dimethyl-	100 (45.4)
Phenol, 2,4-dinitro-	10 (4.54)
Phenol, methyl-	100 (45.4)
Phenol, 2-methyl-4,6-dinitro-	10 (4.54)
Phenol, 2,2'-methylenebis[3,4,6-trichloro-	100 (45.4)
Phenol, 2-(1-methylpropyl)-4,6-dintro	1000 (454)
Phenol, 4-nitro-	100 (45.4)
Phenol, pentachloro-	10 (4.54)
Phenol, 2,3,4,6-tetrachloro-	10 (4.54)
Phenol, 2,4,5-trichloro-	10 (4.54)
Phenol, 2,4,6-trichloro-	10 (4.54)
Phenol, 2,4,6-trinitro-, ammonium salt	10 (4.54)
L-Phenylalanine, 4-[bis(2-chloroethyl)aminol]	1 (0.454)
p-Phenylenediamine	5000 (2270)
1,10-(1,2-Phenylene)pyrene	100 (45.4)
Phenyl mercaptan @	100 (45.4)
Phenylmercuric acetate	100 (45.4)
Phenylthiourea	100 (45.4)

Hazardous Substances	RQ: lbs (kg)
Phorate	10 (4.54)
Phosgene	10 (4.54)
Phosphine	100 (45.4)
Phosphoric acid	5000 (2270)
Phosphoric acid, diethyl 4-nitrophenyl ester	100 (45.4)
Phosphoric acid, lead(2+) salt(2:3)	10 (4.54)
Phosphorodithioic acid, O,O-diethyl S-[2-(ethylthio) ethyl]ester	1 (0.454)
Phosphorodithioic acid, O,O-diethyl S-(ethylthio), methyl ester	10 (4.54)
Phosphorodithioic acid, O,O-diethyl S-methyl ester	5000 (2270)
Phosphorodithioic acid, O,O-dimethyl S-[2(methyl amino)-2-oxoethyl] ester	10 (4.54)
Phosphorofluoridic acid, bis(1-methylethyl) ester	100 (45.4)
Phosphorothioic acid, O,O-diethyl O-(4-nitrophenyl) ester	10 (4.54)
Phosphorothioic acid, O,O-diethyl O-pyrazinyl ester	100 (45.4)
Phosphorothioic acid, O,O-dimethyl O-(4-nitrophenyl) ester	100 (45.4)
Phosphorothioic acid, O,[4-[(dimethylamino)sulfonyl] phenyl] O,O-di-methyl ester	1000 (454)
Phosphorus	1 (0.454)
Phosphorus oxychloride	1000 (454)
Phosphorus pentasulfide	100 (45.4)
Phosphorus sulfide	100 (45.4)
Phosphorus trichloride	1000 (454)
Phthalate anhydride	5000 (2270)
2-Picoline	5000 (2270)
Piperidine, 1-nitroso-	10 (4.54)
Plumbane, tetraethyl-	10 (4.54)
POLYCHLORINATED BIPHENYLS (PCBs)	1 (0.454)
Potassium arsenate	1 (0.454)
Potassium arsenite	1 (0.454)
Potassium bichromate	10 (4.54)
Potassium chromate	10 (4.54)
Postassium cyanide	10 (4.54)
Potassium cyanide K(CN)	10 (4.54)
Potassium hydroxide	1000 (454)
Potassium permanganate	100 (45.4)
Potassium silver cyanide	1 (0.454)
Pronamide	5000 (2270)
Propanal, 2-methyl-2-(methylthio)-,O-[(methylamino) carbonyl]oxime	1 (0.454)
1-Propanamine	5000 (2270)
1-Propanamine, N-nitroso-N-propyl-	10 (4.54)
1-Propanamine, N-propyl-	5000 (2270)
Propane, 1,2-dibromo-3-chloro-	1 (0.454)
Propane, 1,2-dichloro-	1000 (454)
Propane, 2-nitro-	10 (4.54)

Hazardous Substances	RQ: lbs (kg)
Propane, 2,2'-oxybis[2-chloro-	1000 (454)
1,3-Propane sultone	10 (4.54)
Propanedinitrile	1000 (454)
Propanenitrile	10 (4.54)
Propanenitrile, 3-chloro-	1000 (454)
Propanenitrile, 2-hydroxy-2-methyl-	10 (4.54)
1,2,3-Propanetriol, trinitrate-	10 (4.54)
1-Propanol, 2,3-dibromo-, phosphate (3:1)	10 (4.54)
1-Propanol, 2-methyl-	5000 (2270)
2-Propanone	5000 (2270)
2-Propanone, 1-bromo-	1000 (454)
Propargite	10 (4.54)
Propargyl alcohol	1000 (454)
2-Propenal	1 (0.454)
2-Propenamide	5000 (2270)
1-Propene, 1,3-dichloro-	100 (45.4)
1-Propene, 1,1,2,3,3,3-hexachloro-	1000 (454)
2-Propenenitrile	100 (45.4)
2-Propenenitrile, 2-methyl-	1000 (454)
2-Propenoic acid	5000 (2270)
2-Propenoic acid, ethyl ester	1000 (454)
2-Propenoic acid, 2-methyl-, ethyl ester	1000 (454)
2-Propenoic acid, 2-methyl-, methyl ester	1000 (454)
2-Propen-1-ol	100 (45.4)
beta-Propioaldehyde	1000 (454)
Propionic acid	5000 (2270)
Propionic acid, 2-(2,4,5-trichlorophenoxy)-	100 (45.4)
Propionic anhydride	5000 (2270)
Propoxur (baygon)	100 (45.4)
n-Propylamine	5000 (2270)
Propylene dichloride	1000 (454)
Propylene oxide	100 (45.4)
1,2-Propylenimine	1 (0.454)
2-Propyn-1-ol	1000 (454)
Pyrene	5000 (2270)
Pyrethrins	1 (0.454)
3,6-Pyridazinedione, 1,2-dihydro-	5000 (2270)
4-Pyridinamine	1000 (454)
Pyridine	1000 (454)
Pyridine, 2-methyl-	5000 (2270)
Pyridine, 3-(1-methyl-2-pyrrolidinyl)-, (S)	100 (45.4)
2,4-(1H,3H)-Pyrimidinedione, 5-[bis(2-chloroethyl) amino]-	10 (4.54)
4(1H)-Pyrimidinone, 2,3-dihydro-6-methyl-2-thioxo-	10 (4.54)
Pyrrolidine, 1-nitroso-	1 (0.454)

Hazardous Substances	RQ: lbs (kg)
Quinoline	5000 (2270)
RADIONUCLIDES	See Table 2
Reserpine	5000 (2270)
Resorcinol	5000 (2270)
Saccharin and salts	100 (45.4)
Safrole	100 (45.4)
Selenious acid	10 (4.54)
Selenious acid, dithallium(1+)salt	1000 (454)
Selenium ¢	100 (45.4)
Selenium dioxide	10 (4.54)
Selenium oxide	10 (4.54)
Selenium sulfide	10 (4.54)
Selenium sulfide SeS2	10 (4.54)
Selenourea	1000 (454)
L-Serine, diazoacetate (ester)	1 (0.454)
Silver ¢	1000 (454)
Silver cyanide	1 (0.454)
Silver cyanide Ag(CN)	1 (0.454)
Silver nitrate	1 (0.454)
Silvex(2,4,5-TP)	100 (45.4)
Sodium	10 (4.54)
Sodium arsenate	1 (0.454)
Sodium arsenite	1 (0.454)
Sodium azide	1000 (454)
Sodium bichromate	10 (4.54)
Sodium bifluoride	100 (45.4)
Sodium bisulfite	5000 (2270)
Sodium chromate	10 (4.54)
Sodium cyanide	10 (4.54)
Sodium cyanide Na(CN)	10 (4.54)
Sodium dodecylbenzene sulfonate	1000 (454)
Sodium fluoride	1000 (454)
Sodium hydrosulfide	5000 (2270)
Sodium hydroxide	1000 (454)
Sodium hypochlorite	100(45.4)
Sodium methylate	1000 (454)
Sodium nitrite	100 (45.4)
Sodium phosphate, dibasic	5000 (2270)
Sodium phosphate, tribasic	5000 (2270)
Sodium selenite	100 (45.4)
Streptozotocin	1 (0.454)
Strontium chromate	10 (4.54)
Strychnidin-10-one	10 (4.54)
Strychnidin-10-one, 2,3-dimethoxy-	100 (45.4)

Hazardous Substances	RQ: lbs (kg)
Strychnine and salts	10 (4.54)
Styrene	1000 (454)
Styrene oxide	100 (45.4)
Sulfur chloride@	1000 (454)
Sulfur monochloride	1000 (454)
Sulfur phosphide	100 (45.4)
Sulfuric acid	1000 (454)
Sulfuric acid, dimethyl ester	100 (45.4)
Sulfuric acid, dithallium(I+)salt	100 (45.4)
2,4,5-T	1000 (454)
2,4,5-T acid	1000 (454)
2,4,5-T amines	5000 (2270)
2,4,5-T esters	1000 (454)
2,4,5-T salts	1000 (454)
TDE	1 (0.454)
1,2,4,5-Tetrachlorobenzene	5000 (2270)
2,3,7,8-Tetrachlorodibenzo-p-dioxin (TCDD)	1 (0.454)
1,1,1,2-Tetrachloroethane	100 (45.4)
1,1,2,2-Tetrachloroethane	100 (45.4
Tetrachloroethane@	100 (45.4)
Tetrachloroethene	100 (45.4)
Tetrachloroethylene	100 (45.4)
2,3,4,6-Tetrachlorophenol	10 (4.54)
Tetraethyl lead	10 (4.54)
Tetraethyl pyrophosphate	10 (4.54)
Tetraethyldithiopyrophosphate	100 (45.4)
Tetrahydrofuran	1000 (454)
Tetranitromethane	10 (4.54)
Tetraphosphoricacid, hexaethyl ester	100 (45.4)
Thallic oxide	100 (45.4)
Thallium ¢	1000 (454)
Thallium(I) acetate	100 (45.4)
Thallium(I) carbonate	100 (45.4)
Thallium(I) chloride	100 (45.4)
Thallium chloride TlCl	100 (45.4)
Thallium(I) nitrate	100 (45.4)
Thallium oxide T1203	100 (45.4)
Thallium selenite	1000 (454)
Thallium(I) sulfate	100 (45.4)
Thioacetamide	10 (4.54)
Thiodiphosphoric acid, tetraethyl ester	100 (45.4)
Thiofanox	100 (45.4)
Thioimidodicarbonic diamide [(H2N)C(S)]2NH	100 (45.4)
Thiomethanol	100 (45.4)

Hazardous Substances	RQ: lbs (kg)
Thioperoxydicarbonic diamide [(H2N)C(S)]2S2, tetramethyl-	10 (4.54)
Thiophenol	100 (45.4)
Thiosemicarbazide	100 (45.4)
Thiourea	10 (4.54)
Thiourea, (2-chlorophenyl)-	100 (45.4)
Thiourea, 1-naphthalenyl-	100 (45.4)
Thiourea, phenyl-	100 (45.4)
Thiram	10 (4.54)
Titanium tetrachloride	1000 (454)
Toluene	1000 (454)
Toluenediamine	10 (4.54)
Toluene diisocyanate	100 (45.4)
o-Toluidine	100 (45.4)
p-Toluidine	100 (45.4)
o-Toluidine hydrochloride	100 (45.4)
Toxaphene	1 (0.454)
2,4,5-TP acid	100 (45.4)
2,4,5-TP acid esters	100 (45.4)
1H-1,2,4-Triazol-3-amine	10 (4.54)
Trichlorfon	100 (45.4)
1,2,4-Trichlorobenzene	100 (45.4)
1,1,1-Trichloroethane	1000 (454)
1,1,2-Trichloroethane	100 (45.4)
Trichloroethene	100 (45.4)
Trichloroethylene	100 (45.4)
Trichloromethanesulfenyl chloride	100 (45.4)
Trichloromonofluoromethane	5000 (2270)
Trichlorophenol	10 (4.54)
2,3,4-Trichlorophenol	
2,3,5-Trichlorophenol	
2,3,6-Trichlorophenol	
2,4,5-Trichlorophenol	
2,4,6-Trichlorophenol	
3,4,5-Trichlorophenol	
2,4,5-Trichlorophenol	10 (4.54)
2,4,6-Trichlorophenol	10 (4.54)
Triethanolamine dodecylbenzene sulfonate	1000 (454)
Triethylamine	5000 (2270)
Trifluralin	10 (4.54)
Trimethylamine	100 (45.4)
2,2,4-Trimethylpentane	1000 (454)
1,3,5-Trinitrobenzene	10 (4.54)
1,3,5-Trioxane, 2,4,6-trimethyl-	1000 (454)
Tris(2,3-dibromopropyl) phosphate	10 (4.54)

Hazardous Substances	RQ: lbs (kg)
Trypan blue	10 (4.54)
Uracil mustard	10 (4.54)
Uranyl acetate	100 (45.4)
Uranyl nitrate	100 (45.4)
Urea, N-ethyl-N-nitroso-	1 (0.454)
Urea, N-methyl-N-nitroso-	1 (0.454)
Vanadic acid, ammonium salt	1000 (454)
Vanadium oxide V_2O_5	1000 (454)
Vanadium pentoxide	1000 (454)
Vanadyl sulfate	1000 (454)
Vinyl acetate	5000 (2270)
Vinyl acetate monomer	5000 (2270)
Vinylamine, N-methyl-N-nitroso-	10 (4.54)
Vinyl bromide	100 (45.4)
Vinyl chloride	1 (0.454)
Vinylidene chloride	100 (45.4)
Warfarin, & salts, when present at concentrations greater than 0.3%	100 (45.4)
Xylene	100 (45.4)
m-Xylene	1000 (454)
o-Xylene	1000 (454)
p-Xylene	100 (45.4)
Xylene (mixed)	100 (45.4)
Xylenes (isomers and mixture)	100 (45.4)
Xylenol	1000 (454)
Yohimban-16-carboxylic acid, 11,17-dimethoxy-18-[(3,4,5- trimethoxybenzoyl)oxy]-, methyl ester (3beta,16beta, 17alpha,18beta,20alpha)-	5000 (2270)
Zinc ¢	1000 (454)
Zinc acetate	1000 (454)
Zinc ammonium chloride	1000 (454)
Zinc borate	1000 (454)
Zinc bromide	1000 (454)
Zinc carbonate	1000 (454)
Zinc chloride	1000 (454)
Zinc cyanide	10 (4.54)
Zinc cyanide $Zn(CN)_2$	10 (4.54)
Zinc fluoride	1000 (454)
Zinc formate	1000 (454)
Zinc hydrosulfite	1000 (454)
Zinc nitrate	1000 (454)
Zinc phenolsulfonate	5000 (2270)
Zinc phosphide	100 (45.4)
Zinc phosphide Zn_3P_2, when present at concentrations greater than 10%	100 (45.4)

Hazardous Substances	RQ: lbs (kg)
Zinc silicofluoride	5000 (2270)
Zinc sulfate	1000 (454)
Zirconium nitrate	5000 (2270)
Zirconium potassium fluoride	1000 (454)
Zirconium sulfate	5000 (2270)
Zirconium tetrachloride	5000 (2270)
D001 Unlisted Hazardous Wastes Characteristic of Ignitability	100 (45.4)
D002 Unlisted Hazardous Wastes Characteristic of Corrosivity	100 (45.4)
D003 Unlisted Hazardous Wastes Characteristic of Reactivity	100 (45.4)
D004-D043 Unlisted Hazardous Wastes Characteristic of Toxicity	
D004 Arsenic	1 (0.454)
D005 Barium	1000 (454)
D006 Cadmium	10 (4.54)
D007 Chromium	10 (4.54)
D008 Lead	10 (4.54)
D009 Mercury	1 (0.454)
D010 Selenium	10 (4.54)
D011 Silver	1 (0.454)
D012 Endrin	1 (0.454)
D013 Lindane	1 (0.454)
D014 Methoxyclor	1 (0.454)
D015 Toxaphene	1 (0.454)
D016 2,4-D	100 (45.4)
D017 2,4,5-TP	100 (45.4)
D018 Benzene	10 (4.54)
D019 Carbon tetrachloride	10 (4.54)
D020 Chlordane	1 (0.454)
D021 Chlorobenzene	100 (45.4)
D022 Chloroform	10 (4.54)
D023 o-Cresol	100 (45.4)
D024 m-Cresol	100 (45.4)
D025 p-Cresol	100 (45.4)
D026 Cresol	100 (45.4)
D027 1,4-Dichlorobenzene	100 (45.4)
D028 1,2-Dichloroethane	100 (45.4)
D029 1,1-Dichloroethylene	100 (45.4)
D030 2,4-Dinitrotoluene	10 (4.54)
D031 Heptachlor (and hydroxide)	1 (0.454)
D032 Hexachlorobenzene	10 (4.54)
D033 Hexachlorobutadiene	1 (0.454)
D034 Hexachloroethane	100 (45.4)

Hazardous Substances	RQ: lbs (kg)
D035 Methyl ethyl ketone	5000 (2270)
D036 Nitrobenzene	1000 (454)
D037 Pentachlorophenol	10 (4.54)
D038 Pyridine	1000 (454)
D039 Tetrachloroethylene	100 (45.4)
D040 Trichloroethylene	100 (45.4)
D041 2,4,5-Trichlorophenol	10 (4.54)
D042 2,4,6-Trichlorophenol	10 (4.54)
D043 Vinyl Chloride	1 (0.454)
F001	10 (4.54)
The following spent halogenated solvents used in de greasing; all spent, solvent mixtures/blends used in de greasing containing, before use, a total of ten percent or more (by volume) of one or more of the below listed halogenated solvents or those solvents listed in F002, F004, and F005; and stillbottoms from the recovery of these spent solvents and spent solvent mixtures.	
(a) Tetrachloroethylene	100 (45.4)
(b) Trichloroethylene	100 (45.4)
(c) Methylene chloride	1000 (454)
(d) 1,1,1-Trichloroethane	1000 (454)
(e) Carbon tetrachloride	10 (4.54)
(f) Chlorinated fluorocarbons	5000 (2270)
F002	10 (4.54)
The following spent halogenated solvents; all spent sol vent mixtures/blends containing, before use, a total of ten percent or more (by volume) of one or more of the below listed halogenated solvents or those listed in F001, F004, F005; and stillbottoms from the recovery of these spent solvents and spent solvent mixtures.	
(a) Tetrachloroethylene	100 (45.4)
(b) Methylene chloride	1000 (454)
(c) Trichloroethylene	100 (45.4)
(d) 1,1,1-Trichloroethane	1000 (454)
(e) Chlorobenzene	100 (45.4)
(f) 1,1,2-Trichloro-1,2,2- trifluoroethane	5000 (2270)
(g) o-Dichlorobenzene	100 (45.4)
(h) Trichlorofluoromethane	5000 (2270)
(i) 1,1,2 Trichloroethane	100 (45.4)
F003	100 (45.4)
The following spent non-halogenated solvents and solvents:	
(a) Xylene	1000 (454)
(b) Acetone	5000 (2270)
(c) Ethyl acetate	5000 (2270)
(d) Ethylbenzene	1000 (454)
(e) Ethyl ether	100 (45.4)
(f) Methyl isobutyl ketone	5000 (2270)

Hazardous Substances	RQ: lbs (kg)
(g) n-Butyl alcohol	5000 (2270)
(h) Cyclohexanone	5000 (2270)
(i) Methanol	5000 (2270)
F004	100 (45.4)
The following spent non-halogenated solvents and the stillbottoms from the recovery of these solvents:	
(a) Cresols/Cresylic acid	1000 (454)
(b) Nitrobenzene	100 (45.4)
F005	100 (45.4)
The following spent non-halogenated solvents and the stillbottoms from the recovery of these solvents:	
(a) Toluene	1000 (454)
(b) Methyl ethyl ketone	5000 (2270)
(c) Carbon disulfide	100 (45.4)
(d) Isobutanol	5000 (2270)
(e) Pyridine	1000 (454)
F006	10 (4.54)
Wastewater treatment sludges from electroplating operations except from the following processes: (1) sulfuric acid anodizing of aluminum; (2) tin plating on carbon steel; (3) zinc plating (segregated basis) on carbon steel; (4) aluminum or zinc-aluminum plating on carbon steel; (5) cleaning/stripping associated with tin, zinc and aluminum plating on carbon steel; and (6) chemical etching and milling of aluminum.	
F007	10 (4.54)
Spent cyanide plating bath solutions from electroplating operations.	
F008	10 (4.54)
Plating bath residues from the bottom of plating baths from electroplating operations where cyanides are used in the process.	
F009	10 (4.54)
Spent stripping and cleaning bath solutions from electroplating operations where cyanides are used in the process.	
F010	10 (4.54)
Quenching bath residues from oil baths from metal heat treating operations where cyanides are used in the process.	
F011	10 (4.54)
Spent cyanide solutions from salt bath pot cleaning from metal heat treating operations (except for precious metals heat treating spent cyanide solutions from salt bath pot cleaning).	
F012	10 (4.54)
Quenching wastewater treatment sludges from metal heat treating operations where cyanides are used in the process.	

Hazardous Substances	RQ: lbs (kg)
F019	10 (4.54)
Wastewater treatment sludges from the chemical conversion coating of aluminum-except from zirconium phosphating in aluminum can washing when such phosphating is an exclusive conversion coating process.	
F020	1 (0.454)
Wastes (except wastewater and spent carbon from hydrogen chloride purification from the production or manufacturing use (as a reactant, chemical intermediate, or component in a formulating process) of tri- or tetrachlorophenol, or of intermediates used to produce their pesticide derivatives. (This listing does not include wastes from the production of hexachlorophene from highly purified 2,4,5-trichlorophenol.)	
F021	1 (0.454)
Wastes (except wastewater and spent carbon from hydrogen chloride purification) from the production or manufacturing use (as a reactant, chemical intermediate, or component in a formulating process) of pentachlorophenol, or of intermediates used to produce its derivatives.	
F022	1 (0.454)
Wastes (except wastewater and spent carbon from hydrogen chloride purification) from the manufacturing use (as a reactant, chemical intermediate, or component in a formulating process) of tetra-, penta-, or hexachlorobenzenes under alkaline conditions.	
F023	1 (0.454)
Wastes (except wastewater and spent carbon from hydrogen chloride purification) from the production of materials on equipment previously used for the production or manufacturing use (as a reactant, chemical intermediate, or component in a formulating process) of tri- and tetrachlorophenols. (This listing does not include wastes from equipment used only for the production or use of hexachlorophene from highly purified 2,4, 5-trichlorophenol.)	
F024	1 (0.454)
Wastes, including but not limited to distillation residues, heavy ends, tars, and reactor cleanout wastes, from the production of chlorinated aliphatic hydrocarbons, having carbon content from one to five, utilizing free radical catalyzed processes. (This listing does not include light ends, spent filters and filter aids, spent dessicants (sic), wastewater, wastewater treatment sludges, spent catalysts, and wastes listed in Section 261.32.)	
F025	1 (0.454)
Condensed light ends, spent filters and filter aids, and spent desiccant wastes from the production of certain chlorinated aliphatic hydrocarbons, by free radical catalyzed processes. These chlorinated aliphatic hydrocarbons are those having carbon chain lengths ranging from one to and including five, with varying amounts and positions of chlorine substitution.	

Hazardous Substances	RQ: lbs (kg)
F026	1 (0.454)
Wastes (except wastewater and spent carbon from hydrogen chloride purification) from the production of materials on equipment previously used for the manufacturing use (as a reactant, chemical intermediate, or component in a formulating process) of tetra-, penta-, or hexachlorobenzene under alkaline conditions.	
F027	1 (0.454)
Discarded unused formulations containing tri-, tetra-, or pentachlorophenol or discarded unused formulations containing compounds derived from these chlorophenols. (This listing does not include formulations containing hexachlorophene synthesized from prepurified 2,4,5-trichloro phenol as the sole component.)	
F028	1 (0.454)
Residues resulting from the incineration or thermal treatment of soil contaminated with EPA Hazardous Waste Nos. F020, F021, F022, F023, F026, and F027.	
F032	1 (0.454)
F034	1 (0.454)
F035	1 (0.454)
F037	1 (0.454)
F038	1 (0.454)
F039	1 (0.454)
Multi source leachate.	
K001	1 (0.454)
Bottom sediment sludge from the treatment of wastewaters from wood preserving processes that use creosote and/or pentachlorophenol.	
K002	10 (4.54)
Wastewater treatment sludge from the production of chrome yellow and orange pigments.	
K003	10 (4.54)
Wastewater treatment sludge from the production of molybdate orange pigments.	
K004	10 (4.54)
Wastewater treatment sludge from the production of zinc yellow pigments.	
K005	10 (4.54)
Wastewater treatment sludge from the production of chrome green pigments.	
K006	10 (4.54)
Wastewater treatment sludge from the production of chrome oxide green pigments (anhydrous and hydrated).	
K007	10 (4.54)
Wastewater treatment sludge from the production of iron blue pigments.	

Hazardous Substances	RQ: lbs (kg)
K008	10 (4.54)
Oven residue from the production of chrome oxide green pigments.	
K009	10 (4.54)
Distillation bottoms from the production of acetaldehyde from ethylene.	
K010	10 (4.54)
Distillation side cuts from the production of acetaldehyde from ethylene.	
K011	10 (4.54)
Bottom stream from the wastewater stripper in the production of acrylonitrile.	
K013	10 (4.54)
Bottom stream from the acetonitrile column in the production of acrylonitrile.	
K014	5000 (2270)
Bottoms from the acetonitrile purification column in the production of acrylonitrile.	
K015	10 (4.54)
Still bottoms from the distillation of benzyl chloride.	
K016	1 (0.454)
Heavy ends or distillation residues from the production of carbon tetrachloride.	
K017	10 (4.54)
Heavy ends (still bottoms) from the purification column in the production of epichlorohydrin.	
K018	1 (0.454)
Heavy ends from the fractionation column in ethyl chloride production.	
K019	1 (0.454)
Heavy ends from the distillation of ethylene dichloride in ethylene dichloride production.	
K020	1 (0.454)
Heavy ends from the distillation of vinyl chloride in vinyl chloride monomer production.	
K021	10 (4.54)
Aqueous spent antimony catalyst waste from fluoromethanes production.	
K023	5000 (2270)
Distillation light ends from the production of phthalic anhydride from naphthalene.	
K024	5000 (2270)
Distillation bottoms from the production of phthalic anhydride from naphthalene.	

Hazardous Substances	RQ: lbs (kg)
K025	10 (4.54)
Distillation bottoms from the production of nitrobenzene by the nitration of benzene.	
K026	1000 (454)
Stripping still tails from the production of methyl ethyl pyridines.	
K027	10 (4.54)
Centrifuge and distillation residues from toluene diisocyanate production.	
K028	1 (0.454)
Spent catalyst from the hydrochlorinator reactor in the production of 1,1,1-trichloroethane.	
K029	1 (0.454)
Waste from the product steam stripper in the production of 1,1,1-trichloroethane.	
K030	1 (0.454)
Column bottoms or heavy ends from the combined production of trichloroethylene and perchloroethylene.	
K031	1 (0.454)
By-product salts generated in the production of MSMA and cacodylic acid.	
K032	10 (4.54)
Wastewater treatment sludge from the production of chlordane.	
K033	10 (4.54)
Wastewater and scrub water from the chlorination of cyclopentadiene in the production of chlordane.	
K034	10 (4.54)
Filter solids from the filtration of hexachlorocyclopentadiene in the production of chlordane.	
K035	1 (0.454)
Wastewater treatment sludges generated in the production of creosote.	
K036	1 (0.454)
Still bottoms from toluene reclamation distillation in the production of disulfoton.	
K037	1 (0.454)
Wastewater treatment sludges from the production of disulfoton.	
K038	10 (4.54)
Wastewater from the washing and stripping of phorate production.	

Hazardous Substances	RQ: lbs (kg)
K039	10 (4.54)
Filter cake from the filtration of diethylphosphorodithioic acid in the production of phorate.	
K040	10 (4.54)
Wastewater treatment sludge from the production of phorate.	
K041	1 (0.454)
Wastewater treatment sludge from the production of toxaphene.	
K042	10 (4.54)
Heavy ends or distillation residues from the distillation of tetrachlorobenzene in the production of 2,4,5-T.	
K043	10 (4.54)
2,6-Dichlorophenol waste from the production of 2,4-D.	
K044	10 (4.54)
Wastewater treatment sludges from the manufacturing and processing of explosives.	
K045	10 (4.54)
Spent carbon from the treatment of wastewater containing explosives.	
K046	10 (4.54)
Wastewater treatment sludges from the manufacturing, formulation and loading of lead-based initiating compounds.	
K047	10 (4.54)
Pink/red water from TNT operations.	
K048	10 (4.54)
Dissolved air flotation (DAF) float from the petroleum refining industry.	
K049	10 (4.54)
Slop oil emulsion solids from the petroleum refining industry.	
K050	10 (4.54)
Heat exchanger bundle cleaning sludge from the petroleum refining industry.	
K051	10 (4.54)
API separator sludge from the petroleum refining industry.	
K052	10 (4.54)
Tank bottoms (leaded) from the petroleum refining industry.	
K060	1 (0.454)
Ammonia still lime sludge from coking operations.	
K061	10 (4.54)
Emission control dust/sludge from the primary production of steel in electric furnaces.	

Hazardous Substances	RQ: lbs (kg)
K062	10 (4.54)
Spent pickle liquor generated by steel finishing operations of facilities within the iron and steel industry.	
K064	10 (4.54)
Acid plant blowdown slurry/sludge resulting from thickening of blowdown slurry from primary copper production.	
K065	10 (4.54)
Surface impoundment solids contained in and dredged from surface impoundments at primary lead smelting facilities.	
K066	10 (4.54)
Sludge from treatment of process wastewater and/or acid plant blowdown from primary zinc production.	
K069	10 (4.54)
Emission control dust/sludge from secondary lead smelting.	
K071	1 (0.454)
Brine purification muds from the mercury cell process in chlorine production, where separately prepurified brine is not used.	
K073	10 (4.54)
Chlorinated hydrocarbon waste from the purification step of the diaphragm cell process using graphite anodes in chlorine production.	
K083	100 (45.4)
Distillation bottoms from aniline extraction.	
K084	1 (0.454)
Wastewater treatment sludges generated during the production of veterinary pharmaceuticals from arsenic or organo-arsenic compounds.	
K085	10 (4.54)
Distillation or fractionation column bottoms from the production of chlorobenzenes.	
K086	10 (4.54)
Solvent washes and sludges, caustic washes and sludges, or water washes and sludges from cleaning tubs and equipment used in the formulation of ink from pigments, driers, soaps, and stabilizers containing chromium and lead.	
K087	100 (45.4)
Decanter tank tar sludge from coking operations.	
K088	10 (4.54)
Spent potliners from primary aluminum reduction.	
K090	10 (4.54)
Emission control dust or sludge from ferrochromiumsilicon production.	

Hazardous Substances	RQ: lbs (kg)
K091	10 (4.54)
Emission control dust or sludge from ferrochromium pro duction.	
K093	5000 (2270)
Distillation light ends from the production of phthalic anhydride from ortho-xylene.	
K094	5000 (2270)
Distillation bottoms from the production of phthalic anhydride from ortho-xylene.	
K095	100 (45.4)
Distillation bottoms from the production of 1,1,1-trichlo roethane.	
K096	100 (45.4)
Heavy ends from the heavy ends column from the production of 1,1,1-trichloroethane.	
K097	1 (0.454)
Vacuum stripper discharge from the chlordane chlorinator in the production of chlordane.	
K098	1 (0.454)
Untreated process wastewater from the production of toxaphene.	
K099	10 (4.54)
Untreated wastewater from the production of 2,4-D.	
K100	10 (4.54)
Waste leaching solution from acid leaching of emission control dust/sludge from secondary lead smelting.	
K101	1 (0.454)
Distillation tar residues from the distillation of aniline-based compounds in the production of veterinary phamaceuticals from arsenic or organo-arsenic compounds.	
K102	1 (0.454)
Residue from the use of activated carbon for decolorization in the production of veterinary pharmaceuticals from arsenic or organo-arsenic compounds.	
K103	100 (45.4)
Process residues from aniline extraction from the production of aniline.	
K104	10 (4.54)
Combined wastewater streams generated from nitrobenzene/aniline chlorobenzenes.	
K105	10 (4.54)
Separated aqueous stream from the reactor product washing step in the production of chlorobenzenes.	

Hazardous Substances	RQ: lbs (kg)
K106	1 (0.454)
Wastewater treatment sludge from the mercury cell process in chlorine production.	
K107	10 (4.54)
Column bottoms from product seperation from the production of 1,1-dimethylhydrazine (UDMH) from carboxylic acid hydrazines.	
K108	10 (4.54)
Condensed column overheads from product seperation and condensed reactor vent gases from the production of 1,1-dimethylhydrazine (UDMH) from carboxylic acid hydrazides.	
K109	10 (4.54)
Spent filter cartridges from product purification from the production of 1,1-dimethylhydrazine (UDMH), from carboxylic acid hydrazides.	
K110	10 (4.54)
Condensed column overheads from intermediate separation from the production of 1,1-dimethylhydrazines (UDMH) from carboxylic acid hydrazides.	
K111	10 (4.54)
Product washwaters from the production of dinitrotoluene via nitration of toluene.	
K112	10 (4.54)
Reaction by-product water from the drying column in the production of toluenediamine via hydrogenation of dinitrotoluene.	
K113	10 (4.54)
Condensed liquid light ends from the purification of toluenediamine in the production of toluenediamine via hydrogenation of dinitrotoluene.	
K114	10 (4.54)
Vicinals from the purification of toluenediamine in the production of toluenediamine via hydrogenation of dinitrotoluene.	
K115	10 (4.54)
Heavy ends from the purification of toluenediamine in the production of toluenediamine via hydrogenation of dinitrotoluene.	
K116	10 (4.54)
Organic condensate from the solvent recovery column in the production of toluene diisocyanate via phosgenation of toluenediamine.	
K117	1 (0.454)
Wastewater from the reaction vent gas scrubber in the production of ethylene bromide via bromination of ethene.	
K118	1 (0.454)
Spent absorbent solids from purification of ethylene dibromide in the production of ethylene dibromide.	

Hazardous Substances	RQ: lbs (kg)
K123	10 (4.54)
Process wastewater (including supernates, filtrates, and washwaters) from the production of ethylenebisdithiocar bamic acid and its salts.	
K124	10 (4.54)
Reactor vent scrubber water from the production of ethyleneb-isdithiocarbamic acid and it salts.	
K125	10 (4.54)
Filtration, evaporation, and centrifugation solids from the production of ethylenebisdithiocarbamic acid and its salts.	
K126	10 (4.54)
Baghouse dust and floor sweepings in milling and pack aging operations from the production or formulation of ethylenebis-dithiocarbamic acid and its salts.	
K131	100 (45.4)
Waste water from the reactor and spent sulfuric acid from the acid dryer in the production of methyl bromide.	
K132	1000 (454)
Spent absorbent and wastewater solids from the production of methyl bromide.	
K136	1 (0.454)
Still bottoms from the purification of ethylene dibromide in the production of ethylene dibromide via bromination of ethene.	
K141	1 (0.454)
K142	1 (0.454)
K143	1 (0.454)
K144	1 (0.454)
K145	1 (0.454)
K147	1 (0.454)
K148	1 (0.454)
K149	10 (4.54)
K150	10 (4.54)
K151	10 (4.54)
K156	1 (0.454)
K157	1 (0.454)
K158	1 (0.454)
K169	10 (4.54)
K170	1 (0.454)
K171	1 (0.454)
K172	1 (0.454)
K174	1 (0.454)
K175	1 (0.454)
K176	1 (0.454)
K177	5000 (2270)
K178	1 (0.454)

Footnotes:

¢ the RQ for these hazardous substances is limited to those pieces of the metal having a diameter smaller than 100 micrometers (0.004 inches)

¢¢ the RQ for asbestos is limited to friable forms only

@ indicates that the name was added by RSPA because (1) the name is a synonym for a specific hazardous substance and (2) the name appears in the Hazardous Materials Table as a proper shipping name.

Radionuclide	Atomic Number	RQ: Ci (TBq)
Actinium-224	89	100 (3.7)
Actinium-225	89	1 (.037)
Actinium-226	89	10 (.37)
Actinium-227	89	0.001 (.000037)
Actinium-228	89	10 (.37)
Aluminum-26	13	10 (.37)
Americium-237	95	1000 (37)
Americium-238	95	100 (3.7)
Americium-239	95	100 (3.7)
Americium-240	95	10 (.37)
Americium-241	95	0.01 (.00037)
Americium-242	95	100 (3.7)
Americium-242m	95	0.01 (.00037)
Americium-243	95	0.01 (.00037)
Americium-244	95	10 (.37)
Americium-244m	95	1000 (37)
Americium-245	95	1000 (37)
Americium-246	95	1000 (37)
Americium-246m	95	1000 (37)
Antimony-115	51	1000 (37)
Antimony-116	51	1000 (37)
Antimony-116m	51	100 (3.7)
Antimony-117	51	1000 (37)
Antimony-118m	51	10 (.37)
Antimony-119	51	1000 (37)
Antimony-120 (16 min)	51	1000 (37)
Antimony-120 (5.76 day	51	10 (.37)
Antimony-122	51	10 (.37)
Antimony-124	51	10 (.37)
Antimony-124m	51	1000 (37)
Antimony-125	51	10 (.37)
Antimony-126	51	10 (.37)
Antimony-126m	51	1000 (37)
Antimony-127	51	10 (.37)
Antimony-128 (10.4 min)	51	1000 (37)
Antimony-128 (9.01 hr)	51	10 (.37)
Antimony-129	51	100 (3.7)
Antimony-130	51	100 (3.7)
Antimony-131	51	1000 (37)
Argon-39	18	1000 (37)
Argon-41	18	10 (.37)
Arsenic-69	33	1000 (37)
Arsenic-70	33	100 (3.7)
Arsenic-71	33	100 (3.7)

Radionuclide	Atomic Number	RQ: Ci (TBq)
Arsenic-72	33	10 (.37)
Arsenic-73	33	100 (3.7)
Arsenic-74	33	10 (.37)
Arsenic-76	33	100 (3.7)
Arsenic-77	33	1000 (37)
Arsenic-78	33	100 (3.7)
Astatine-207	85	100 (3.7)
Astatine-211	85	100 (3.7)
Barium-126	56	1000 (37)
Barium-128	56	10 (.37)
Barium-131	56	10 (.37)
Barium-131m	56	1000 (37)
Barium-133	56	10 (.37)
Barium-133m	56	100 (3.7)
Barium-135m	56	1000 (37)
Barium-139	56	1000 (37)
Barium-140	56	10 (.37)
Barium-141	56	1000 (37)
Barium-142	56	1000 (37)
Berkelium-245	97	100 (3.7)
Berkelium-246	97	10 (.37)
Berkelium-247	97	0.01 (.00037)
Berkelium-249	97	1 (.037)
Berkelium-250	97	100 (3.7)
Beryllium-7	4	100 (3.7)
Beryllium-10	4	1 (.037)
Bismuth-200	83	100 (3.7)
Bismuth-201	83	100 (3.7)
Bismuth-202	83	1000 (37)
Bismuth-203	83	10 (.37)
Bismuth-205	83	10 (.37)
Bismuth-206	83	10 (.37)
Bismuth-207	83	10 (.37)
Bismuth-210	83	10 (.37)
Bismuth-210m	83	0.1 (.0037)
Bismuth-212	83	100 (3.7)
Bismuth-213	83	100 (3.7)
Bismuth-214	83	100 (3.7)
Bromine-74	35	100 (3.7)
Bromine-74m	35	100 (3.7)
Bromine-75	35	100 (3.7)
Bromine-76	35	10 (.37)
Bromine-77	35	100 (3.7)
Bromine-80m	35	1000 (37)

Radionuclide	Atomic Number	RQ: Ci (TBq)
Bromine-80	35	1000 (37)
Bromine-82	35	10 (.37)
Bromine-83	35	1000 (37)
Bromine-84	35	100 (3.7)
Cadmium-104	48	1000 (37)
Cadmium-107	48	1000 (37)
Cadmium-109	48	1 (.037)
Cadmium-113	48	0.1 (.0037)
Cadmium-113m	48	0.1 (.0037)
Cadmium-115	48	100 (3.7)
Cadmium-115m	48	10 (.37)
Cadmium-117	48	100 (3.7)
Cadmium-117m	48	10 (.37)
Calcium-41	20	10 (.37)
Calcium-45	20	10 (.37)
Calcium-47	20	10 (.37)
Californium-244	98	1000 (37)
Californium-246	98	10 (.37)
Californium-248	98	0.1 (.0037)
Californium-249	98	0.01 (.00037)
Californium-250	98	0.01 (.00037)
Californium-251	98	0.01 (.00037)
Californium-252	98	0.1 (.0037)
Californium-253	98	10 (.37)
Californium-254	98	0.1 (.0037)
Carbon-11	6	1000 (37)
Carbon-14	6	10 (.37)
Cerium-134	58	10 (.37)
Cerium-135	58	10 (.37)
Cerium-137	58	1000 (37)
Cerium-137m	58	100 (3.7)
Cerium-139	58	100 (3.7)
Cerium-141	58	10 (.37)
Cerium-143	58	100 (3.7)
Cerium-144	58	1 (.037)
Cesium-125	55	1000 (37)
Cesium-127	55	100 (3.7)
Cesium-129	55	100 (3.7)
Cesium-130	55	1000 (37)
Cesium-131	55	1000 (37)
Cesium-132	55	10 (.37)
Cesium-134	55	1 (.037)
Cesium-134m	55	1000 (37)
Cesium-135	55	10 (.37)

Radionuclide	Atomic Number	RQ: Ci (TBq)
Cesium-135m	55	100 (3.7)
Cesium-136	55	10 (.37)
Cesium-137	55	1 (.037)
Cesium-138	55	100 (3.7)
Chlorine-36	17	10 (.37)
Chlorine-38	17	100 (3.7)
Chlorine-39	17	100 (3.7)
Chromium-48	24	100 (3.7)
Chromium-49	24	1000 (37)
Chromium-49	24	1000 (37)
Chromium-51	24	1000 (37)
Cobalt-55	27	10 (.37)
Cobalt-56	27	10 (.37)
Cobalt-57	27	100 (3.7)
Cobalt-58	27	10 (.37)
Cobalt-58m	27	1000 (37)
Cobalt-60	27	10 (.37)
Cobalt-60m	27	1000 (37)
Cobalt-61	27	1000 (37)
Cobalt-62m	27	1000 (37)
Copper-60	29	100 (3.7)
Copper-61	29	100 (3.7)
Copper-64	29	1000 (37)
Copper-67	29	100 (3.7)
Curium-238	96	1000 (37)
Curium-240	96	1 (.037)
Curium-241	96	10 (.37)
Curium-242	96	1 (.037)
Curium-243	96	0.01 (.00037)
Curium-244	96	0.01 (.00037)
Curium-245	96	0.01 (.00037)
Curium-246	96	0.01 (.00037)
Curium-247	96	0.01 (.00037)
Curium-248	96	0.001 (.000037)
Curium-249	96	1000 (37)
Dysprosium-155	66	100 (3.7)
Dysprosium-157	66	100 (3.7)
Dysprosium-159	66	100 (3.7)
Dysprosium-165	66	1000 (37)
Dysprosium-166	66	10 (.37)
Einsteinium-250	99	10 (.37)
Einsteinium-251	99	1000 (37)
Einsteinium-253	99	10 (.37)
Einsteinium-254	99	0.1 (.0037)

Radionuclide	Atomic Number	RQ: Ci (TBq)
Einsteinium-254m	99	1 (.037)
Erbium-161	68	100 (3.7)
Erbium-165	68	1000 (37)
Erbium-169	68	100 (3.7)
Erbium-171	68	100 (3.7)
Erbium-172	68	10 (.37)
Europium-145	63	10 (.37)
Europium-146	63	10 (.37)
Europium-147	63	10 (.37)
Europium-148	63	10 (.37)
Europium-149	63	100 (3.7)
Europium-150 (12.6 hr)	63	1000 (37)
Europium-150 (34.2 yr)	63	10 (.37)
Europium-152	63	10 (.37)
Europium-152m	63	100 (3.7)
Europium-154	63	10 (.37)
Europium-155	63	10 (.37)
Europium-156	63	10 (.37)
Europium-157	63	10 (.37)
Europium-158	63	1000 (37)
Fermium-252	100	10 (.37)
Fermium-253	100	10 (.37)
Fermium-254	100	100 (3.7)
Fermium-255	100	100 (3.7)
Fermium-257	100	1 (.037)
Fluorine-18	9	1000 (37)
Francium-222	87	100 (3.7)
Francium-223	87	100 (3.7)
Gadolinium-145	64	100 (3.7)
Gadolinium-146	64	10 (.37)
Gadolinium-147	64	10 (.37)
Gadolinium-148	64	0.001 (.000037)
Gadolinium-149	64	100 (3.7)
Gadolinium-151	64	100 (3.7)
Gadolinium-152	64	0.001 (.000037)
Gadolinium-153	64	10 (.37)
Gadolinium-159	64	1000 (37)
Gallium-65	31	1000 (37)
Gallium-66	31	10 (.37)
Gallium-67	31	100 (3.7)
Gallium-68	31	1000 (37)
Gallium-70	31	1000 (37)
Gallium-72	31	10 (.37)
Gallium-73	31	100 (3.7)

Radionuclide	Atomic Number	RQ: Ci (TBq)
Germanium-66	32	100 (3.7)
Germanium-67	32	1000 (37)
Germanium-68	32	10 (.37)
Germanium-69	32	10 (.37)
Germanium-71	32	1000 (37)
Germanium-75	32	1000 (37)
Germanium-77	32	10 (.37)
Germanium-78	32	1000 (37)
Gold-193	79	100 (3.7)
Gold-194	79	10 (.37)
Gold-195	79	100 (3.7)
Gold-198	79	100 (3.7)
Gold-198m	79	10 (.37)
Gold-199	79	100 (3.7)
Gold-200	79	1000 (37)
Gold-200m	79	10 (.37)
Gold-201	79	1000 (37)
Hafnium-170	72	100 (3.7)
Hafnium-172	72	1 (.037)
Hafnium-173	72	100 (3.7)
Hafnium-175	72	100 (3.7)
Hafnium-177m	72	1000 (37)
Hafnium-178m	72	0.1 (.0037)
Hafnium-179m	72	100 (3.7)
Hafnium-180m	72	100 (3.7)
Hafnium-181	72	10 (.37)
Hafnium-182	72	0.1 (.0037)
Hafnium-182m	72	100 (3.7)
Hafnium-183	72	100 (3.7)
Hafnium-184	72	100 (3.7)
Holmium-155	67	1000 (37)
Holmium-157	67	1000 (37)
Holmium-159	67	1000 (37)
Holmium-161	67	1000 (37)
Holmium-162	67	1000 (37)
Holmium-162m	67	1000 (37)
Holmium-164	67	1000 (37)
Holmium-164m	67	1000 (37)
Holmium-166	67	100 (3.7)
Holmium-166m	67	1 (.037)
Holmium-167	67	100 (3.7)
Hydrogen-3	1	100 (3.7)
Indium-109	49	100 (3.7)
Indium-110 (69.1 min)	49	100 (3.7)

Radionuclide	Atomic Number	RQ: Ci (TBq)
Indium-110 (4.9 hr)	49	10 (.37)
Indium-111	49	100 (3.7)
Indium-112	49	1000 (37)
Indium-113m	49	1000 (37)
Indium-114m	49	10 (.37)
Indium-115	49	0.1 (.0037)
Indium-115m	49	100 (3.7)
Indium-116m	49	100 (3.7)
Indium-117	49	1000 (37)
Indium-117m	49	100 (3.7)
Indium-119m	49	1000 (37)
Iodine-120	53	10 (.37)
Iodine-120m	53	100 (3.7)
Iodine-121	53	100 (3.7)
Iodine-123	53	10 (.37)
Iodine-124	53	0.1 (.0037)
Iodine-125	53	0.01 (.00037)
Iodine-126	53	0.01 (.00037)
Iodine-128	53	1000 (37)
Iodine-129	53	0.001 (.000037)
Iodine-130	53	1 (.037)
Iodine-131	53	0.01 (.00037)
Iodine-132	53	10 (.37)
Iodine-132m	53	10 (.37)
Iodine-133	53	0.1 (.0037)
Iodine-134	53	100 (3.7)
Iodine-135	53	10 (.37)
Iridium-182	77	1000 (37)
Iridium-184	77	100 (3.7)
Iridium-185	77	100 (3.7)
Iridium-186	77	10 (.37)
Iridium-187	77	100 (3.7)
Iridium-188	77	10 (.37)
Iridium-189	77	100 (3.7)
Iridium-190	77	10 (.37)
Iridium-190m	77	1000 (37)
Iridium-192	77	10 (.37)
Iridium-192m	77	100 (3.7)
Iridium-194	77	100 (3.7)
Iridium-194m	77	10 (.37)
Iridium-195	77	1000 (37)
Iridium-195m	77	100 (3.7)
Iron-52	26	100 (3.7)
Iron-55	26	100 (3.7)

Radionuclide	Atomic Number	RQ: Ci (TBq)
Iron-59	26	10 (.37)
Iron-60	26	0.1 (.0037)
Krypton-74	36	10 (.37)
Krypton-76	36	10 (.37)
Krypton-77	36	10 (.37)
Krypton-79	36	100 (3.7)
Krypton-81	36	1000 (37)
Krypton-83m	36	1000 (37)
Krypton-85	36	1000 (37)
Krypton-85m	36	100 (3.7)
Krypton-87	36	10 (.37)
Krypton-88	36	10 (.37)
Lanthanum-131	57	1000 (37)
Lanthanum-132	57	100 (3.7)
Lanthanum-135	57	1000 (37)
Lanthanum-137	57	10 (.37)
Lanthanum-138	57	1 (.037)
Lanthanum-140	57	10 (.37)
Lanthanum-141	57	1000 (37)
Lanthanum-142	57	100 (3.7)
Lanthanum-143	57	1000 (37)
Lead-195m	82	1000 (37)
Lead-198	82	100 (3.7)
Lead-199	82	100 (3.7)
Lead-200	82	100 (3.7)
Lead-201	82	100 (3.7)
Lead-202	82	1 (.037)
Lead-202m	82	10 (.37)
Lead-203	82	100 (3.7)
Lead-205	82	100 (3.7)
Lead-209	82	1000 (37)
Lead-210	82	0.01 (.00037)
Lead-211	82	100 (3.7)
Lead-212	82	10 (.37)
Lead-214	82	100 (3.7)
Lutetium-169	71	10 (.37)
Lutetium-170	71	10 (.37)
Lutetium-171	71	10 (.37)
Lutetium-172	71	10 (.37)
Lutetium-173	71	100 (3.7)
Lutetium-174	71	10 (.37)
Lutetium-174m	71	10 (.37)
Lutetium-176	71	1 (.037)
Lutetium-176m	71	1000 (37)

Radionuclide	Atomic Number	RQ: Ci (TBq)
Lutetium-177	71	100 (3.7)
Lutetium-177m	71	10 (.37)
Lutetium-178	71	1000 (37)
Lutetium-178m	71	1000 (37)
Lutetium-179	71	1000 (37)
Magnesium-28	12	10 (.37)
Manganese-51	25	1000 (37)
Manganese-52	25	10 (.37)
Manganese-52m	25	1000 (37)
Manganese-53	25	1000 (37)
Manganese-54	25	10 (.37)
Manganese-56	25	100 (3.7)
Mendelevium-257	101	100 (3.7)
Mendelevium-258	101	1 (.037)
Mercury-193	80	100 (3.7)
Mercury-193m	80	10 (.37)
Mercury-194	80	0.1 (.0037)
Mercury-195	80	100 (3.7)
Mercury-195m	80	100 (3.7)
Mercury-197	80	1000 (37)
Mercury-197m	80	1000 (37)
Mercury-199m	80	1000 (37)
Mercury-203	80	10 (.37)
Molybdenum-90	42	100 (3.7)
Molybdenum-93	42	100 (3.7)
Molybdenum-93m	42	10 (.37)
Molybdenum-99	42	100 (3.7)
Molybdenum-101	42	1000 (37)
Neodymium-136	60	1000 (37)
Neodymium-138	60	1000 (37)
Neodymium-139	60	1000 (37)
Neodymium-139m	60	100 (3.7)
Neodymium-141	60	1000 (37)
Neodymium-147	60	10 (.37)
Neodymium-149	60	100 (3.7)
Neodymium-151	60	1000 (37)
Neptunium-232	93	1000 (37)
Neptunium-233	93	1000 (37)
Neptunium-234	93	10 (.37)
Neptunium-235	93	1000 (37)
Neptunium-236 (1.2 E 5 yr)	93	0.1 (.0037)
Neptunium-236 (22.5 hr)	93	100 (3.7)
Neptunium-237	93	0.01 (.00037)
Neptunium-238	93	10 (.37)

Radionuclide	Atomic Number	RQ: Ci (TBq)
Neptunium-239	93	100 (3.7)
Neptunium-240	93	100 (3.7)
Nickel-56	28	10 (.37)
Nickel-57	28	10 (.37)
Nickel-59	28	100 (3.7)
Nickel-63	28	100 (3.7)
Nickel-65	28	100 (3.7)
Nickel-66	28	10 (.37)
Niobium-88	41	100 (3.7)
Niobium-89 (66 min)	41	100 (3.7)
Niobium-89 (122 min)	41	100 (3.7)
Niobium-90	41	10 (.37)
Niobium-93m	41	100 (3.7)
Niobium-94	41	10 (.37)
Niobium-95	41	10 (.37)
Niobium-95m	41	100 (3.7)
Niobium-96	41	10 (.37)
Niobium-97	41	100 (3.7)
Niobium-98	41	1000 (37)
Osmium-180	76	1000 (37)
Osmium-181	76	100 (3.7)
Osmium-182	76	100 (3.7)
Osmium-185	76	10 (.37)
Osmium-189m	76	1000 (37)
Osmium-191	76	100 (3.7)
Osmium-191m	76	1000 (37)
Osmium-193	76	100 (3.7)
Osmium-194	76	1 (.037)
Palladium-100	46	100 (3.7)
Palladium-101	46	100 (3.7)
Palladium-103	46	100 (3.7)
Palladium-107	46	100 (3.7)
Palladium-109	46	1000 (37)
Phosphorus-32	15	0.1 (.0037)
Phosphorus-33	15	1 (.037)
Platinum-186	78	100 (3.7)
Platinum-188	78	100 (3.7)
Platinum-189	78	100 (3.7)
Platinum-191	78	100 (3.7)
Platinum-193	78	1000 (37)
Platinum-193m	78	100 (3.7)
Platinum-195m	78	100 (3.7)
Platinum-197	78	1000 (37)
Platinum-197m	78	1000 (37)

Radionuclide	Atomic Number	RQ: Ci (TBq)
Platinum-199	78	1000 (37)
Platinum-200	78	100 (3.7)
Plutonium-234	94	1000 (37)
Plutonium-235	94	1000 (37)
Plutonium-236	94	0.1 (.0037)
Plutonium-237	94	1000 (37)
Plutonium-238	94	0.01 (.00037)
Plutonium-239	94	0.01 (.00037)
Plutonium-240	94	0.01 (.00037)
Plutonium-241	94	1 (.037)
Plutonium-242	94	0.01 (.00037)
Plutonium-243	94	1000 (37)
Plutonium-244	94	0.01 (.00037)
Plutonium-245	94	100 (3.7)
Polonium-203	84	100 (3.7)
Polonium-205	84	100 (3.7)
Polonium-207	84	10 (.37)
Polonium-210	84	0.01 (.00037)
Potassium-40	19	1 (.037)
Potassium-42	19	100 (3.7)
Potassium-43	19	10 (.37)
Potassium-44	19	100 (3.7)
Potassium-45	19	1000 (37)
Praseodymium-136	59	1000 (37)
Praseodymium-137	59	1000 (37)
Praseodymium-138m	59	100 (3.7)
Praseodymium-139	59	1000 (37)
Praseodymium-142	59	100 (3.7)
Praseodymium-142m	59	1000 (37)
Praseodymium-143	59	10 (.37)
Praseodymium-144	59	1000 (37)
Praseodymium-145	59	1000 (37)
Praseodymium-147	59	1000 (37)
Promethium-141	61	1000 (37)
Promethium-143	61	100 (3.7)
Promethium-144	61	10 (.37)
Promethium-145	61	100 (3.7)
Promethium-146	61	10 (.37)
Promethium-147	61	10 (.37)
Promethium-148	61	10 (.37)
Promethium-148m	61	10 (.37)
Promethium-149	61	100 (3.7)
Promethium-150	61	100 (3.7)
Promethium-151	61	100 (3.7)

Radionuclide	Atomic Number	RQ: Ci (TBq)
Protactinium-227	91	100 (3.7)
Protactinium-228	91	10 (.37)
Protactinium-230	91	10 (.37)
Protactinium-231	91	0.01 (.00037)
Protactinium-232	91	10 (.37)
Protactinium-233	91	100 (3.7)
Protactinium-234	91	10 (.37)
RADIONUCLIDES§†		1 (.037)
Radium-223	88	1 (.037)
Radium-224	88	10 (.37)
Radium-225	88	1 (.037)
Radium-226**	88	0.1 (.0037)
Radium-227	88	1000 (37)
Radium-228	88	0.1 (.0037)
Radon-220	86	0.1 (.0037)
Radon-222	86	0.1 (.0037)
Rhenium-177	75	1000 (37)
Rhenium-178	75	1000 (37)
Rhenium-181	75	100 (3.7)
Rhenium-182 (12.7 hr)	75	10 (.37)
Rhenium-182 (64.0 hr)	75	10 (.37)
Rhenium-184	75	10 (.37)
Rhenium-184m	75	10 (.37)
Rhenium-186	75	100 (3.7)
Rhenium-186m	75	10 (.37)
Rhenium-187	75	1000 (37)
Rhenium-188	75	1000 (37)
Rhenium-188m	75	1000 (37)
Rhenium-189	75	1000 (37)
Rhodium-99	45	10 (.37)
Rhodium-99m	45	100 (3.7)
Rhodium-100	45	10 (.37)
Rhodium-101	45	10 (.37)
Rhodium-101m	45	100 (3.7)
Rhodium-102	45	10 (.37)
Rhodium-102m	45	10 (.37)
Rhodium-103m	45	1000 (37)
Rhodium-105	45	100 (3.7)
Rhodium-106m	45	10 (.37)
Rhodium-107	45	1000 (37)
Rubidium-79	37	1000 (37)
Rubidium-81	37	100 (3.7)
Rubidium-81m	37	1000 (37)
Rubidium-82m	37	10 (.37)

Radionuclide	Atomic Number	RQ: Ci (TBq)
Rubidium-83	37	10 (.37)
Rubidium-84	37	10 (.37)
Rubidium-86	37	10 (.37)
Rubidium-88	37	1000 (37)
Rubidium-89	37	1000 (37)
Rubidium-87	37	10 (.37)
Ruthenium-94	44	1000 (37)
Ruthenium-97	44	100 (3.7)
Ruthenium-103	44	10 (.37)
Ruthenium-105	44	100 (3.7)
Ruthenium-106	44	1 (.037)
Samarium-141	62	1000 (37)
Samarium-141m	62	1000 (37)
Samarium-142	62	1000 (37)
Samarium-145	62	100 (3.7)
Samarium-146	62	0.01 (.00037)
Samarium-147	62	0.01 (.00037)
Samarium-151	62	10 (.37)
Samarium-153	62	100 (3.7)
Samarium-155	62	1000 (37)
Samarium-156	62	100 (3.7)
Scandium-43	21	1000 (37)
Scandium-44	21	100 (3.7)
Scandium-44m	21	10 (.37)
Scandium-46	21	10 (.37)
Scandium-47	21	100 (3.7)
Scandium-48	21	10 (.37)
Scandium-49	21	1000 (37)
Selenium-70	34	1000 (37)
Selenium-73	34	10 (.37)
Selenium-73m	34	100 (3.7)
Selenium-75	34	10 (.37)
Selenium-79	34	10 (.37)
Selenium-81	34	1000 (37)
Selenium-81m	34	1000 (37)
Selenium-83	34	1000 (37)
Silicon-31	14	1000 (37)
Silicon-32	14	1 (.037)
Silver-102	47	100 (3.7)
Silver-103	47	1000 (37)
Silver-104	47	1000 (37)
Silver-104m	47	1000 (37)
Silver-105	47	10 (.37)
Silver-106	47	1000 (37)

Radionuclide	Atomic Number	RQ: Ci (TBq)
Silver-106m	47	10 (.37)
Silver-108m	47	10 (.37)
Silver-110m	47	10 (.37)
Silver-111	47	10 (.37)
Silver-112	47	100 (3.7)
Silver-115	47	1000 (37)
Sodium-22	11	10 (.37)
Sodium-24	11	10 (.37)
Strontium-80	38	100 (3.7)
Strontium-81	38	1000 (37)
Strontium-83	38	100 (3.7)
Strontium-85	38	10 (.37)
Strontium-85m	38	1000 (37)
Strontium-87m	38	100 (3.7)
Strontium-89	38	10 (.37)
Strontium-90	38	0.1 (.0037)
Strontium-91	38	10 (.37)
Strontium-92	38	100 (3.7)
Sulfur-35	16	1 (.037)
Tantalum-172	73	100 (3.7)
Tantalum-173	73	100 (3.7)
Tantalum-174	73	100 (3.7)
Tantalum-175	73	100 (3.7)
Tantalum-176	73	10 (.37)
Tantalum-177	73	1000 (37)
Tantalum-178	73	1000 (37)
Tantalum-179	73	1000 (37)
Tantalum-180	73	100 (3.7)
Tantalum-180m	73	1000 (37)
Tantalum-182	73	10 (.37)
Tantalum-182m	73	1000 (37)
Tantalum-183	73	100 (3.7)
Tantalum-184	73	10 (.37)
Tantalum-185	73	1000 (37)
Tantalum-186	73	1000 (37)
Technetium-93	43	100 (3.7)
Technetium-93m	43	1000 (37)
Technetium-94	43	10 (.37)
Technetium-94m	43	100 (3.7)
Technetium-96	43	10 (.37)
Technetium-96m	43	1000 (37)
Technetium-97	43	100 (3.7)
Technetium-97m	43	100 (3.7)
Technetium-98	43	10 (.37)

Radionuclide	Atomic Number	RQ: Ci (TBq)
Technetium-99	43	10 (.37)
Technetium-99m	43	100 (3.7)
Technetium-101	43	1000 (37)
Technetium-104	43	1000 (37)
Tellurium-116	52	1000 (37)
Tellurium-121	52	10 (.37)
Tellurium-121m	52	10 (.37)
Tellurium-123	52	10 (.37)
Tellurium-123m	52	10 (.37)
Tellurium-125m	52	10 (.37)
Tellurium-127	52	1000 (37)
Tellurium-127m	52	10 (.37)
Tellurium-129	52	1000 (37)
Tellurium-129m	52	10 (.37)
Tellurium-131	52	1000 (37)
Tellurium-131m	52	10 (.37)
Tellurium-132	52	10 (.37)
Tellurium-133	52	1000 (37)
Tellurium-133m	52	1000 (37)
Tellurium-134	52	1000 (37)
Terbium-147	65	100 (3.7)
Terbium-149	65	100 (3.7)
Terbium-150	65	100 (3.7)
Terbium-151	65	10 (.37)
Terbium-153	65	100 (3.7)
Terbium-154	65	10 (.37)
Terbium-155	65	100 (3.7)
Terbium-156m (5.0 hr)	65	1000 (37)
Terbium-156m (24.4 hr)	65	1000 (37)
Terbium-156	65	10 (.37)
Terbium-157	65	100 (3.7)
Terbium-158	65	10 (.37)
Terbium-160	65	10 (.37)
Terbium-161	65	100 (3.7)
Thallium-194	81	1000 (37)
Thallium-194m	81	100 (3.7)
Thallium-195	81	100 (3.7)
Thallium-197	81	100 (3.7)
Thallium-198	81	10 (.37)
Thallium-198m	81	100 (3.7)
Thallium-199	81	100 (3.7)
Thallium-200	81	10 (.37)
Thallium-201	81	1000 (37)
Thallium-202	81	10 (.37)

Radionuclide	Atomic Number	RQ: Ci (TBq)
Thallium-204	81	10 (.37)
Thorium (Irradiated)	90	***
Thorium (Natural)	90	**
Thorium-226	90	100 (3.7)
Thorium-227	90	1 (.037)
Thorium-228	90	0.01 (.00037)
Thorium-229	90	0.001 (.000037)
Thorium-230	90	0.01 (.00037)
Thorium-231	90	100 (3.7)
Thorium-232**	90	0.001 (.000037)
Thorium-234	90	100 (3.7)
Thulium-162	69	1000 (37)
Thulium-166	69	10 (.37)
Thulium-167	69	100 (3.7)
Thulium-170	69	10 (.37)
Thulium-171	69	100 (3.7)
Thulium-172	69	100 (3.7)
Thulium-173	69	100 (3.7)
Thulium-175	69	1000 (37)
Tin-110	50	100 (3.7)
Tin-111	50	1000 (37)
Tin-113	50	10 (.37)
Tin-117m	50	100 (3.7)
Tin-119m	50	10 (.37)
Tin-121	50	1000 (37)
Tin-121m	50	10 (.37)
Tin-123	50	10 (.37)
Tin-123m	50	1000 (37)
Tin-125	50	10 (.37)
Tin-126	50	1 (.037)
Tin-127	50	100 (3.7)
Tin-128	50	1000 (37)
Titanium-44	22	1 (.037)
Titanium-45	22	1000 (37)
Tungsten-176	74	1000 (37)
Tungsten-177	74	100 (3.7)
Tungsten-178	74	100 (3.7)
Tungsten-179	74	1000 (37)
Tungsten-181	74	100 (3.7)
Tungsten-185	74	10 (.37)
Tungsten-187	74	100 (3.7)
Tungsten-188	74	10 (.37)
Uranium (Depleted)	92	***
Uranium (Irradiated)	92	***

Radionuclide	Atomic Number	RQ: Ci (TBq)
Uranium (Natural)	92	**
Uranium Enriched 20% or greater	92	***
Uranium Enriched less than 20%	92	***
Uranium-230	92	1 (.037)
Uranium-231	92	1000 (37)
Uranium-232	92	0.01 (.00037)
Uranium-233	92	0.1 (.0037)
Uranium-234**	92	0.1 (.0037)
Uranium-235**	92	0.1 (.0037)
Uranium-236	92	0.1 (.0037)
Uranium-237	92	100 (3.7)
Uranium-238**	92	0.1 (.0037)
Uranium-239	92	1000 (37)
Uranium-240	92	1000 (37)
Vanadium-47	23	1000 (37)
Vanadium-48	23	10 (.37)
Vanadium-49	23	1000 (37)
Xenon-120	54	100 (3.7)
Xenon-121	54	10 (.37)
Xenon-122	54	100 (3.7)
Xenon-123	54	10 (.37)
Xenon-125	54	100 (3.7)
Xenon-127	54	100 (3.7)
Xenon-129m	54	1000 (37)
Xenon-131m	54	1000 (37)
Xenon-133	54	1000 (37)
Xenon-133m	54	1000 (37)
Xenon-135	54	100 (3.7)
Xenon-135m	54	10 (.37)
Xenon-138	54	10 (.37)
Ytterbium-162	70	1000 (37)
Ytterbium-166	70	10 (.37)
Ytterbium-167	70	1000 (37)
Ytterbium-169	70	10 (.37)
Ytterbium-175	70	100 (3.7)
Ytterbium-177	70	1000 (37)
Ytterbium-178	70	1000 (37)
Yttrium-86	39	10 (.37)
Yttrium-86m	39	1000 (37)
Yttrium-87	39	10 (.37)
Yttrium-88	39	10 (.37)
Yttrium-90	39	10 (.37)
Yttrium-90m	39	100 (3.7)
Yttrium-91	39	10 (.37)

Radionuclide	Atomic Number	RQ: Ci (TBq)
Yttrium-91m	39	1000 (37)
Yttrium-92	39	100 (3.7)
Yttrium-93	39	100 (3.7)
Yttrium-94	39	1000 (37)
Yttrium-95	39	1000 (37)
Zinc-62	30	100 (3.7)
Zinc-63	30	1000 (37)
Zinc-65	30	10 (.37)
Zinc-69	30	1000 (37)
Zinc-69m	30	100 (3.7)
Zinc-71m	30	100 (3.7)
Zinc-72	30	100 (3.7)
Zirconium-86	40	100 (3.7)
Zirconium-88	40	10 (.37)
Zirconium-89	40	100 (3.7)
Zirconium-93	40	1 (.037)
Zirconium-95	40	10 (.37)
Zirconium-97	40	10 (.37)

§ The RQs for all radionuclides apply to chemical compounds containing the radionuclides and elemental forms regardless of the diameter of pieces of solid material.

† The RQ of one curie applies to all radionuclides not otherwise listed. Whenever the RQs in TABLE 1—HAZARDOUS SUBSTANCES OTHER THAN RADIONUCLIDES and this table conflict, the lowest RQ shall apply. For example, uranyl acetate and uranyl nitrate have RQs shown in TABLE 1 of 100 pounds, equivalent to about one-tenth the RQ level for uranium-238 in this table.

** The method to determine the RQs for mixtures or solutions of radionuclides can be found in paragraph 7 of the note preceding TABLE 1 of this appendix. RQs for the following four common radionuclide mixtures are provided: radium-226 in secular equilibrium with its daughters (0.053 curie); natural uranium (0.1 curie); natural uranium in secular equilibrium with its daughters (0.052 curie); and natural thorium in secular equilibrium with its daughters (0.011 curie).

*** Indicates that the name was added by RSPA because it appears in the list of radionuclides in 49 CFR 173.435. The reportable quantity (RQ), if not specifically listed elsewhere in this appendix, shall be determined in accordance with the procedures in paragraph 7 of this appendix.

Appendix B to §172.101 – List of Marine Pollutants

1. See §171.4 of this subchapter for applicability to marine pollutants. This appendix lists potential marine pollutants as defined in §171.8 of this subchapter.

2. Marine pollutants listed in this appendix are not necessarily listed by name in the §172.101 Table. If a marine pollutant not listed by name or by synonym in the §172.101 Table meets the definition of any hazard Class 1 through 8, then you must determine the class and division of the material in accordance with §173.2a of this subchapter. You must also select the most appropriate hazardous material description and proper shipping name. If a marine pollutant not listed by name or by synonym in the §172.101 Table does not meet the definition of any Class 1 through 8, then you must offer it for transportation under the most appropriate of the following two Class 9 entries: "Environmentally hazardous substances, liquid, n.o.s." UN 3028, or "Environmentally hazardous substances, solid, n.o.s." UN3077.

3. This appendix contains two columns. The first column, entitled "S.M.P." (for severe marine pollutants), identifies whether a material is a severe marine pollutant. If the letters "PP" appear in this column for a material, the material is a severe marine pollutant, otherwise it is not. The second column, entitled "Marine Pollutant", lists the marine pollutants.

4. If a material is not listed in this appendix and meets the criteria for a marine pollutant as provided in Chapter 2.10 of the IMDG Code, Guidelines for the Identification of Harmful Substances in Packaged Form, (incorporated by reference; see §171.7 of this subchapter), the material may be transported as a marine pollutant in accordance with the applicable requirements of this subchapter.

5. If a material listed in this appendix does not meet the criteria for a marine pollutant as provided in Chapter 2.10 of the IMDG Code, Guidelines for the Identification of Harmful Substances in Packaged Form, (incorporated by reference; see §171.7 of this

subchapter), it may be excepted from the requirements of this subchapter as a marine pollutant if that exception is approved by the Associate Administrator.

LIST OF MARINE POLLUTANTS

S.M.P.	Marine Pollutant
....	Acetone cyanohydrin, stabilized
....	Acetylene tetrabromide
....	Acetylene tetrachloride
....	Acraldehyde, inhibited
....	Acrolein, inhibited
....	Acrolein stabilized
....	Acrylic aldehyde, inhibited
....	Alcohol C-12 - C-16 poly(1-6) ethoxylate
....	Alcohol C-13 - C-16 poly (1-6) ethoxylate
....	Alcohol C-6 C-17 (secondary)poly(3-6) ethoxylate
....	Aldicarb
PP........	Aldrin
....	Alkybenzenesulphonates, branched and straight chain *(excluding C11-C13 straight chain or branched chain homologues)*
....	Alkyl (C12-C14) dimethylamine
....	Alkyl (C7-C9) nitrates
....	Allyl bromide
....	ortho-Aminoanisole
....	Aminocarb
....	Ammonium dinitro-o-cresolate
....	n-Amylbenzene
PP........	Azinphos-ethyl
PP........	Azinphos-methyl
....	Barium cyanide
....	Bendiocarb
....	Benomyl
....	Benquinox
....	Benzyl chlorocarbonate
....	Benzyl chloroformate
PP........	Binapacryl

S.M.P.	Marine Pollutant
....	*N,N-Bis* (2-hydroxyethyl) oleamide (LOA)
PP.........	Brodifacoum
....	Bromine cyanide
....	Bromoacetone
....	Bromoallylene
....	Bromobenzene
....	ortho-Bromobenzyl cyanide
....	Bromocyane
....	Bromoform
PP.........	Bromophos-ethyl
....	3-Bromopropene
....	Bromoxynil
....	Butanedione
....	2-Butenal, stabilized
....	Butyl benzyl phthalate
....	*N-tert*-butyl-*N*-cyclopropyl-6-methylthio-1,3,5-triazine-2,4-diamine
....	para-tertiary-butyltoluene
PP.........	Cadmium compounds
....	Cadmium sulphide
....	Calcium arsenate
....	Calcium arsenate and calcium arsenite, mixtures, solid
....	Calcium cyanide
PP.........	Camphechlor
....	Carbaryl
....	Carbendazim
....	Carbofuran
....	Carbon tetrabromide
....	Carbon tetrachloride
PP.........	Carbophenothion
....	Cartap hydrochloride
PP.........	Chlordane
....	Chlorfenvinphos
PP.........	Chlorinated paraffins (C-10 – C-13)
PP.........	Chlorinated paraffins (C14 – C17), with more than 1% shorter chain length

S.M.P.	Marine Pollutant
....	Chlorine
....	Chlorine cyanide, inhibited
....	Chlomephos
....	Chloroacetone, stabilized
....	1-Chloro-2,3-Epoxypropane
....	2-Chloro-6-nitrotoluene
....	4-Chloro-2-nitrotoluene
....	Chloro-ortho-nitrotoluene
....	2-Chloro-5-trifluoromethylnitrobenzene
....	para-Chlorobenzyl chloride, liquid or solid
....	Chlorodinitrobenzenes, liquid or solid
....	1-Chloroheptane
....	1-Chlorohexane
....	Chloronitroanilines
....	Chloronitrotoluenes, *liquid*
....	Chloronitrotoluenes, *solid*
....	1-Chlorooctane
PP........	Chlorophenolates, liquid
PP........	Chlorophenolates, solid
....	Chlorophenyltrichlorosilane
....	Chloropicrin
....	Chlorotoluenes (metȧ-; para-)
PP........	Chlorpyriphos
PP........	Chlorthiophos
....	Cocculus
....	Coconitrile
....	Copper acetoarsenite
....	Copper arsenite
....	Copper chloride
PP........	Copper chloride (solution)
PP........	Copper cyanide
PP........	Copper metal powder
PP........	Copper sulphate, anhydrous, hydrates
....	Coumachlor
PP........	Coumaphos

S.M.P.	Marine Pollutant
PP	Cresyl diphenyl phosphate
	Crotonaldehyde, stabilized
	Crotonic aldehyde, stabilized
	Crotoxyphos
	Cupric arsenite
PP	Cupric chloride
PP	Cupric cyanide
PP	Cupric sulfate
	Cupriethylenediamine solution
PP	Cuprous chloride
	Cyanide mixtures
	Cyanide solutions
	Cyanides, inorganic, n.o.s.
	Cyanogen bromide
	Cyanogen chloride, inhibited
	Cyanogen chloride, stabilized
	Cyanophos
PP	1,5,9-Cyclododecatriene
PP	Cyhexatin
PP	Cymenes (o-;m-;p-)
PP	Cypermethrin
PP	DDT
	Decycloxytetrahydrothiophene dioxide
	Decyl acrylate
	DEF
	Desmedipham
	Di-allate
	Di-n-Butyl phthalate
	1,4-Di-tert-butylbenzene
PP	Dialifos
	4,4´-Diaminodiphenylmethane
PP	Diazinon
	1,3-Dibromobenzene
PP	Dichlofenthion
	Dichloroanilines

S.M.P.	Marine Pollutant
....	1,3-Dichlorobenzene
....	1,4-Dichlorobenzene
....	Dichlorobenzene (meta-; para-)
....	2,2-Dichlorodiethyl ether
....	Dichlorodimethyl ether, symmetrical
....	Di-(2-chloroethyl) ether
....	1,1-Dichloroethylene, inhibited
....	1,6-Dichlorohexane
....	Dichlorophenyltrichlorosilane
PP........	Dichlorvos
PP........	Dichlofop-methyl
....	Dicrotophos
PP........	Dieldrin
....	Diisopropylbenzenes
....	Diisopropylnaphthalenes, mixed isomers
PP........	Dimethoate
PP........	N,N-Dimethyldodecylamine
....	Dimethylhydrazine, symmetrical
....	Dimethylhydrazine, unsymmetrical
....	Dinitro-o-cresol, *solid*
....	Dinitro-o-cresol, *solution*
....	Dinitrochlorobenzenes, liquid or solid
....	Dinitrophenol, *dry or wetted with less than 15 percent water, by mass*
....	Dinitrophenol solutions
....	Dinitrophenol, wetted *with not less than 15 percent water, by mass*
....	Dinitrophenolates *alkali metals, dry or wetted with less than 15 per cent water, by mass*
....	Dinitrophenolates, wetted *with not less than 15 percent water, by mass*
....	Dinobuton
....	Dinoseb
....	Dinoseb acetate
....	Dioxacarb
....	Dioxathion

S.M.P.	Marine Pollutant
....	Dipentene
....	Diphacinone
....	Diphenyl
PP.........	Diphenylamine chloroarsine
PP.........	Diphenylchloroarsine, solid *or* liquid
....	2,4-Di-tert-butylphenol
PP.........	2,6-Di-tert-Butylphenol
....	Disulfoton
....	DNOC
....	DNOC (pesticide)
....	Dodecyl diphenyl oxide disulphonate
PP.........	Dodecyl hydroxypropyl sulfide
....	1-Dodecylamine
PP.........	Dodecylphenol
....	Drazoxolon
....	Edifenphos
PP.........	Endosulfan
PP.........	Endrin
....	Epibromohydrin
....	Epichlorohydrin
PP.........	EPN
PP.........	Esfenvalerate
PP.........	Ethion
....	Ethoprophos
....	Ethyl fluid
....	Ethyl mercaptan
....	5-Ethyl-2-picoline
....	Ethyl propenoate, inhibited
....	2-Ethyl-3-propylacrolein
....	Ethyl tetraphosphate
....	Ethyldichloroarsine
....	2-Ethylhexaldehyde
....	Ethylene dibromide and methyl bromide mixtures, liquid
....	2-Ethylhexyl nitrate
....	Fenamiphos

S.M.P.	Marine Pollutant
PP........	Fenbutatin oxide
PP........	Fenchlorazole-ethyl
PP........	Fenitrothion
PP........	Fenoxapro-ethyl
PP........	Fenoxaprop-P-ethyl
PP........	Fenpropathrin
....	Fensulfothion
PP........	Fenthion
PP........	Fentin acetate
PP........	Fentin hydroxide
....	Ferric arsenate
....	Ferric arsenite
....	Ferrous arsenate
PP........	Fonofos
....	Formetanate
PP........	Furathiocarb (ISO)
PP........	gamma-BHC
....	Gasoline, leaded
PP........	Heptachlor
....	n-Heptaldehyde
....	Heptenophos
....	normal-Heptyl chloride
....	n-Heptylbenzene
PP........	Hexachlorobutadiene
PP........	1,3-Hexachlorobutadiene
....	Hexaethyl tetraphosphate, *liquid*
....	Hexaethyl tetraphosphate, *solid*
....	normal-Hexyl chloride
....	n-Hexylbenzene
....	Hydrocyanic acid, anhydrous, stabilized containing less than 3% water
....	Hydrocyanic acid, anhydrous, stabilized, containing less than 3% water and absorbed in a porous inert material
....	Hydrocyanic acid, aqueous solutions *not more than 20% hydrocyanic acid*

S.M.P.	Marine Pollutant
....	Hydrogen cyanide solution in alcohol, *with not more than* 45% hydrogen cyanide
....	Hydrogen cyanide, stabilized *with less than 3% water*
....	Hydrogen cyanide, stabilized *with less than 3% water and absorbed in a porous inert material*
....	Hydroxydimethylbenzenes, liquid or solid
....	Ioxynil
....	Isobenzan
....	Isobutyl butyrate
....	Isobutylbenzene
....	Isodecyl acrylate
....	Isodecyl diphenyl phosphate
....	Isofenphos
....	Isooctyl nitrate
....	Isoprocarb
....	Isopropenylbenzene
....	Isotetramethylbenzene
PP.........	Isoxathion
....	Lead acetate
....	Lead arsenates
....	Lead arsenites
....	Lead compounds, soluble, n.o.s.
....	Lead cyanide
....	Lead nitrate
....	Lead perchlorate, solid or solution
....	Lead tetraethyl
....	Lead tetramethyl
PP.........	Lindane
....	Linuron
....	London Purple
....	Magnesium arsenate
....	Malathion
....	Mancozeb (ISO)
....	Maneb
....	Maneb preparation, stabilized against self-heating
....	Maneb preparations *with not less than 60% maneb*

S.M.P.	Marine Pollutant
....	Maneb stabilized *or* Maneb preparations, stabilized *against self-heating*
....	Manganese ethylene-1,2-bisdithiocarbamate
....	Manganeseethylene-1,2-bisdithiocarbamate, stabilized against self-heating
....	Mecarbam
....	Mephosfolan
....	Mercaptodimethur
PP........	Mercuric acetate
PP........	Mercuric ammonium chloride
PP........	Mercuric arsenate
PP........	Mercuric benzoate
PP........	Mercuric bisulphate
PP........	Mercuric bromide
PP........	Mercuric chloride
PP........	Mercuric cyanide
PP........	Mercuric gluconate
....	Mercuric iodide
PP........	Mercuric nitrate
PP........	Mercuric oleate
PP........	Mercuric oxide
PP........	Mercuric oxycyanide, desensitized
PP........	Mercuric potassium cyanide
PP........	Mercuric Sulphate
PP........	Mercuric thiocyanate
PP........	Mercurol
PP........	Mercurous acetate
PP........	Mercurous bisulphate
PP........	Mercurous bromide
PP........	Mercurous chloride
PP........	Mercurous nitrate
PP........	Mercurous salicylate
PP........	Mercurous sulphate
PP........	Mercury acetates
PP........	Mercury ammonium chloride
PP........	Mercury based pesticide, liquid, flammable, toxic

S.M.P.	Marine Pollutant
PP.........	Mercury based pesticide, liquid, toxic, flammable
PP.........	Mercury based pesticide, liquid, toxic
PP.........	Mercury based pesticide, solid, toxic
PP.........	Mercury benzoate
PP.........	Mercury bichloride
PP.........	Mercury bisulphates
PP.........	Mercury bromides
PP.........	Mercury compounds, liquid, n.o.s.
PP.........	Mercury compounds, solid, n.o.s.
PP.........	Mercury cyanide
PP.........	Mercury gluconate
PP.........	NMercury (I) (mercurous) compounds (pesticides)
PP.........	NMercury (II) (mercuric) compounds (pesticides)
....	Mercury iodide
PP.........	Mercury nucleate
PP.........	Mercury oleate
PP.........	Mercury oxide
PP.........	Mercury oxycyanide, desensitized
PP.........	Mercury potassium cyanide
PP.........	Mercury potassium iodide
PP.........	Mercury salicylate
PP.........	Mercury sulfates
PP.........	Mercury thiocyanate
....	Metam-sodium
....	Methamidophos
....	Methanethiol
....	Methidathion
....	Methomyl
....	ortho-Methoxyaniline
....	Methyl bromide and ethylene dibromide mixtures, liquid
....	1-Methyl-2-ethylbenzene
....	Methyl mercaptan
....	3-Methylacrolein, stabilized
....	Methylchlorobenzenes
....	Methylnitrophenols

S.M.P.	Marine Pollutant
....	alpha-Methylstyrene
....	Methyltrithion
....	Methylvinylbenzenes, inhibited
PP........	Mevinphos
....	Mexacarbate
....	Mirex
....	Monocratophos
....	Motor fuel anti-knock mixtures
....	Motor fuel anti-knock mixtures or compunds
....	Nabam
....	Naled
PP........	Nickel carbonyl
PP........	Nickel cyanide
PP........	Nickel tetracarbonyl
....	3-Nitro-4-chlorobenzotrifluoride
....	Nitrobenzene
....	Nitrobenzotrifluorides, liquid or solid
....	Nitroxylenes, liquid or solid
....	Nonylphenol
....	*normal*-Octaldehyde
....	Oleylamine
PP........	Organotin compounds, liquid, n.o.s.
PP........	Organotin compounds, (pesticides)
PP........	Organotin compounds, solid, n.o.s.
PP........	Organotin pesticides, liquid, flammable, toxic, n.o.s. *flash point less than 23 deg.C*
PP........	Organotin pesticides, liquid, toxic, flam-mable, n.o.s.
PP........	Organotin pesticides, liquid, toxic, n.o.s.
PP........	Organotin pesticides, solid, toxic, n.o.s.
....	Orthoarsenic acid
PP........	Osmium tetroxide
....	Oxamyl
....	Oxydisulfoton
....	Paraoxon
PP........	Parathion

S.M.P.	Marine Pollutant
PP.	Parathion-methyl
PP.	PCBs
. . . .	Pentachloroethane
PP.	Pentachlorophenol
. . . .	Pentalin
. . . .	n-Pentylbenzene
. . . .	Perchloroethylene
. . . .	Perchloromethylmercaptan
. . . .	Petrol, leaded
PP.	Phenarsazine chloride
. . . .	d-Phenothrin
PP.	Phenthoate
. . . .	1-Phenylbutane
. . . .	2-Phenylbutane
. . . .	Phenylcyclohexane
PP.	Phenylmercuric acetate
PP.	Phenylmercuric compounds, n.o.s.
PP.	Phenylmercuric hydroxide
PP.	Phenylmercuric nitrate
. . . .	2-Phenylpropene
PP.	Phorate
PP.	Phosaione
. . . .	Phosmet
PP.	Phosphamidon
PP.	Phosphorus, white, molten
PP.	Phosphorus, white *or* yellow dry *or* under water *or* in solution
PP.	Phosphorus white, or yellow, molten
PP.	Phosphorus, yellow, molten
. . . .	Pindone (and salts of)
. . . .	Pirimicarb
PP.	Pirimiphos-ethyl
PP.	Polychlorinated biphenyls
PP.	Polyhalogenated biphenyls, liquid *or* Ter-phenyls liquid
PP.	Polyhalogenated biphenyls, solid *or* Ter-phenyls solid

S.M.P.	Marine Pollutant
PP	Potassium cuprocyanide
	Potassium cyanide, solid
	Potassium cyanide, solution
PP	Potassium cyanocuprate (I)
PP	Potassium cyanomercurate
PP	Potassium mercuric iodide
	Promecarb
	Propachlor
	Propaphos
	Propenal, inhibited
	Propoxur
	Prothoate
	Prussic acid, anhydrous, stabilized
	Prussic acid, anhydrous, stabilized, absorbed in a porous inert material
PP	Pyrazophos
	Quinalphos
PP	Quizalofop
PP	Quizalofop-p-ethyl
	Rotenone
	Salithion
PP	Silafluofen
	Silver arsenite
	Silver cyanide
	Silver orthoarsenite
PP	Sodium copper cyanide, solid
PP	Sodium copper cyanide solution
PP	Sodium cuprocyanide, solid
PP	Sodium cuprocyanide, solution
	Sodium cyanide, solid
	Sodium cyanide, solution
	Sodium dinitro-o-cresolate, *dry or wetted* with less than 15 percent water, by mass
	Sodium dinitro-ortho-cresolate, wetted *with not less than 15 percent water, by mass*
PP	Sodium pentachlorophenate

S.M.P.	Marine Pollutant
....	Strychnine *or* Strychnine salts
....	Sulfotep
PP.........	Sulprophos
....	Tallow nitrile
....	Temephos
....	TEPP
PP.........	Terbufos
....	Tetrabromoethane
....	Tetrabromomethane
....	1,1,2,2-Tetrachloroethane
....	Tetrachloroethylene
....	Tetrachloromethane
....	Tetraethyl dithiopyrophosphate
PP.........	Tetraethyl lead, liquid
....	Tetramethrin
....	Tetramethyllead
....	Thallium chlorate
....	Thallium compounds, n.o.s.
....	Thallium compounds (pesticides)
....	Thallium nitrate
....	Thallium sulfate
....	Thallous chlorate
....	Thiocarbonyl tetrachloride
....	Triaryl phosphates, isopropylated
PP.........	Triaryl phosphates, n.o.s.
....	Triazophos
....	Tribromomethane
PP.........	Tributyltin compounds
....	Trichlorfon
PP.........	1,2,3-Trichlorobenzene
....	Trichlorobenzenes, liquid
....	Trichlorobutene
....	Trichlorobutylene
....	Trichloromethane sulphuryl chloride
....	Trichloromethyl sulphochloride

S.M.P.	Marine Pollutant
....	Trichloronat
....	Tricresyl phosphate (less than 1% ortho-isomer)
PP........	Tricresyl phosphate, not less than 1% ortho-isomer but not more than 3% orthoisomer
PP........	Tricresyl phosphate *with more than 3 per cent ortho isomer*
....	Triethylbenzene
....	Triisopropylated phenyl phosphates
....	Trimethylene dichloride
....	Triphenyl phosphate/tert-butylated triphenyl phosphates mixtures containing 5% to 10% triphenyl phosphates
PP........	Triphenyl phosphate/tert-butylated triphenyl phosphates mixtures containing 10% to 48% triphenyl phosphates
PP........	Triphenylphosphate
PP........	Triphenyltin compounds
....	Tritolyl phosphate (less than 1% ortho-isomer)
PP........	Tritolyl phosphate (not less than 1% ortho-isomer)
....	Trixylenyl phosphate
....	Vinylidene chloride, inhibited
....	Vinylidene chloride, stabilized
....	Warfarin (and salts of)
PP........	White phosphorus, dry
PP........	White phosphorus, wet
....	White spirit, low (15-20%) aromatic
PP........	Yellow phosphorus, dry
PP........	Yellow phosphorus, wet
....	Zinc bromide
....	Zinc cyanide

Special Provisions

§172.102 Special provisions.

(a) *General.* When Column 7 of the §172.101 Table refers to a special provision for a hazardous material, the meaning and requirements of that provision are as set forth in this section. When a special provision specifies packaging or packaging requirements—

(1) The special provision is in addition to the standard requirements for all packagings prescribed in §173.24 of this subchapter and any other applicable packaging requirements in subparts A and B of part 173 of this subchapter; and

(2) To the extent a special provision imposes limitations or additional requirements on the packaging provisions set forth in Column 8 of the §172.101 Table, packagings must conform to the requirements of the special provision.

(b) *Description of codes for special provisions.* Special provisions contain packaging provisions, prohibitions, exceptions from requirements for particular quantities or forms of materials and requirements or prohibitions applicable to specific modes of transportation, as follows:

(1) A code consisting only of numbers (for example, "11") is multi-modal in application and may apply to bulk and non-bulk packagings.

(2) A code containing the letter "A" refers to a special provision which applies only to transportation by aircraft.

(3) A code containing the letter "B" refers to a special provision that applies only to bulk packaging requirements. Unless otherwise provided in this subchapter, these special provisions do not apply to UN, IM Specification portable tanks or IBCs.

(4) A code containing the letters "IB" or "IP" refers to a special provision that applies only to transportation in IBCs.

(5) A code containing the letter "N" refers to a special provision which applies only to non-bulk packaging requirements.

(6) A code containing the letter "R" refers to a special provision which applies only to transportation by rail.

(7) A code containing the letter "T" refers to a special provision which applies only to transportation in UN or IM Specification portable tanks.

(8) A code containing the letters "TP" refers to a portable tank special provision for UN or IM Specification portable tanks that is in addition to those provided by the portable tank instructions or the requirements in part 178 of this subchapter.

(9) A code containing the letter "W" refers to a special provision that applies only to transportation by water.

(c) *Tables of special provisions.* The following tables list, and set forth the requirements of, the special provisions referred to in Column 7 of the §172.101 Table.

(1) *Numeric provisions.* These provisions are multi-modal and apply to bulk and non-bulk packagings:

Code/Special Provisions

1 This material is poisonous by inhalation (see §171.8 of this subchapter) in Hazard Zone A (see §173.116(a) or §173.133(a) of this subchapter), and must be described as an inhalation hazard under the provisions of this subchapter.

2 This material is poisonous by inhalation (see §171.8 of this subchapter) in Hazard Zone B (see §173.116(a) or §173.133(a) of this subchapter), and must be described as an inhalation hazard under the provisions of this subchapter.

3 This material is poisonous by inhalation (see §171.8 of this subchapter) in Hazard Zone C (see §173.116(a) of this subchapter), and must be described as an inhalation hazard under the provisions of this subchapter.

4 This material is poisonous by inhalation (see §171.8 of this subchapter) in Hazard Zone D (see §173.116(a) of this subchapter), and must be described as an inhalation hazard under the provisions of this subchapter.

5 If this material meets the definition for a material poisonous by inhalation (see §171.8 of this subchapter), a shipping name must be selected which identifies the inhalation hazard, in Division 2.3 or Division 6.1, as appropriate.

6 This material is poisonous-by-inhalation and must be described as an inhalation hazard under the provisions of this subchapter.

8 A hazardous substance that is not a hazardous waste may be shipped under the shipping description "Other regulated substances, liquid *or* solid, n.o.s.", as appropriate. In addition, for solid materials, special provision B54 applies.

9 Packaging for certain PCBs for disposal and storage is prescribed by EPA in 40 CFR 761.60 and 761.65.

11 The hazardous material must be packaged as either a liquid or a solid, as appropriate, depending on its physical form at 55°C (131°F) at atmospheric pressure.

12 In concentrations greater than 40 percent, this material has strong oxidizing properties and is capable of starting fires in contact with combustible materials. If appropriate, a package containing this material must conform to the additional labeling requirements of §172.402 of this subchapter.

13 The words "Inhalation Hazard" shall be entered on each shipping paper in association with the shipping description, shall be marked on each non-bulk package in association with the proper shipping name and identification number, and shall be marked on two opposing sides of each bulk package. Size of marking on bulk package must conform to §172.302(b) of this subchapter. The requirements of §§172.203(m) and 172.505 of this subchapter do not apply.

14 Motor fuel antiknock mixtures are:

a. Mixtures of one or more organic lead mixtures (such as tetraethyl lead, triethylmethyl lead, diethyldimethyl lead, ethyltrimethyl lead, and tetramethyl lead) with one or more halogen compounds (such as ethylene dibromide and ethylene dichloride), hydrocarbon solvents or other equally efficient stabilizers; or

b. tetraethyl lead.

15 This entry applies to "Chemical kits" and "First aid kits" containing one or more compatible items of hazardous materials in boxes, cases, etc. that are used for medical, analytical, diagnostic or testing purposes. For transportation by aircraft, materials forbidden for transportation by passenger aircraft or cargo aircraft may not be included in the kits. Chemical kits and first aid kits are excepted from the specification packaging requirements of this subchapter when packaged in combination packagings. Chemical kits and first aid kits are also excepted from the labeling and placarding requirements of this subchapter, except when offered for transportation or transported by air. Chemical and first aid kits may be transported in accordance with the consumer commodity and ORM exceptions in §173.156, provided they meet all required conditions. Kits that are carried on board transport vehicles for first aid or operating purposes are not subject to the requirements of this subchapter.

16 This description applies to smokeless powder and other solid propellants that are used as powder for small arms and have been classed as Division 1.3 and 4.1 in accordance with §173.56 of this subchapter.

18 This description is authorized only for fire extinguishers listed in §173.309(b) of this subchapter meeting the following conditions:

a. Each fire extinguisher may only have extinguishing contents that are nonflammable, non-poisonous, non-corrosive and commercially free from corroding components.

b. Each fire extinguisher must be charged with a nonflammable, non-poisonous, dry gas that has a dew-point at or below minus 46.7°C (minus 52°F) at 101kPa (1 atmosphere) and is free of corroding components, to not more than the service pressure of the cylinder.

c. A fire extinguisher may not contain more than 30% carbon dioxide by volume or any other corrosive extinguishing agent.

d. Each fire extinguisher must be protected externally by suitable corrosion-resisting coating.

19 For domestic transportation only, the identification number "UN1075" may be used in place of the identification number specified in Column (4) of the §172.101 Table. The identification number used must be consistent on package markings, shipping papers and emergency response information.

21 This material must be stabilized by appropriate means (e.g., addition of chemical inhibitor, purging to remove oxygen) to prevent dangerous polymerization (see §173.21(f) of this subchapter).

22 If the hazardous material is in dispersion in organic liquid, the organic liquid must have a flash point above 50°C (122°F).

23 This material may be transported under the provisions of Division 4.1 only if it is so packed that the percentage of diluent will not fall below that stated in the shipping description at any time during transport. Quantities of not more than 500 g per package with not less than 10 percent water by mass may also be classed in Division 4.1, provided a negative test result is obtained when tested in accordance with test series 6(c) of the UN Manual of Tests and Criteria (IBR, see §171.7 of this subchapter).

24 Alcoholic beverages containing more than 70 percent alcohol by volume must be transported as materials in Packing Group II. Alcoholic beverages containing more than 24 percent but not more than 70 percent alcohol by volume must be transported as materials in Packing Group III.

26 This entry does not include ammonium permanganate, the transport of which is prohibited except when approved by the Associate Administrator.

28 The dihydrated sodium salt of dichloroisocyanuric acid is not subject to the requirements of this subchapter.

29 Lithium cells and batteries and equipment containing or packed with lithium cells and batteries which do not comply with the provisions of §173.185 of this subchapter may be transported only if they are approved by the Associate Administrator.

30 Sulfur is not subject to the requirements of this subchapter if transported in a non-bulk packaging or if formed to a specific shape (for example, prills, granules, pellets, pastilles, or flakes). A bulk packaging containing sulfur is not subject to the placarding requirements of subpart F of this part, if it is marked with the appropriate identification number as required by subpart D of this part. Molten sulfur must be marked as required by §172.325 of this subchapter.

31 Materials which have undergone sufficient heat treatment to render them non-hazardous are not subject to the requirements of this subchapter.

32 Polymeric beads and molding compounds may be made from polystyrene, poly(methyl methacrylate) or other polymeric material.

33 Ammonium nitrates and mixtures of an inorganic nitrite with an ammonium salt are prohibited.

34 The commercial grade of calcium nitrate fertilizer, when consisting mainly of a double salt (calcium nitrate and ammonium nitrate) containing not more than 10 percent ammonium nitrate and at least 12 percent water of crystallization, is not subject to the requirements of this subchapter.

35 Antimony sulphides and oxides which do not contain more than 0.5 percent of arsenic calculated on the total mass do not meet the definition of Division 6.1.

36 The maximum net quantity per package is 5 L (1 gallon) or 5 kg (11 pounds).

37 Unless it can be demonstrated by testing that the sensitivity of the substance in its frozen state is no greater than in its liquid state, the substance must remain liquid during normal transport conditions. It must not freeze at temperatures above -15°C (5°F).

38 If this material shows a violent effect in laboratory tests involving heating under confinement, the labeling requirements of Special Provision 53 apply, and the material must be packaged in accordance with packing method OP6 in §173.225 of this subchapter. If the SADT of the technically pure substance is higher than 75°C, the technically pure substance and formulations derived from it are not self-reactive materials and, if not meeting any other hazard class, are not subject to the requirements of this subchapter.

39 This substance may be carried under provisions other than those of Class 1 only if it is so packed that the percentage of water will not fall below that stated at any time during transport. When phlegmatized with water and inorganic inert material, the content of urea nitrate must not exceed 75 percent by mass and the mixture should not be capable of being detonated by test 1(a)(i) or test 1(a) (ii) in the UN Manual of Tests and Criteria (IBR, see §171.7 of this subchapter).

40 Polyester resin kits consist of two components: a base material (Class 3, Packing Group II or III) and an activator (organic peroxide), each separately packed in an inner packaging. The organic peroxide must be type D, E, or F, not requiring temperature control, and be limited to a quantity of 125 mL (4.22 ounces) per inner packaging if liquid, and 500 g (1 pound) if solid. The components may be placed in the same outer packaging provided they will not interact dangerously in the event of leakage. Packing group will be II or III, according to the criteria for Class 3, applied to the base material.

43 The membrane filters, including paper separators and coating or backing materials, that are present in transport, must not be able to propagate a detonation as tested by one of the tests de scribed in the UN Manual of Tests and Criteria, Part I, Test series 1(a) (IBR, see §171.7 of this subchapter). On the basis of the results of suitable burning rate tests, and taking into account the standard tests in the UN Manual of Tests and Criteria, Part III, subsection 33.2.1 (IBR, see §171.7 of this subchapter), nitrocellulose membrane filters in the form in which they are to be transported that do not meet the criteria for a Division 4.1 material are not subject to the requirements of this subchapter. Packagings must be so constructed that explosion is not possible by reason of increased internal pressure. Nitrocellulose membrane filters covered by this entry, each with a mass not exceeding 0.5 g, are not subject to the requirements of this subchapter when contained individually in an article or a sealed packet.

44 The formulation must be prepared so that it remains homogeneous and does not separate during transport. Formulations with low nitrocellulose contents and neither showing dangerous properties when tested for their ability to detonate, deflagrate or explode when heated under defined confinement by the appropriate test methods and criteria in the UN Manual of Tests and Criteria (IBR, see §171.7 of this subchapter), nor classed as a Division 4.1 (flammable solid) when tested in accordance with the procedures specified in §173.124 of this subchapter (chips, if necessary, crushed and sieved to a particle size of less than 1.25 mm), are not subject to the requirements of this subchapter.

45 Temperature should be maintained between 18 °C (64.4 °F) and 40 °C (104 °F). Tanks containing solidified methacrylic acid must not be reheated during transport.

46 This material must be packed in accordance with packing method OP6 (see §173.225 of this subchapter). During transport, it must be protected from direct sunshine and stored (or kept) in a cool and well-ventilated place, away from all sources of heat.

47 Mixtures of solids that are not subject to this subchapter and flammable liquids may be transported under this entry without first applying the classification criteria of Division 4.1, provided there is no free liquid visible at the time the material is loaded or at the time the packaging or transport unit is closed. Except when the liquids are fully absorbed in solid material contained in sealed bags, each packaging must correspond to a design type that has passed a leakproofness test at the Packing Group II level. Small inner packagings consisting of sealed packets containing less than 10 mL of a Class 3 liquid in Packing Group II or III absorbed onto a solid material are not subject to this subchapter provided there is no free liquid in the packet.

48 Mixtures of solids which are not subject to this subchapter and toxic liquids may be transported under this entry without first applying the classification criteria of Division 6.1, provided there is no free liquid visible at the time the material is loaded or at the time the packaging or transport unit is closed. Each packaging must correspond to a design type that has passed a leakproofness test at the Packing Group II level. This entry may not be used for solids containing a Packing Group I liquid.

49 Mixtures of solids which are not subject to this subchapter and corrosive liquids may be transported under this entry without first applying the classification criteria of Class 8, provided there is no free liquid visible at the time the material is loaded or at the time the packaging or transport unit is closed. Each packaging must correspond to a design type that has passed a leakproofness test at the Packing Group II level.

50 Cases, cartridge, empty with primer which are made of metallic or plastic casings and meeting the classification criteria of Division 1.4 are not regulated for domestic transportation.

51 This description applies to items previously described as "Toy propellant devices, Class C" and includes reloadable kits. Model rocket motors containing 30 grams or less propellant are classed as Division 1.4S and items containing more than 30 grams of propellant but not more than 62.5 grams of propellant are classed as Division 1.4C.

52 This entry may only be used for substances that do not exhibit explosive properties of Class 1 (explosive) when tested in accordance with Test Series 1 and 2 of Class 1 (explosive) in the UN Manual of Tests and Criteria, Part I (incorporated by reference; see §171.7 of this subchapter).

53 Packages of these materials must bear the subsidiary risk label, "EXPLOSIVE", and the subsidiary hazard class/division must be entered in parentheses immediately following the primary hazard class in the shipping description, unless otherwise provided in this subchapter or through an approval issued by the Associate Administrator, or the competent authority of the country of origin. A copy of the approval shall accompany the shipping papers.

54 Maneb or maneb preparations not meeting the definition of Division 4.3 or any other hazard class are not subject to the requirements of this subchapter when transported by motor vehicle, rail car, or aircraft.

55 This device must be approved in accordance with §173.56 of this subchapter by the Associate Administrator.

56 A means to interrupt and prevent detonation of the detonator from initiating the detonating cord must be installed between each electric detonator and the detonating cord ends of the jet perforating guns before the charged jet perforating guns are offered for transportation.

57 Maneb or Maneb preparations stabilized against self-heating need not be classified in Division 4.2 when it can be demonstrated by testing that a volume of 1 m3 of substance does not self-ignite and that the temperature at the center of the sample does not exceed 200°C, when the sample is maintained at a temperature of not less than 75°C ± 2°C for a period of 24 hours, in accordance with procedures set forth for testing self-heating materials in the UN Manual of Tests and Criteria (IBR, see §171.7 of this subchapter).

58 Aqueous solutions of Division 5.1 inorganic solid nitrate substances are considered as not meeting the criteria of Division 5.1 if the concentration of the substances in solution at the minimum temperature encountered in transport is not greater than 80% of the saturation limit.

59 Ferrocerium, stabilized against corrosion, with a minimum iron content of 10 percent is not subject to the requirements of this subchapter.

60 After September 30, 1997, an oxygen generator, chemical, that is shipped with its means of initiation attached must incorporate at least two positive means of preventing unintentional actuation of the generator, and be classed and approved by the Associate Administrator. The procedures for approval of a chemical oxygen generator that contains an explosive means of initiation (e.g., a primer or electric match) are specified in §173.56 of this subchapter. Each person who offers a chemical oxygen generator for transportation after September 30, 1997, shall: (1) ensure that it is offered in conformance with the conditions of the approval; (2) maintain a copy of the approval at each facility where the chemical oxygen generator is packaged; and (3) mark the approval number on the outside of the package.

61 A chemical oxygen generator is spent if its means of ignition and all or a part of its chemical contents have been expended.

64 The group of alkali metals includes lithium, sodium, potassium, rubidium, and caesium.

65 The group of alkaline earth metals includes magnesium, calcium, strontium, and barium.

66 Formulations of these substances containing not less than 30 percent non-volatile, non-flammable phlegmatizer are not subject to this subchapter.

70 Black powder that has been classed in accordance with the requirements of §173.56 of this subchapter may be reclassed and offered for domestic transportation as a Division 4.1 material if it is offered for transportation and transported in accordance with the limitations and packaging requirements of §173.170 of this subchapter.

74 During transport, this material must be protected from direct sunshine and stored or kept in a cool and well-ventilated place, away from all sources of heat.

77 For domestic transportation, a Division 5.1 subsidiary risk label is required only if a carbon dioxide and oxygen mixture contains more than 23.5% oxygen.

78 This entry may not be used to describe compressed air which contains more than 23.5 percent oxygen. An oxidizer label is not required for any oxygen concentration of 23.5 percent or less.

79 This entry may not be used for mixtures that meet the definition for oxidizing gas.

81 Polychlorinated biphenyl items, as defined in 40 CFR 761.3, for which specification packagings are impractical, may be packaged in non-specification packagings meeting the general packaging requirements of subparts A and B of part 173 of this subchapter. Alternatively, the item itself may be used as a packaging if it meets the general packaging requirements of subparts A and B of part 173 of this subchapter.

101 The name of the particular substance or article must be specified.

102 The ends of the detonating cord must be tied fast so that the explosive cannot escape. The articles may be transported as in Division 1.4 Compatibility Group D (1.4D) if all of the conditions specified in §173.63(a) of this subchapter are met.

103 Detonators which will not mass detonate and undergo only limited propagation in the shipping package may be assigned to 1.4B classification code. Mass detonate means that more than 90 percent of the devices tested in a package explode practically simultaneously. Limited propagation means that if one detonator near the center of a shipping package is exploded, the aggregate weight of explosives, excluding ignition and delay charges, in this and all additional detonators in the outside packaging that explode may not exceed 25 grams.

105 The word "Agents" may be used instead of "Explosives" when approved by the Associate Administrator.

106 The recognized name of the particular explosive may be specified in addition to the type.

107 The classification of the substance is expected to vary especially with the particle size and packaging but the border lines have not been experimentally determined; appropriate classifications should be verified following the test procedures in §§173.57 and 173.58 of this subchapter.

108 Fireworks must be so constructed and packaged that loose pyrotechnic composition will not be present in packages during transportation.

109 Rocket motors must be nonpropulsive in transportation unless approved in accordance with §173.56 of this subchapter. A rocket motor to be considered "nonpropulsive" must be capable of unrestrained burning and must not appreciably move in any direction when ignited by any means.

110 Fire extinguishers transported under UN1044 may include installed actuating cartridges (cartridges, power device of Division 1.4C or 1.4S), without changing the classification of Division 2.2, provided the aggregate quantity of deflagrating (propellant) explosives does not exceed 3.2 grams per extinguishing unit.

111 Explosive substances of Division 1.1 Compatibility Group A (1.1A) are forbidden for transportation if dry or not desensitized, unless incorporated in a device.

113 The sample must be given a tentative approval by an agency or laboratory in accordance with §173.56 of this subchapter.

114 Jet perforating guns, charged, oil well, without detonator may be reclassed to Division 1.4 Compatibility Group D (1.4D) if the following conditions are met:

a. The total weight of the explosive contents of the shaped charges assembled in the guns does not exceed 90.5 kg (200 pounds) per vehicle; and

b. The guns are packaged in accordance with Packing Method US1 as specified in §173.62 of this subchapter.

115 Boosters with detonator, detonator assemblies and boosters with detonators in which the total explosive charge per unit does not exceed 25 g, and which will not mass detonate and undergo only limited propagation in the shipping package may be assigned to 1.4B classification code. Mass detonate means more than 90 percent of the devices tested in a package explode practically simultaneously. Limited propagation means that if one booster near the center of the package is exploded, the aggregate weight of explosives, excluding ignition and delay charges, in this and all additional boosters in the outside packaging that explode may not exceed 25 g.

116 Fuzes, detonating may be classed in Division 1.4 if the fuzes do not contain more than 25 g of explosive per fuze and are made and packaged so that they will not cause functioning of other fuzes, explosives or other explosive devices if one of the fuzes detonates in a shipping packaging or in adjacent packages.

117 If shipment of the explosive substance is to take place at a time that freezing weather is anticipated, the water contained in the explosive substance must be mixed with denatured alcohol so that freezing will not occur.

118 This substance may not be transported under the provisions of Division 4.1 unless specifically authorized by the Associate Administrator.

119 This substance, when in quantities of not more than 11.5 kg (25.3 pounds), with not less than 10 percent water, by mass, also may be classed as Division 4.1, provided a negative test result is obtained when tested in accordance with test series 6(c) of the UN Manual of Tests and Criteria (IBR, see §171.7 of this subchapter).

120 The phlegmatized substance must be significantly less sensitive than dry PETN.

121 This substance, when containing less alcohol, water or phlegmatizer than specified, may not be transported unless approved by the Associate Administrator.

123 Any explosives, blasting, type C containing chlorates must be segregated from explosives containing ammonium nitrate or other ammonium salts.

125 Lactose or glucose or similar materials may be used as a phlegmatizer provided that the substance contains not less than 90%, by mass, of phlegmatizer. These mixtures may be classified in Division 4.1 when tested in accordance with test series 6(c) of the UN Manual of Tests and Criteria (IBR, see §171.7 of this subchapter) and approved by the Associate Administrator. Testing must be conducted on at least three packages as prepared for transport. Mixtures containing at least 98%, by mass, of phlegmatizer are not subject to the requirements of this subchapter. Packages containing mixtures with not less than 90% by mass, of phlegmatizer need not bear a POISON subsidiary risk label.

127 Mixtures containing oxidizing and organic materials transported under this entry may not meet the definition and criteria of a Class 1 material. (See §173.50 of this subchapter.)

128 Regardless of the provisions of §172.101(c)(12), aluminum smelting by-products and aluminum remelting by-products described under this entry, meeting the definition of Class 8, Packing Group II and III may be classed as a Division 4.3 material and transported under this entry. The presence of a Class 8 hazard must be communicated as required by this Part for subsidiary hazards.

129 These materials may not be classified and transported unless authorized by the Associate Administrator on the basis of results from Series 2 Test and a Series 6(c) Test from the UN Manual of Tests and Criteria (IBR, see §171.7 of this subchapter) on packages as prepared for transport. The packing group assignment and packaging must be approved by the Associate Administrator on the basis of the criteria in §173.21 of this subchapter and the package type used for the Series 6(c) test.

130 For other than a dry battery specifically covered by another entry in the §172.101 Table, "Batteries, dry" are not subject to the requirements of this subchapter when they are securely packaged and offered for transportation in a manner that prevents the dangerous evolution of heat (for example, by the effective insulation of exposed terminals) and protects against short circuits.

131 This material may not be offered for transportation unless approved by the Associate Administrator.

132 This entry may only be used for uniform, ammonium nitrate-base fertilizer mixtures, containing nitrogen, phosphate or potash, meeting the following criteria: (1) Contains not more than 70% ammonium nitrate; and (2) Contains not more than 0.4% total combustible, organic material calculated as carbon or with not more than 45% ammonium nitrate and unrestricted combustible material. Fertilizers within these composition limits are only subject to the requirements of this subchapter when transported by aircraft or vessel, and are not subject to the requirements of this subchapter if shown by a trough test, as specified in the UN Manual of Tests and Criteria, Part III, Sub-section 38.2 (IBR, see §171.7 of this subchapter), not to be liable to self-sustaining decomposition.

134 This entry only applies to vehicles, machinery and equipment powered by wet batteries, sodium batteries, or lithium batteries that are transported with these batteries installed. Examples of such items are electrically-powered cars, lawn mowers, wheelchairs, and other mobility aids. Self-propelled vehicles that also contain an internal combustion engine must be consigned under the entry "Vehicle, flammable gas powered" or "Vehicle, flammable liquid powered", as appropriate. Except as provided in Special Provision A102, vehicles, machinery and equipment powered by primary lithium batteries that are transported with these batteries installed are forbidden aboard passenger-carrying aircraft.

135 The entries "Vehicle, flammable gas powered" or "Vehicle, flammable liquid powered," as appropriate, must be used when internal combustion engines are installed in a vehicle. These entries include hybrid electric vehicles powered by both an internal combustion engine and batteries

136 This entry only applies to machinery and apparatus containing hazardous materials as in integral element of the machinery or apparatus. It may not be used to describe machinery or apparatus for which a proper shipping name exists in the §172.101 Table. Except when approved by the Associate Administrator, machinery or apparatus may only contain hazardous materials for which exceptions are referenced in Column (8) of the §172.101 Table and are provided in part 173, subpart D, of this subchapter. Hazardous materials shipped under this entry are excepted from the labeling requirements of this subchapter unless offered for transportation or transported by aircraft and are not subject to the placarding requirements of part 172, subpart F, of this subchapter. Orientation markings as described in §172.312(a)(2) are required when liquid hazardous materials may escape due to incorrect orientation. The machinery or apparatus, if unpackaged, or the packaging in which it is contained shall be marked "Dangerous goods in machinery" or "Dangerous goods in apparatus", as appropriate, with the identification number UN3363. For transportation by aircraft, machinery or apparatus may not contain any material forbidden for transportation by passenger or cargo aircraft. The Associate Administrator may except from the requirements of this subchapter, equipment, machinery and apparatus provided:

a. It is shown that it does not pose a significant risk in transportation;

b. The quantities of hazardous materials do not exceed those specified in §173.4 of this subchapter; and

c. The equipment, machinery or apparatus conforms with §173.222 of this subchapter.

137 Cotton, dry; flax, dry; and sisal, dry are not subject to the requirements of this subchapter when they are baled in accordance with ISO 8115, "Cotton Bales-Dimensions and Density" (IBR, see §171.7 of this subchapter) to a density of not less than 360 kg/m^3 (22.1 lb/ft^3) for cotton, 400 kg/m^3 (24.97 lb/ft^3) for flax and 620 kg/m^3 (38.71 lb/ft^3) for sisal and transported in a freight container or closed transport vehicle.

138 Lead compounds which, when mixed in a ratio of 1:1000 with 0.07M (Molar concentration) hydrochloric acid and stirred for one hour at a temperature of 23°C ± 2°C, exhibit a solubility of 5% or less are considered insoluble.

139 Use of the "special arrangement" proper shipping names for international shipments must be made under an IAEA Certificate of Competent Authority issued by the Associate Administrator in accordance with the requirements in §173.471, §173.472, or §173.473 of this subchapter. Use of these proper shipping names for domestic shipments may be made only under a DOT exemption, as defined in, and in accordance with the requirements of subpart B of part 107 of this subchapter.

140 This material is regulated only when it meets the defining criteria for a hazardous substance or a marine pollutant. In addition, the column 5 reference is modified to read "III" on those occasions when this material is offered for transportation or transported by highway or rail.

141 A toxin obtained from a plant, animal, or bacterial source containing an infectious substance, or a toxin contained in an infectious substance, must be classed as Division 6.2, described as an infectious substance, and assigned to UN 2814 or UN 2900, as appropriate.

142 These hazardous materials may not be classified and transported unless authorized by the Associate Administrator. The Associate Administrator will base the authorization on results from Series 2 tests and a Series 6(c) test from the UN Manual of Tests and Criteria (IBR, see §171.7 of this subchapter) on packages as prepared for transport in accordance with the requirements of this subchapter.

144 If transported as a residue in an underground storage tank (UST), as defined in 40 CFR 180.12, that has been cleaned and purged or rendered inert according to the American Petroleum Institute (API) Standard 1604 (IBR, see §171.7 of this subchapter), then the tank and this material are not subject to any other requirements of this subchapter. However, sediments remaining in the tank that meet the definition for a hazardous material are subject to the applicable regulations of this subchapter.

145 This entry applies to formulations that neither detonate in the cavitated state nor deflagrate in laboratory testing, show no effect when heated under confinement, exhibit no explosive power, and are thermally stable (self-accelerating decomposition temperature (SADT) at 60°C (140°F) or higher for a 50 kg (110.2 lbs.) package). Formulations not meeting these criteria must be transported under the provisions applicable to the appropriate entry in the Organic Peroxide Table in §173.225 of this subchapter.

146 This description may be used for a material that poses a hazard to the environment but does not meet the definition for a hazardous waste or a hazardous substance, as defined in §171.8 of this subchapter, or any hazard class as defined in Part 173 of this subchapter, if it is designated as environmentally hazardous by the Competent Authority of the country of origin, transit or destination.

147 This entry applies to non-sensitized emulsions, suspensions and gels consisting primarily of a mixture of ammonium nitrate and a fuel intended to produce a Type E blasting explosive only after further processing. The mixture typically has the following composition: 60-85% ammonium nitrate; 5-30% water; 2-8% fuel; 0.5-4% emulsifier or thickening agent; 0-10% soluble flame suppressants; and trace additives. Other inorganic nitrate salts may replace part of the ammonium nitrate. These substances may not be classified and transported unless approved by the Associate Administrator.

149 When transported as a limited quantity or a consumer commodity, the maximum net capacity specified in §173.150(b)(2) of this subchapter for inner packagings may be increased to 5 L (1.3 gallons).

150 This description may be used only for uniform mixtures of fertilizers containing ammonium nitrate as the main ingredient within the following composition limits:

a. Not less than 90% ammonium nitrate with not more than 0.2% total combustible, organic material calculated as carbon, and with added matter, if any, that is inorganic and inert when in contact with ammonium nitrate; or

b. Less than 90% but more than 70% ammonium nitrate with other inorganic materials, or more than 80% but less than 90% ammonium nitrate mixed with calcium carbonate and/or dolomite, and not more than 0.4% total combustible, organic material calculated as carbon; or

c. Ammonium nitrate-based fertilizers containing mixtures of ammonium nitrate and ammonium sulphate with more than 45% but less than 70% ammonium nitrate, and not more than 0.4% total combustible, organic material calculated as carbon such that the sum of the percentage of compositions of ammonium nitrate and ammonium sulphate exceeds 70%.

151 If this material meets the definition of a flammable liquid in §173.120 of this subchapter, a FLAMMABLE LIQUID label is also required and the basic description on the shipping paper must indicate the Class 3 subsidiary hazard.

155 Fish meal or fish scrap may not be transported if the temperature at the time of loading either exceeds 35°C (95°F), or exceeds 5°C (41°F) above the ambient temperature, whichever is higher.

156 Asbestos that is immersed or fixed in a natural or artificial binder material, such as cement, plastic, asphalt, resins or mineral ore, or contained in manufactured products is not subject to the requirements of this subchapter.

157 This entry includes hybrid electric vehicles powered by both an internal combustion engine and wet, sodium or lithium batteries installed. Vehicles containing an internal combustion engine must be consigned under the entry "Vehicle, flammable gas powered" or "Vehicle, flammable liquid powered", as appropriate. Except as provided in Special Provision A102, vehicles powered by primary lithium batteries, that are transported with these batteries installed are forbidden aboard passenger-carrying aircraft.

159 This material must be protected from direct sunshine and kept in a cool, well-ventilated place away from sources of heat.

160 This entry applies to articles that are used as life-saving vehicle air bag inflators, air bag modules or seat-belt pretensioners containing Class 1 (explosive) materials or materials of other hazard classes. Air bag inflators and modules must be tested in accordance with Test series 6(c) of Part I of the UN Manual of Tests and Criteria (incorporated by reference; see §171.7 of this subchapter), with no explosion of the device, no fragmentation of device casing or pressure vessel, and no projection hazard or thermal effect that would significantly hinder fire-fighting or other emergency response efforts in the immediate vicinity. If the air bag inflator unit satisfactorily passes the series 6(c) test, it is not necessary to repeat the test on the air bag module.

161 For domestic transport, air bag inflators, air bag modules or seat belt pretensioners that meet the criteria for a Division 1.4G explosive must be transported using the description, "Articles, pyrotechnic *for technical purposes*," UN0431.

162 This material may be transported under the provisions of Division 4.1 only if it is packed so that at no time during transport will the percentage of diluent fall below the percentage that is stated in the shipping description.

163 Substances must satisfactorily pass Test Series 8 of the UN Manual of Tests and Criteria, Part I, Section 18 (IBR, see §171.7 of this subchapter).

164 Substances must not be transported under this entry unless approved by the Associate Administrator on the basis of the results of appropriate tests according to Part I of the UN Manual of Tests and Criteria (IBR, see §171.7 of this subchapter). The material must be packaged so that the percentage of diluent does not fall below that stated in the approval at any time during transportation.

165 These substances are susceptible to exothermic decomposition at elevated temperatures. Decomposition can be initiated by heat, moisture or by impurities (e.g., powdered metals (iron, manganese, cobalt, magnesium)). During the course of transportation, these substances must be shaded from direct sunlight and all sources of heat and be placed in adequately ventilated areas.

166 When transported in non-friable tablet form calcium hypochlorite, dry or hydrated, may be transported as a Packing Group III material.

167 These storage systems shall always be considered as containing hydrogen.

170 Air must be eliminated from the vapor space by nitrogen or other means.

171 This entry may only be used when the material is transported in non-friable tablet form or for granular or powered mixtures that have been shown to meet the PG III criteria in §173.127.

172 This entry includes alcohol mixtures containing up to 5% petroleum products.

173 An appropriate generic entry may be used for this material.

(2) *"A" codes.* These provisions apply only to transportation by aircraft:

Code/Special Provisions

A1 Single packagings are not permitted on passenger aircraft.

A2 Single packagings are not permitted on aircraft.

A3 For combination packagings, if glass inner packagings (including ampoules) are used, they must be packed with absorbent material in tightly closed metal receptacles before packing in outer packagings.

A4 Liquids having an inhalation toxicity of Packing Group I are not permitted on aircraft.

A5 Solids having an inhalation toxicity of Packing Group I are not permitted on passenger aircraft and may not exceed a maximum net quantity per package of 15 kg (33 pounds) on cargo aircraft.

A6 For combination packagings, if plastic inner packagings are used, they must be packed in tightly closed metal receptacles before packing in outer packagings.

A7 Steel packagings must be corrosion-resistant or have protection against corrosion.

A8 For combination packagings, if glass inner packagings (including ampoules) are used, they must be packed with cushioning material in tightly closed metal receptacles before packing in outer packagings.

A9 For combination packagings, if plastic bags are used, they must be packed in tightly closed metal receptacles before packing in outer packagings.

A10 When aluminum or aluminum alloy construction materials are used, they must be resistant to corrosion.

A11 For combination packagings, when metal inner packagings are permitted, only specification cylinders constructed of metals which are compatible with the hazardous material may be used.

A13 Bulk packagings are not authorized for transportation by aircraft.

A14 This material is not authorized to be transported as a limited quantity or consumer commodity in accordance with §173.306 of this subchapter when transported aboard an aircraft.

A19 Combination packagings consisting of outer fiber drums or plywood drums, with inner plastic packagings, are not authorized for transportation by aircraft

A20 Plastic bags as inner receptacles of combination packagings are not authorized for transportation by aircraft.

A29 Combination packagings consisting of outer expanded plastic boxes with inner plastic bags are not authorized for transportation by aircraft.

A30 Ammonium permanganate is not authorized for transportation on aircraft.

A34 Aerosols containing a corrosive liquid in Packing Group II charged with a gas are not permitted for transportation by aircraft.

A35 This includes any material which is not covered by any of the other classes but which has an anesthetic, narcotic, noxious or other similar properties such that, in the event of spillage or leakage on an aircraft, extreme annoyance or discomfort could be caused to crew members so as to prevent the correct performance of assigned duties.

A37 This entry applies only to a material meeting the definition in §171.8 of this subchapter for self-defense spray.

A51 When transported by cargo-only aircraft, an oxygen generator must conform to the provisions of an approval issued under Special Provision 60 and be contained in a packaging prepared and originally offered for transportation by the approval holder.

A52 A cylinder containing Oxygen, compressed, may not be loaded into a passenger-carrying aircraft or into an inaccessible cargo location on a cargo-only aircraft unless it is placed in an overpack or outer packaging that conforms to the performance criteria of Air Transport Association (ATA) Specification No. 300 (IBR, see §171.7 of this subchapter) for Category I shipping containers.

A53 Refrigerating machines and refrigerating machine components are not subject to the requirements of this subchapter when containing less than 12 kg (26.4 pounds) of a non-flammable gas or when containing 12 L (3 gallons) or less of ammonia solution (UN2672) (see §173.307 of this subchapter).

A54 Lithium batteries or lithium batteries contained or packed with equipment that exceed the maximum gross weight allowed by Column (9B) of the §172.101 Table may only be transported on cargo aircraft if approved by the Associate Administrator.

A55 Prototype lithium batteries and cells that are packed with not more than 24 cells or 12 batteries per packaging that have not completed the test requirements in Sub-section 38.3 of the UN Manual of Tests and Criteria (incorporated by reference; see §171.7 of this subchapter) may be transported by cargo aircraft if approved by the Associate Administrator and provided the following requirements are met:

a. The cells and batteries must be transported in rigid outer packagings that conform to the requirements of Part 178 of this subchapter at the Packing Group I performance level; and

b. Each cell and battery must be protected against short circuiting, must be surrounded by cushioning material that is non-combustible and non-conductive, and must be individually packed in an inner packaging that is placed inside an outer specification packaging.

A56 Radioactive material with a subsidiary hazard of Division 4.2, Packing Group I, must be transported in Type B packages when offered for transportation by aircraft. Radioactive material with a subsidiary hazard of Division 2.1 is forbidden from transport on passenger aircraft.

A81 The quantity limits in columns (9A) and (9B) do not apply to body fluids known to contain or suspected of containing an infectious substance when transported in primary receptacles not exceeding 1,000 mL (34 ounces) and in outer packagings not exceeding 4 L (1 gallon) and packaged in accordance with §173.196 of this subchapter.

A82 The quantity limits in columns (9A) and (9B) do not apply to human or animal body parts, whole organs or whole bodies known to contain or suspected of containing an infectious substance.

A100 Primary (non-rechargeable) lithium batteries and cells are forbidden for transport aboard passenger carrying aircraft. Secondary (rechargeable) lithium batteries and cells are authorized aboard passenger carrying aircraft in packages that do not exceed a gross weight of 5 kg.

A101 A primary (non-rechargeable) lithium battery or cell packed with equipment is forbidden for transport aboard a passenger carrying aircraft unless:

a. The battery or cell complies with the requirements and limitations of §173.185(b)(1), (b)(2), (b)(3), (b)(4) and (b)(6) or §173.185(c)(1), (c)(2), (c)(3) and (c)(5) of this subchapter;

b. The package contains no more than the number of lithium batteries or cells necessary to power the intended piece of equipment;

c. The equipment and the battery or cell are packed in a strong packaging;

d. The gross weight of the package does not exceed 5 kg. Packages complying with the requirements of this special provision are excepted from all other requirements of this subchapter.

A102 A primary (non-rechargeable) lithium battery or cell contained in equipment is forbidden for transport aboard a passenger carrying aircraft unless:

a. The battery or cell complies with the requirements and limitations of §173.185(b)(1), (b)(2), (b)(3), (b)(4) and (b)(6) or §173.185(c)(1), (c)(2), (c)(3) and (c)(5) of this subchapter;

b. The package contains no more than the number of lithium batteries or cells necessary to power the intended piece of equipment;

c. The equipment containing the battery or cell is packed in strong packagings; and

d. The net weight of the package does not exceed 5 kg. Packages complying with the requirements of this special provision are excepted from all other requirements of this subchapter.

A103 A secondary (rechargeable) lithium battery or cell packed with equipment is authorized aboard passenger carrying aircraft in packages that do not exceed a gross weight of 5 kg.

A104 A secondary (rechargeable) lithium battery or cell packed in equipment is authorized aboard passenger carrying aircraft in packages that do not exceed a net weight of 5 kg.

(3) *"B" codes.* These provisions apply only to bulk packagings. Except as otherwise provided in this subchapter, these special provisions do not apply to UN portable tanks or IBCs:

Code/Special Provisions

B1 If the material has a flash point at or above 38°C (100°F) and below 93°C (200°F), then the bulk packaging requirements of §173.241 of this subchapter are applicable. If the material has a flash point of less than 38°C (100°F), then the bulk packaging requirements of §173.242 of this subchapter are applicable.

B2 MC 300, MC 301, MC 302, MC 303, MC 305, and MC 306, and DOT 406 cargo tanks are not authorized.

B3 MC 300, MC 301, MC 302, MC 303, MC 305, and MC 306, and DOT 406 cargo tanks and DOT 57 portable tanks are not authorized.

B4 MC 300, MC 301, MC 302, MC 303, MC 305, and MC 306, and DOT 406 cargo tanks are not authorized.

B5 Only ammonium nitrate solutions with 35 percent or less water that will remain completely in solution under all conditions of transport at a maximum lading temperature of 116°C (240°F) are authorized for transport in the following bulk packagings: MC 307, MC 312, DOT 407 and DOT 412 cargo tanks with at least 172 kPa (25 psig) design pressure. The packaging shall be designed for a working temperature of at least 121°C (250°F). Only Specifications

MC 304, MC 307 or DOT 407 cargo tank motor vehicles are authorized for transportation by vessel.

B6 Packagings shall be made of steel.

B7 Safety relief devices are not authorized on multi-unit tank car tanks. Openings for safety relief devices on multi-unit tank car tanks shall be plugged or blank flanged.

B8 Packagings shall be made of nickel, stainless steel, or steel with nickel, stainless steel, lead or other suitable corrosion resistant metallic lining.

B9 Bottom outlets are not authorized.

B10 MC 300, MC 301, MC 302, MC 303, MC 305 and MC 306 and DOT 406 cargo tanks, and DOT 57 portable tanks are not authorized.

B11 Tank car tanks must have a test pressure of at least 2,068.5 kPa (300 psig). Cargo and portable tanks must have a design pressure of at least 1,207 kPa (175 psig).

B13 A nonspecification cargo tank motor vehicle authorized in §173.247 of this subchapter must be at least equivalent in design and in construction to a DOT 406 cargo tank or MC 306 cargo tank (if constructed before August 31, 1995), except as follows:

a. Packagings equivalent to MC 306 cargo tanks are excepted from the certification, venting, and emergency flow requirements of the MC 306 specification.

b. Packagings equivalent to DOT 406 cargo tanks are excepted from §§178.345-7(d)(5), circumferential reinforcements; 178.345-10, pressure relief; 178.345-11, outlets; 178.345-14, marking, and 178.345-15, certification.

c. Packagings are excepted from the design stress limits at elevated temperatures, as described in Section VIII of the ASME Code (IBR, see §171.7 of this subchapter). However, the design stress limits may not exceed 25 percent of the stress for 0 temper at the maximum design temperature of the cargo tank, as specified in the Aluminum Association's "Aluminum Standards and Data" (IBR, see §171.7 of this subchapter).

B14 Each bulk packaging, except a tank car or a multi-unit-tank car tank, must be insulated with an insulating material so that the overall thermal conductance at 15.5°C (60°F) is no more than 1.5333 kilojoules per hour per square meter per degree Celsius (0.075 Btu per hour per square foot per degree Fahrenheit) temperature differential. Insulating materials must not promote corrosion to steel when wet.

B15 Packagings must be protected with non-metallic linings impervious to the lading or have a suitable corrosion allowance.

B16 The lading must be completely covered with nitrogen, inert gas or other inert materials.

B18 Open steel hoppers or bins are authorized.

B23 Tanks must be made of steel that is rubber lined or unlined. Unlined tanks must be passivated before being placed in service. If unlined tanks are washed out with water, they must be repassivated prior to return to service. Lading in unlined tanks must be inhibited so that the corrosive effect on steel is not greater than that of hydrofluoric acid of 65 percent concentration.

B25 Packagings must be made from monel or nickel or monel-lined or nickel-lined steel.

B26 Tanks must be insulated. Insulation must be at least 100 mm (3.9 inches) except that the insulation thickness may be reduced to 51 mm (2 inches) over the exterior heater coils. Interior heating coils are not authorized. The packaging may not be loaded with a material outside of the packaging's design temperature range. In addition, the material also must be covered with an inert gas or the container must be filled with water to the tank's capacity. After unloading, the residual material also must be covered with an inert gas or the container must be filled with water to the tank's capacity.

B27 Tanks must have a service pressure of 1,034 kPa (150 psig). Tank car tanks must have a test pressure rating of 1,379 kPa (200 psig). Lading must be blanketed at all times with a dry inert gas at a pressure not to exceed 103 kPa (15 psig).

B28 Packagings must be made of stainless steel.

B30 MC 312, MC 330, MC 331 and DOT 412 cargo tanks and DOT 51 portable tanks must be made of stainless steel, except that steel other than stainless steel may be used in accordance with the provisions of §173.24b(b) of this subchapter. Thickness of stainless steel for tank shell and heads for cargo tanks and portable tanks must be the greater of 7.62 mm (0.300 inch) or the thickness required for a tank with a design pressure at least equal to 1.5 times the vapor pressure of the lading at 46°C (115°F). In addition, MC 312 and DOT 412 cargo tank motor vehicles must:

a. Be ASME Code (U) stamped for 100% radiography of all pressure-retaining welds;

b. Have accident damage protection which conforms with §178.345-8 of this subchapter;

c. Have a MAWP or design pressure of at least 87 psig: and

d. Have a bolted manway cover.

B32 MC 312, MC 330, MC 331, DOT 412 cargo tanks and DOT 51 portable tanks must be made of stainless steel, except that steel other than stainless steel may be used in accordance with the provisions of §173.24b(b) of this subchapter. Thickness of stainless steel for tank shell and heads for cargo tanks and portable tanks must be the greater of 6.35 mm (0.250 inch) or the thickness required for a tank with a design pressure at least equal to 1.3 times the vapor pressure of the lading at 46°C

(115°F). In addition, MC 312 and DOT 412 cargo tank motor vehicles must:

a. Be ASME Code (U) stamped for 100% radiography of all pressure-retaining welds;

b. Have accident damage protection which conforms with §178.345–8 of this subchapter;

c. Have a MAWP or design pressure of at least 87 psig; and

d. Have a bolted manway cover.

B33 MC 300, MC 301, MC 302, MC 303, MC 305, MC 306, and DOT 406 cargo tanks equipped with a 1 psig normal vent used to transport gasoline must conform to Table I of this Special Provision. Based on the volatility class determined by using ASTM D439 and the Reid vapor pressure (RVP) of the particular gasoline, the maximum lading pressure and maximum ambient temperature permitted during the loading of gasoline may not exceed that listed in Table I.

TABLE I—MAXIMUM AMBIENT TEMPERATURE—GASOLINE

ASTM D439 volatility class	Maximum lading and ambient temperature (see note 1)
A. (RVP<=9.0 psia)	131°F
B. (RVP<=10.0 psia)	124°F
C. (RVP<=11.5 psia)	116°F
D. (RVP<=13.5 psia)	107°F
E. (RVP<=15.0 psia)	100°F

Note 1: Based on maximum lading pressure of 1 psig at top of cargo tank.

B35 Tank cars containing hydrogen cyanide may be alternatively marked "Hydrocyanic acid, liquefied" if otherwise conforming to marking requirements in subpart D of this part. Tank cars marked “HYDROCYANIC ACID” prior to October 1, 1991 do not need to be remarked.

B37 The amount of nitric oxide charged into any tank car tank may not exceed 1,379 kPa (200 psig) at 21°C (70°F).

B42 Tank cars must have a test pressure of 34.47 Bar (500 psig) or greater and conform to Class 105J. Each tank car must have a reclosing pressure relief device having a start-to-discharge pressure of 10.34 Bar (150 psig). The tank car specification may be marked to indicate a test pressure of 13.79 Bar (200 psig).

B44 All parts of valves and safety relief devices in contact with lading must be of a material which will not cause formation of acetylides.

B45 Each tank must have a reclosing combination pressure relief device equipped with stainless steel or platinum rupture discs approved by the AAR Tank Car Committee.

B46 The detachable protective housing for the loading and unloading valves of multi-unit tank car tanks must withstand tank test pressure and must be approved by the Associate Administrator.

B47 Each tank may have a reclosing pressure relief device having a start-to-discharge pressure setting of 310 kPa (45 psig).

B48 Portable tanks in sodium metal service may be visually inspected at least once every 5 years instead of being retested hydrostatically. Date of the visual inspection must be stenciled on the tank near the other required markings.

B49 Tanks equipped with interior heater coils are not authorized. Single unit tank car tanks must have a reclosing pressure relief device having a start-to-discharge pressure set at no more than 1551 kPa (225 psig).

B50 Each valve outlet of a multi-unit tank car tank must be sealed by a threaded solid plug or a threaded cap with inert luting or gasket material. Valves must be of stainless steel and the caps, plugs, and valve seats must be of a material that will not deteriorate as a result of contact with the lading.

B52 Notwithstanding the provisions of §173.24b of this subchapter, non-reclosing pressure relief devices are authorized on DOT 57 portable tanks.

B53 Packagings must be made of either aluminum or steel.

B54 Open-top, sift-proof rail cars are also authorized.

B55 Water-tight, sift-proof, closed-top, metal-covered hopper cars, equipped with a venting arrangement (including flame arrestors) approved by the Associate Administrator are also authorized.

B56 Water-tight, sift-proof, closed-top, metal-covered hopper cars also authorized if the particle size of the hazardous material is not less than 149 microns.

B57 Class 115A tank car tanks used to transport chloroprene must be equipped with a non-reclosing pressure relief device of a diameter not less than 305 mm (12 inches) with a maximum rupture disc burst pressure of 310 kPa (45 psig).

B59 Water-tight, sift-proof, closed-top, metal-covered hopper cars are also authorized provided that the lading is covered with a nitrogen blanket.

B60 DOT Specification 106A500X multi-unit tank car tanks that are not equipped with a pressure relief device of any type are authorized. For the transportation of phosgene, the outage must be sufficient to prevent tanks from becoming liquid full at 55°C (130°F).

B61 Written procedures covering details of tank car appurtenances, dome fittings, safety devices, and marking, loading, handling, inspection, and testing practices must be approved by the Associate Administrator before any single unit tank car tank is offered for transportation.

B64 Each single unit tank car tank built after December 31, 1990 must be equipped with a tank head puncture resistance system that conforms to §179.16 of this subchapter.

B65 Tank cars must have a test pressure of 34.47 Bar (500 psig) or greater and conform to Class 105A. Each tank car must have a pressure relief device having a start-to-discharge pressure of 15.51 Bar (225 psig). The tank car specification may be marked to indicate a test pressure of 20.68 Bar (300 psig).

B66 Each tank must be equipped with gas tight valve protection caps. Outage must be sufficient to prevent tanks from becoming liquid full at 55°C (130°F). Specification 110A500W tanks must be stainless steel.

B67 All valves and fittings must be protected by a securely attached cover made of metal not subject to deterioration by the lading, and all valve openings, except safety valve, must be fitted with screw plugs or caps to prevent leakage in the event of valve failure.

B68 Sodium must be in a molten condition when loaded and allowed to solidify before shipment. Outage must be at least 5 percent at 98°C (208°F). Bulk packagings must have exterior heating coils fusion welded to the tank shell which have been properly stress relieved. The only tank car tanks authorized are Class DOT 105 tank cars having a test pressure of 2,069 kPa (300 psig) or greater.

B69 Dry sodium cyanide or potassium cyanide may be shipped in sift-proof weather-resistant metal covered hopper cars, covered motor vehicles, portable tanks or non-specification bins. Bins must be approved by the Associate Administrator.

B70 If DOT 103ANW tank car tank is used: All cast metal in contact with the lading must have 96.7 percent nickel content; and the lading must be anhydrous and free from any impurities.

B71 Tank cars must have a test pressure of 20.68 Bar (300 psig) or greater and conform to Class 105, 112, 114 or 120.

B72 Tank cars must have a test pressure of 34.47 Bar (500 psig) or greater and conform to Class 105J, 106, or 110.

B74 Tank cars must have a test pressure of 20.68 Bar (300 psig) or greater and conform to Class 105S, 106, 110, 112J, 114J or 120S.

B76 Tank cars must have a test pressure of 20.68 Bar (300 psig) or greater and conform to Class 105S, 112J, 114J or 120S. Each tank car must have a reclosing pressure relief device having a start-to-discharge pressure of 10.34 Bar (150 psig). The tank car specification may be marked to indicate a test pressure of 13.79 Bar (200 psig).

B77 Other packaging are authorized when approved by the Associate Administrator.

B78 Tank cars must have a test pressure of 4.14 Bar (60 psig) or greater and conform to Class 103, 104, 105, 109, 111, 112, 114 or 120. Heater pipes must be of welded construction designed for a test pressure of 500 pounds per square inch. A 25 mm (1 inch) woven lining of asbestos or other approved material must be placed between the bolster slabbing and the bottom of the tank. If a tank car tank is equipped with a non-reclosing pressure relief device, the rupture disc must be perforated with a 3.2 mm (0.13 inch) diameter hole. If a tank car tank is equipped with a reclosing pressure relief valve, the tank must also be equipped with a vacuum relief valve.

B80 Each cargo tank must have a minimum design pressure of 276 kPa (40 psig).

B81 Venting and pressure relief devices for tank car tanks and cargo tanks must be approved by the Associate Administrator.

B82 Cargo tanks and portable tanks are not authorized.

B83 Bottom outlets are prohibited on tank car tanks transporting sulfuric acid in concentrations over 65.25 percent.

B84 Packagings must be protected with non-metallic linings impervious to the lading or have a suitable corrosion allowance for sulfuric acid or spent sulfuric acid in concentration up to 65.25 percent.

B85 Cargo tanks must be marked with the name of the lading accordance with the requirements of §172.302(b).

B90 Steel tanks conforming or equivalent to ASME specifications which contain solid or semisolid residual motor fuel antiknock mixture (including rust, scale, or other contaminants) may be shipped by rail freight or highway. The tank must have been designed and constructed to be capable of withstanding full vacuum. All openings must be closed with gasketed blank flanges or vapor tight threaded closures.

B115 Rail cars, highway trailers, roll-on/roll-off bins, or other non-specification bulk packagings are authorized. Packagings must be sift-proof, prevent liquid water from reaching the hazardous material, and be provided with sufficient venting to preclude dangerous accumulation of flammable, corrosive, or toxic gaseous emissions such as methane, hydrogen, and ammonia. The material must be loaded dry.

(4) *Table 1, and Table 2-IB Codes and IP Special IBC Packing Provisions.* These provisions apply only to transportation in IBCs. When no IBC code is assigned in the §172.101 Table for a specific proper shipping name, or in §173.255(e) for Type F organic peroxides, an IBC may not be used unless authorized by the Associate Administrator. The letter "Z" shown in the marking code for composite IBCs must be replaced with a capital code letter designation found in §178.702(a)(2) of this subchapter to specify the material used for the outer packaging. Tables 1 and 2 follow:

TABLE 1.—IB CODES (IBC CODES)

IBC Code	Authorized IBCs
IB1	*Authorized IBCs:* Metal (31A, 31B and 31N). *Additional Requirement:* Only liquids with a vapor pressure less than or equal to 110 kPa at 50°C (1.1 bar at 122°F), or 130 kPa at 55°C (1.3 bar at 131°F) are authorized.
IB2	*Authorized IBCs:* Metal (31A, 31B and 31N); Rigid plastics (31H1 and 31H2); Composite (31HZ1). *Additional Requirement:* Only liquids with a vapor pressure less than or equal to 110 kPa at 50°C (1.1 bar at 122°F), or 130 kPa at 55°C (1.3 bar at 131°F) are authorized.
IB3	*Authorized IBCs:* Metal (31A, 31B and 31N); Rigid plastics (31H1 and 31H2); Composite (31HZ1 and 31HA2, 31HB2, 31HN2, 31HD2 and 31HH2). *Additional Requirement:* Only liquids with a vapor pressure less than or equal to 110 kPa at 50°C (1.1 bar at 122°F), or 130 kPa at 55°C (1.3 bar at 131°F) are authorized, except for UN 2672 (also see Special Provision IP8 in Table 2 for UN2672).
IB4	*Authorized IBCs:* Metal (11A, 11B, 11N, 21A, 21B, 21N, 31A, 31B and 31N).
IB5	*Authorized IBCs:* Metal (11A, 11B, 11N, 21A, 21B, 21N, 31A, 31B and 31N); Rigid plastics (11H1, 11H2, 21H1, 21H2, 31H1 and 31H2); Composite (11HZ1, 21HZ1 and 31HZ1).
IB6	*Authorized IBCs*: Metal (11A, 11B, 11N, 21A, 21B, 21N, 31A, 31B and 31N); Rigid plastics (11H1, 11H2, 21H1, 21H2, 31H1 and 31H2); Composite (11HZ1, 11HZ2, 21HZ1, 21HZ2, 31HZ1 and 31HZ2). *Additional Requirement:* Composite IBCs 11HZ2 and 21HZ2 may not be used when the hazardous materials being transported may become liquid during transport.
IB7	*Authorized IBCs:* Metal (11A, 11B, 11N, 21A, 21B, 21N, 31A, 31B and 31N); Rigid plastics (11H1, 11H2, 21H1, 21H2, 31H1 and 31H2); Composite (11HZ1, 11HZ2, 21HZ1, 21HZ2, 31HZ1 and 31HZ2); Wooden (11C, 11D and 11F). *Additional Requirement:* Liners of wooden IBCs must be sift-proof.
IB8	*Authorized IBCs:* Metal (11A, 11B, 11N, 21A, 21B, 21N, 31A, 31B and 31N); Rigid plastics (11H1, 11H2, 21H1, 21H2, 31H1 and 31H2); Composite (11HZ1, 11HZ2, 21HZ1, 21HZ2, 31HZ1 and 31HZ2); Fiberboard (11G); Wooden (11C, 11D and 11F); Flexible (13H1, 13H2, 13H3, 13H4, 13H5, 13L1, 13L2, 13L3, 13L4, 13M1 or 13M2).
IB9	IBCs are only authorized if approved by the Associate Administrator.

TABLE 2.—IP CODES

IP1	IBCs must be packed in closed freight containers or a closed transport vehicle.
IP2	When IBCs other than metal or rigid plastics IBCs are used, they must be offered for transportation in a closed freight container or a closed transport vehicle.
IP3	Flexible IBCs must be sift-proof and water-resistant or must be fitted with a sift-proof and water-resistant liner.
IP4	Flexible, fiberboard or wooden IBCs must be sift-proof and water-resistant or be fitted with a sift-proof and water-resistant liner.
IP5	IBCs must have a device to allow venting. The inlet to the venting device must be located in the vapor space of the IBC under maximum filling conditions.
IP6	Non-specification bulk bins are authorized.
IP7	For UN identification numbers 1327, 1363, 1364, 1365, 1386, 1841, 2211, 2217, 2793 and 3314, IBCs are not required to meet the IBC performance tests specified in part 178, subpart N of this subchapter.
IP8	Ammonia solutions may be transported in rigid or composite plastic IBCs (31H1, 31H2 and 31HZ1) that have successfully passed, without leakage or permanent deformation, the hydrostatic test specified in §178.814 of this subchapter at a test pressure that is not less than 1.5 times the vapor pressure of the contents at 55°C (131°F).
IP13	Transportation by vessel in IBCs is prohibited.
IP14	Air shall be eliminated from the vapor space by nitrogen or other means.
IP20	Dry sodium cyanide or potassium cyanide is also permitted in siftproof, water-resistant, fiberboard IBCs when transported in closed freight containers or transport vehicles.

(5) *"N" codes.* These provisions apply only to non-bulk packagings:

Code/Special Provisions

N3 Glass inner packagings are permitted in combination or composite packagings only if the hazardous material is free from hydrofluoric acid.

N4 For combination or composite packagings, glass inner packagings, other than ampoules, are not permitted.

N5 Glass materials of construction are not authorized for any part of a packaging which is normally in contact with the hazardous material.

N6 Battery fluid packaged with electric storage batteries, wet or dry, must conform to the packaging provisions of §173.159(g) or (h) of this subchapter.

N7 The hazard class or division number of the material must be marked on the package in accordance with §172.302 of this subchapter. However, the hazard label corresponding to the hazard class or division may be substituted for the marking.

N8 Nitroglycerin solution in alcohol may be transported under this entry only when the solution is packed in metal cans of not more than 1 L capacity each, overpacked in a wooden box containing not more than 5 L. Metal cans must be completely surrounded with absorbent cushioning material. Wooden boxes must be completely lined with a suitable material impervious to water and nitroglycerin.

N10 Lighters and their inner packagings, which have been approved by the Associate Administrator (see §173.21(i) of this subchapter), must be packaged in one of the following outer packagings at the Packing Group II level: 4C1 or 4C2 wooden boxes; 4D plywood boxes; 4F reconstituted wood boxes; 4G fiberboard boxes; or 4H1 or 4H2 plastic boxes. The approval number (*e.g.,* T-* * *) must be marked on each outer package and on the shipping paper.

N11 This material is excepted for the specification packaging requirements of this subchapter if the material is packaged in strong, tight non-bulk packaging meeting the requirements of subparts A and B of part 173 of this subchapter.

N12 Plastic packagings are not authorized.

N20 A 5M1 multi-wall paper bag is authorized if transported in a closed transport vehicle.

N25 Steel single packagings are not authorized.

N32 Aluminum materials of construction are not authorized for single packagings.

N33 Aluminum drums are not authorized.

N34 Aluminum construction materials are not authorized for any part of a packaging which is normally in contact with the hazardous material.

N36 Aluminum or aluminum alloy construction materials are permitted only for halogenated hydrocarbons that will not react with aluminum.

N37 This material may be shipped in an integrally-lined fiber drum (1G) which meets the general packaging requirements of subpart B of part 173 of this subchapter, the requirements of part 178 of this subchapter at the packing group assigned for the material and to any other special provisions of column 7 of the §172.101 table.

N40 This material is not authorized in the following packagings:

a. A combination packaging consisting of a 4G fiberboard box with inner receptacles of glass or earthenware;

b. A single packaging of a 4C2 sift-proof, natural wood box; or

c. A composite packaging 6PG2 (glass, porcelain or stoneware receptacles within a fiberboard box).

N41 Metal construction materials are not authorized for any part of a packaging which is normally in contact with the hazardous material.

N42 1A1 drums made of carbon steel with thickness of body and heads of not less than 1.3 mm (0.050 inch) and with a corrosion-resistant phenolic lining are authorized for stabilized benzyl chloride if tested and certified to the Packing Group I performance level at a specific gravity of not less than 1.8.

N43 Metal drums are permitted as single packagings only if constructed of nickel or monel.

N45 Copper cartridges are authorized as inner packagings if the hazardous material is not in dispersion.

N46 Outage must be sufficient to prevent cylinders or spheres from becoming liquid full at 55°C (130°F). The vacant space (outage) may be charged with a nonflammable nonliquefied compressed gas if the pressure in the cylinder or sphere at 55°C (130°F) does not exceed 125 percent of the marked service pressure.

N72 Packagings must be examined by the Bureau of Explosives and approved by the Associate Administrator.

N73 Packagings consisting of outer wooden or fiberboard boxes with inner glass, metal or other strong containers; metal or fiber drums; kegs or barrels; or strong metal cans are authorized and need not conform to the requirements of part 178 of this subchapter.

N74 Packages consisting of tightly closed inner containers of glass, earthenware, metal or polyethylene, capacity not over 0.5 kg (1.1 pounds) securely cushioned and packed in outer wooden barrels or wooden or fiberboard boxes, not over 15 kg (33 pounds) net weight, are authorized and need not conform to the requirements of part 178 of this subchapter.

N75 Packages consisting of tightly closed inner packagings of glass, earthenware or metal, securely cushioned and packed in outer wooden barrels or wooden or fiberboard boxes, capacity not over 2.5 kg (5.5 pounds) net weight, are authorized and need not conform to the requirements of part 178 of this subchapter.

N76 For materials of not more than 25 percent active ingredient by weight, packages consisting of inner metal packagings not greater than 250 mL (8 ounces) capacity each, packed in strong outer packagings together with sufficient absorbent material to completely absorb the liquid contents are authorized and need not conform to the requirements of part 178 of this subchapter.

N77 For materials of not more than two percent active ingredients by weight, packagings need not conform to the requirements of part 178 of this subchapter, if liquid contents are absorbed in an inert material.

N78 Packages consisting of inner glass, earthenware, or polyethylene or other nonfragile plastic bottles or jars not over 0.5 kg (1.1 pounds) capacity each, or metal cans not over five pounds capacity each, packed in outer wooden boxes, barrels or kegs, or fiberboard boxes are authorized and need not conform to the requirements of part 178 of this subchapter. Net weight of contents in fiberboard boxes may not exceed 29 kg (64 pounds). Net weight of contents in wooden boxes, barrels or kegs may not exceed 45 kg (99 pounds).

N79 Packages consisting of tightly closed metal inner packagings not over 0.5 kg (1.1 pounds) capacity each, packed in outer wooden or fiberboard boxes, or wooden barrels, are authorized and need not conform to the requirements of part 178 of this subchapter. Net weight of contents may not exceed 15 kg (33 pounds).

N80 Packages consisting of one inner metal can, not over 2.5 kg (5.5 pounds) capacity, packed in an outer wooden or fiberboard box, or a wooden barrel, are authorized and need not conform to the requirements of part 178 of this subchapter.

N82 See §173.306 of this subchapter for classification criteria for flammable aerosols.

N83 This material may not be transported in quantities of more than 11.5 kg (25.4 lbs) per package.

N84 The maximum quantity per package is 500 g (1.1 lbs.).

N85 Packagings certified at the Packing Group I performance level may not be used.

(6) *"R" codes.* These provisions apply only to transportation by rail.

[Reserved]

(7) *"T" codes.* (i) These provisions apply to the transportation of hazardous materials in UN portable tanks. Portable tank instructions specify the requirements applicable to a portable tank when used for the transportation of a specific hazardous material. These requirements must be met in addition to the design and construction specifications in part 178 of this subchapter. Portable tank instructions T1 through T22 specify the applicable minimum test pressure, the mini mum shell thickness (in reference steel), bottom opening requirements and pressure relief requirements. Liquefied compressed gases are assigned to portable tank instruction T50. Refrigerated liquefied gases that are authorized to be transported in portable tanks are specified in tank instruction T75.

(ii) The following table specifies the portable tank requirements applicable to "T" Codes T1 through T22. Column 1 specifies the "T" Code. Column 2 specifies the minimum test pressure, in bar (1 bar = 14.5 psig), at which the periodic hydrostatic testing required by §180.605 of this subchapter must be conducted. Column 3 specifies the section reference for minimum shell thickness or, alternatively, the minimum shell thickness value. Column 4 specifies the applicability of §178.275(g)(3) of this subchapter for the pressure relief devices. When the word "Normal" is indicated, §178.275(g)(3) of this subchapter does not apply. Column 5 references the applicable requirements for bottom openings in part 178 of this subchapter or references "Prohibited" which means bottom openings are prohibited. The table follows:

TABLE OF PORTABLE TANK T CODER T1—T22
[Portable tank codes T1—T22 apply to liquid and solid hazardous materials of Classes 3 through 9 which are transported in portable tanks.]

Portable tank instruction (1)	Minimum test pressure (bar) (2)	Minimum shell thickness (in mm-reference steel) (*See* §178.274(d)) (3)	Pressure-relief requirements (*See* §178.275(g)) (4)	Bottom opening requirements (*See* §178.275(d)) (5)
T1	1.5	§178.274(d)(2)	Normal	§178.275(d)(2).
T2	1.5	§178.274(d)(2)	Normal	§178.275(d)(3).
T3	2.65	§178.274(d)(2)	Normal	§178.275(d)(2).
T4	2.65	§178.274(d)(2)	Normal	§178.275(d)(3).
T5	2.65	§178.274(d)(2)	§178.275(g)(3)	Prohibited.
T6	4	§178.274(d)(2)	Normal	§178.275(d)(2).
T7	4	§178.274(d)(2)	Normal	§178.275(d)(3).
T8	4	§178.274(d)(2)	Normal	Prohibited.
T9	4	6 mm	Normal	Prohibited.
T10	4	6 mm	§178.275(g)(3)	Prohibited.
T11	6	§178.274(d)(2)	Normal	§178.275(d)(3).
T12	6	§178.274(d)(2)	§178.275(g)(3)	§178.275(d)(3).
T13	6	6 mm	Normal	Prohibited.
T14	6	6 mm	§178.275(g)(3)	Prohibited.
T15	10	§178.274(d)(2)	Normal	§178.275(d)(3).
T16	10	§178.274(d)(2)	§178.275(g)(3)	§178.275(d)(3).
T17	10	6 mm	Normal	§178.275(d)(3).
T18	10	6 mm	§178.275(g)(3)	§178.275(d)(3).
T19	10	6 mm	§178.275(g)(3)	Prohibited.
T20	10	8 mm	§178.275(g)(3)	Prohibited.
T21	10	10 mm	Normal	Prohibited.
T22	10	10 mm	§178.275(g)(3)	Prohibited.

(iii) *T50.* When portable tank instruction T50 is referenced in Column (7) of the §172.101 Table, the applicable liquefied compressed gases are authorized to be transported in portable tanks in accordance with the requirements of §173.313 of this subchapter.

(iv) *T75.* When portable tank instruction T75 is referenced in Column (7) of the §172.101 Table, the applicable refrigerated liquefied gases are authorized to be transported in portable tanks in accordance with the requirements of §178.277 of this subchapter.

(v) *UN and IM portable tank codes/special provisions.* When a specific portable tank instruction is specified by a "T" Code in Column (7) of the §172.101 Table for a specific hazardous material, a specification portable tank conforming to an alternative tank instruction may be used if:

(A) The alternative portable tank has a higher or equivalent test pressure (for example, 4 bar when 2.65 bar is specified);

(B) The alternative portable tank has greater or equivalent wall thickness (for example, 10 mm when 6 mm is specified);

(C) The alternative portable tank has a pressure relief device as specified in the "T" Code. If a frangible disc is required in series with the reclosing pressure relief device for the specified portable tank, the alternative portable tank must be fitted with a frangible disc in series with the reclosing pressure relief device; and

(D) With regard to bottom openings—

(1) When two effective means are specified, the alternative portable tank is fitted with bottom openings having two or three effective means of closure or no bottom openings; or

(2) When three effective means are specified, the portable tank has no bottom openings or three effective means of closure; or

(3) When no bottom openings are authorized, the alternative portable tank must not have bottom openings.

(vi) Except when an organic peroxide is authorized under §173.225(g), if a hazardous material is not assigned a portable tank "T" Code, the hazardous material may not be transported in a portable tank unless approved by the Associate Administrator.

(8) *"TP" codes.* (i) These provisions apply to the transportation of hazardous materials in IM and UN Specification portable tanks. Portable tank special provisions are assigned to certain hazardous materials to specify requirements that are in addition to those provided by the portable tank instructions or the requirements in part 178 of this subchapter. Portable tank special provisions are designated with the abbreviation TP (tank provision) and are assigned to specific hazardous materials in Column (7) of the §172.101 Table.

(ii) The following is a list of the portable tank special provisions:

Code/Special Provisions

TP1 The maximum degree of filling must not exceed the degree of filling determined by the following:

$$\left(\text{Degree of filling} = \frac{97}{1 + \alpha(t_r - t_f)}\right)$$

Where:

t_r is the maximum mean bulk temperature during transport, and t_f is the temperature in degrees celsius of the liquid during filling.

TP2 a. The maximum degree of filling must not exceed the degree of filling determined by the following:

$$\left(\text{Degree of filling} = \frac{95}{1 + \alpha(t_r - t_f)}\right)$$

Where:

t_r is the maximum mean bulk temperature during transport,

t_f is the temperature in degrees celsius of the liquid during filling, and

α is the mean coefficient of cubical expansion of the liquid between the mean temperature of the liquid during filling (t_f) and the maximum mean bulk temperature during transportation (t_r) both in degrees celsius.

b. For liquids transported under ambient conditions α may be calculated using the formula:

$$\alpha = \frac{d_{15} - d_{50}}{35d_{50}}$$

Where:

d_{15} and d_{50} are the densities (in units of mass per unit volume) of the liquid at 15°C (59°F) and 50°C (122°F), respectively.

TP3 The maximum degree of filling (in %) for solids transported above their melting points and for elevated temperature liquids shall be determined by the following:

$$\left(\text{Degree of filling} = 95\frac{d_r}{d_f}\right).$$

Where: d_f and d_r are the mean densities of the liquid at the mean temperature of the liquid during filling and the maximum mean bulk temperature during transport respectively.

TP4 The maximum degree of filling for portable tanks must not exceed 90%.

TP5 For a portable tank used for the transport of flammable refrigerated liquefied gases or refrigerated liquefied oxygen, the maximum rate at which the portable tank may be filled must not exceed the liquid flow capacity of the primary pressure relief system rated at a pressure not exceeding 120 percent of the portable tank's design pressure. For portable tanks used for the transport of refrigerated liquefied helium and refrigerated liquefied atmospheric gas (except oxygen), the maximum rate at which the tank is filled must not exceed the liquid flow capacity of the pressure relief device rated at 130 percent of the portable tank's design pressure. Except for a portable tank containing refrigerated liquefied helium, a portable tank shall have an outage of at least two percent below the inlet of the pressure relief device or pressure control valve, under conditions of incipient opening, with the portable tank in a level attitude. No outage is required for helium.

TP6 The tank must be equipped with a pressure release device which prevent a tank from bursting under fire engulfment conditions (the conditions prescribed in CGA pamphlet S-1.2 (see §171.7 of this subchapter) or alternative conditions approved by the Associate Administrator may be used to consider the fire engulfment condition), taking into account the properties of the hazardous material to be transported.

TP7 The vapor space must be purged of air by nitrogen or other means.

TP8 A portable tank having a minimum test pressure of 1.5 bar (150 kPa) may be used when the flash point of the hazardous material transported is greater than 0°C (32°F).

TP9 A hazardous material assigned to special provision TP9 in Column (7) of the §172.101 Table may only be transported in a portable tank if approved by the Associate Administrator.

TP10 The portable tank must be fitted with a lead lining at least 5 mm (0.2 inches) thick. The lead lining must be tested annually to ensure that it is intact and functional. Another suitable lining material may be used if approved by the Associate Administrator.

TP12 This material is considered highly corrosive to steel.

TP13 Self-contained breathing apparatus must be provided when this hazardous material is transported by sea.

TP16 The portable tank must be protected against over and under pressurization which may be experienced during transportation. The means of protection must be approved by the approval agency designated to approve the portable tank in accordance with the procedures in part 107, subpart E, of this subchapter. The pressure relief device must be preceded by a frangible disk in accordance with the requirements in §178.275(g)(3) of this subchapter to prevent crystallization of the product in the pressure relief device.

TP17 Only inorganic non-combustible materials may be used for thermal insulation of the tank.

TP18 The temperature of this material must be maintained between 18°C (64.4°F) and 40°C (104°F) while in transportation. Portable tanks containing solidified methacrylic acid must not be re heated during transportation.

TP19 The calculated wall thickness must be increased by 3 mm at the time of construction. Wall thickness must be verified ultrasonically at intervals midway between periodic hydraulic tests (every 2.5 years). The portable tank must not be used if the wall thickness is less than that prescribed by the applicable T code in Column (7) of the Table for this material.

TP20 This hazardous material must only be transported in insulated tanks under a nitrogen blanket.

TP21 The wall thickness must not be less than 8 mm. Portable tanks must be hydraulically tested and internally inspected at intervals not exceeding 2.5 years.

TP22 Lubricants for portable tank fittings (for example, gaskets, shut-off valves, flanges) must be oxygen compatible.

TP24 The portable tank may be fitted with a device to prevent the build up of excess pressure due to the slow decomposition of the hazardous material being transported. The device must be in the vapor space when the tank is filled under maximum filling conditions. This device must also prevent an unacceptable amount of leakage of liquid in the case of overturning.

TP25 Sulphur trioxide 99.95% pure and above may be transported in tanks without an inhibitor provided that it is maintained at a temperature equal to or above 32.5°C (90.5°F).

TP26 The heating device must be exterior to the shell. For UN3176, this requirement only applies when the hazardous material reacts dangerously with water.

TP27 A portable tank having a minimum test pressure of 4 bar (400 kPa) may be used provided the calculated test pressure is 4 bar or less based on the MAWP of the hazardous material, as defined in §178.275 of this subchapter, where the test pressure is 1.5 times the MAWP.

TP28 A portable tank having a minimum test pressure of 2.65 bar (265 kPa) may be used provided the calculated test pressure is 2.65 bar or less based on the MAWP of the hazardous material, as defined in §178.275 of this subchapter, where the test pressure is 1.5 times the MAWP.

TP29 A portable tank having a minimum test pressure of 1.5 bar (150.0 kPa) may be used provided the calculated test pressure is 1.5 bar or less based on the MAWP of the hazardous materials, as defined in §178.275 of this subchapter, where the test pressure is 1.5 times the MAWP.

TP30 This hazardous material may only be transported in insulated tanks.

TP31 This hazardous material may only be transported in tanks in the solid state.

TP32 Portable tanks may be used subject to the following conditions:

a. Each portable tank constructed of metal must be fitted with a pressure-relief device consisting of a reclosing spring loaded type, a frangible disc or a fusible element. The set to discharge for the spring loaded pressure relief device and the burst pressure for the frangible disc, as applicable, must not be greater than 2.65 bar for portable tanks with minimum test pressures greater than 4 bar;

b. The suitability for transport in tanks must be demonstrated using test 8(d) in Test Series 8 (see UN Manual of Tests and Criteria, Part 1, Subsection 18.7) (IBR, see §171.7 of this subchapter) or an alternative means approved by the Associate Administrator.

TP33 The portable tank instruction assigned for this substance applies for granular and powdered solids and for solids which are filled and discharged at temperatures above their melting point which are cooled and transported as a solid mass. Solid substances transported or offered for transport above their melting point are authorized for transportation in portable tanks conforming to the provisions of portable tank instruction T4 for solid substances of packing group III or T7 for solid substances of packing group II, unless a tank with more stringent requirements for minimum shell thickness, maximum allowable working pressure, pressure-relief devices or bottom outlets are assigned in which case the more stringent tank instruction and special provisions shall apply. Filling limits must be in accordance with portable tank special provision TP3. Solids meeting the definition of an elevated temperature material must be transported in accordance with the applicable requirements of this subchapter.

TP37 IM portable tanks are only authorized for the shipment of hydrogen peroxide solutions in water containing 72% or less hydrogen peroxide by weight. Pressure relief devices shall be designed to prevent the entry of foreign matter, the leak age of liquid and the development of any dangerous excess pressure. In addition, the portable tank must be designed so that internal surfaces may be effectively cleaned and passivated. Each tank must be equipped with pressure relief de vices conforming to the following requirements:

Concentration of hydrogen per peroxide solution	Total[1]
52% or less	11
Over 52%, but not greater than 60%	22
Over 60%, but not greater than 72%	32

[1]Total venting capacity in standard cubic feet hour (S.C.F.H.) per pound of hydrogen peroxide solution.

TP38 Each portable tank must be insulated with an insulating material so that the overall thermal conductance at 15.5°C (60°F) is no more than 1.5333 kilojoules per hour per square meter per degree Celsius (0.075 Btu per hour per square foot per degree Fahrenheit) temperature differential. Insulating materials may not promote corrosion to steel when wet.

TP44 Each portable tank must be made of stainless steel, except that steel other than stainless steel may be used in accordance with the provisions of §173.24b(b) of this subchapter. Thickness of stainless steel for tank shell and heads must be the greater of 7.62 mm (0.300 inch) or the thickness required for a portable tank with a design pressure at least equal to 1.5 times the vapor pressure of the hazardous material at 46°C (115°F).

TP45 Each portable tank must be made of stainless steel, except that steel other than stainless steel may be used in accordance with the provisions of 173.24b(b) of this subchapter. Thickness of stainless steel for portable tank shells and heads must be the greater of 6.35 mm (0.250 inch) or the thickness required for a portable tank with a design pressure at least equal to 1.3 times the vapor pressure of the hazardous material at 46°C (115°F).

TP46 Portable tanks in sodium metal service are not required to be hydrostatically retested.

(9) *"W" codes.* These provisions apply only to transportation by water:

Code/Special Provisions

W7 Vessel stowage category for uranyl nitrate hexahydrate solution is "D" as defined in §172.101(k)(4).

W8 Vessel stowage category for pyrophoric thorium metal or pyrophoric uranium metal is "D" as defined in §172.101(k)(4).

W9 When offered for transportation by water, the following Specification packagings are not authorized unless approved by the Associate Administrator: woven plastic bags, plastic film bags, textile bags, paper bags, IBCs and bulk packagings.

W41 When offered for transportation by water, this material must be packaged in bales and be securely and tightly bound with rope, wire or similar means.

Part 397 — Transportation of Hazardous Materials: Driving and Parking Rules

Subpart A — General

Sections

Subpart C — Routing of Non-Radioactive Hazardous Materials

Subpart D — Routing of Class 7 (Radioactive) Materials

AUTHORITY: 49 U.S.C. 322; 49 CFR 1.48. Subpart A also issued under 49 U.S.C. 31136, 31502. Subparts C, D, and E also issued under 49 U.S.C. 5112, 5125.

Subpart A — General

§397.1 Application of the rules in this part.

(a) The rules in this part apply to each motor carrier engaged in the transportation of hazardous materials by a motor vehicle which must be marked or placarded in accordance with §177.823 of this title and to—

(1) Each officer or employee of the motor carrier who performs supervisory duties related to the transportation of hazardous materials; and

(2) Each person who operates or who is in charge of a motor vehicle containing hazardous materials.

(b) Each person designated in paragraph (a) of this section must know and obey the rules in this part.

§397.2 Compliance with Federal motor carrier safety regulations.

A motor carrier or other person to whom this part is applicable must comply with the rules in Part 390 through 397, inclusive, of this subchapter when he/she is transporting hazardous materials by a motor vehicle which must be marked or placarded in accordance with §177.823 of this title.

§397.3 State and local laws, ordinances and regulations.

Every motor vehicle containing hazardous materials must be driven and parked in compliance with the laws, ordinances, and regulations of the jurisdiction in which it is being operated, unless they are at variance with specific regulations of the Department of Transportation which are applicable to the operation of that vehicle and which impose a more stringent obligation or restraint.

§397.5 Attendance and surveillance of motor vehicles.

(a) Except as provided in paragraph (b) of this section, a motor vehicle which contains a Division 1.1, 1.2, or 1.3 (explosive) material must be attended at all times by its driver or a qualified representative of the motor carrier that operates it.

(b) The rules in paragraph (a) of this section do not apply to a motor vehicle which contains Division 1.1, 1.2, or 1.3 material if all the following conditions exist—

(1) The vehicle is located on the property of a motor carrier, on the property of a shipper or consignee of the explosives, in a safe haven, or, in the case of a vehicle containing 50 pounds or less of Division 1.1, 1.2, or 1.3 material, on a construction or survey site; and

(2) The lawful bailee of the explosives is aware of the nature of the explosives the vehicle contains and has been instructed in the procedures which must be followed in emergencies; and

(3) The vehicle is within the bailee's unobstructed field of view or is located in a safe haven.

(c) A motor vehicle which contains hazardous materials other than Division 1.1, 1.2, or 1.3 materials, and which is located on a public street or highway, or the shoulder of a public highway, must be attended by its driver. However, the vehicle need not be attended while its driver is performing duties which are incident and necessary to the driver's duties as the operator of the vehicle.

(d) For purposes of this section—

(1) A motor vehicle is attended when the person in charge of the vehicle is on the vehicle, awake, and not in a sleeper berth, or is within 100 feet of the vehicle and has it within his/her unobstructed field of view.

(2) A qualified representative of a motor carrier is a person who—

(i) Has been designated by the carrier to attend the vehicle;

(ii) Is aware of the nature of the hazardous materials contained in the vehicle he/she attends.

(iii) Has been instructed in the procedures he/she must follow in emergencies; and

(iv) Is authorized to move the vehicle and has the means and ability to do so.

(3) A safe haven is an area specifically approved in writing by local, State, or Federal governmental authorities for the parking of unattended vehicles containing Division 1.1, 1.2, or 1.3 materials.

(e) The rules in this section do not relieve the driver from any obligation imposed by law relating to the placing of warning devices when a motor vehicle is stopped on a public street or highway.

§397.7 Parking.

(a) A motor vehicle which contains Division 1.1, 1.2, or 1.3 materials must not be parked under any of the following circumstances —

(1) On or within 5 feet of the traveled portion of a public street or highway;

(2) On private property (including premises of a fueling or eating facility) without the knowledge and consent of the person who is in charge of the property and who is aware of the nature of the hazardous materials the vehicle contains; or

(3) Within 300 feet of a bridge, tunnel, dwelling, building, or place where people work, congregate, or assemble, except for brief periods when the necessities of operation require the vehicle to be parked and make it impracticable to park the vehicle in any other place.

(b) A motor vehicle which contains hazardous materials other than Division 1.1, 1.2, or 1.3 materials must not be parked on or within five feet of the traveled portion of public street or highway except for brief periods when the necessities of operation require the vehicle to be parked and make it impracticable to park the vehicle in any other place.

§397.9 [Reserved]

§397.11 Fires.

(a) A motor vehicle containing hazardous materials must not be operated near an open fire unless its driver has first taken precautions to ascertain that the vehicle can safely pass the fire without stopping.

(b) A motor vehicle containing hazardous materials must not be parked within 300 feet of an open fire.

§397.13 Smoking.

No person may smoke or carry a lighted cigarette, cigar, or pipe on or within 25 feet of—

(a) A motor vehicle which contains Class 1 materials, Class 5 materials, or flammable materials classified as Division 2.1, Class 3, Divisions 4.1 and 4.2; or

(b) An empty tank motor vehicle which has been used to transport Class 3, flammable materials, or Division 2.1 flammable gases, which, when so used, was required to be marked or placarded in accordance with the rules in §177.823 of this title.

§397.15 Fueling.

When a motor vehicle which contains hazardous materials is being fueled—

(a) Its engine must not be operating; and

(b) A person must be in control of the fueling process at the point where the fuel tank is filled.

§397.17 Tires.

(a) A driver must examine each tire on a motor vehicle at the beginning of each trip and each time the vehicle is parked.

(b) If, as the result of an examination pursuant to paragraph (a) of this section, or otherwise, a tire is found to be flat, leaking, or improperly inflated, the driver must cause the tire to be repaired, replaced, or properly inflated before the vehicle is driven. However, the vehicle may be driven to the nearest safe place to perform the required repair, replacement, or inflation.

(c) If, as the result of an examination pursuant to paragraph (a) of this section, or otherwise, a tire is found to be overheated, the driver shall immediately cause the overheated tire to be removed and placed at a safe distance from the vehicle. The driver shall not operate the vehicle until the cause of the overheating is corrected.

(d) Compliance with the rules in this section does not relieve a driver from the duty to comply with the rules in §§397.5 and 397.7.

§397.19 Instructions and documents.

(a) A motor carrier that transports Division 1.1, 1.2, or 1.3 (explosive) materials must furnish the driver of each motor vehicle in which the explosives are transported with the following documents:

(1) A copy of the rules in this part;

(2) [Reserved]

(3) A document containing instructions on procedures to be followed in the event of accident or delay. The documents must include the names and telephone numbers of persons (including representatives of carriers or shippers) to be contacted, the nature of the explosives being transported, and the precautions to be taken in emergencies such as fires, accidents, or leakages.

(b) A driver who receives documents in accordance with paragraph (a) of this section must sign a receipt for them. The motor carrier shall maintain the receipt for a period of one year from the date of signature.

(c) A driver of a motor vehicle which contains Division 1.1, 1.2, or 1.3 materials must be in possession of, be familiar with, and be in compliance with

(1) The documents specified in paragraph (a) of this section;

(2) The documents specified in §177.817 of this title; and

(3) The written route plan specified in §397.67.

Subpart C — Routing Of Non-Radioactive Hazardous Materials

§397.61 Purpose and scope.

This subpart contains routing requirements and procedures that States and Indian tribes are required to follow if they establish, maintain, or enforce routing designations over which a non-radioactive hazardous material (NRHM) in a quantity which requires placarding may or may not be transported by a motor vehicle. It also provides regulations for motor carriers transporting placarded or marked NRHM and procedures for dispute resolutions regarding NRHM routing designations.

§397.63 Applicability.

The provisions of this subpart apply to any State or Indian tribe that establishes, maintains, or enforces any routing designations over which NRHM may or may not be transported by motor vehicle. They also apply to any motor carrier that transports or causes to be transported placarded or marked NRHM in commerce.

§397.65 Definitions.

For purposes of this subpart, the following definitions apply:

Administrator. The Federal Highway Administrator, who is the chief executive of the Federal Highway Administration, an agency within the United States Department of Transportation, or his/her designate.

Commerce. Any trade, traffic, or transportation in the United States which:

(1) is between a place under the jurisdiction of a State or Indian tribe and any place outside of such jurisdiction; or

(2) is solely within a place under the jurisdiction of a State or Indian tribe but which affects trade, traffic, or transportation described in subparagraph (a).

FHWA. The Federal Highway Administration, an agency within the Department of Transportation.

Hazardous material. A substance or material, including a hazardous substance, which has been determined by the Secretary of Transportation to be capable of posing an unreasonable risk to health, safety, or property when transported in commerce, and which has been so designated.

Indian tribe. Has the same meaning as contained in §4 of the Indian Self-Determination and Education Act, 25 U.S.C. 450b.

Motor carrier. A for-hire motor carrier or a private motor carrier of property. The term includes a motor carrier's agents, officers and representatives as well as employees responsible for hiring, supervising, training, assigning, or dispatching of drivers.

Motor vehicle. Any vehicle, machine, tractor, trailer, or semitrailer propelled or drawn by mechanical power and used upon the highways in the transportation of passengers or property, or any combination thereof.

NRHM. A non-radioactive hazardous material transported by motor vehicle in types and quantities which require placarding, pursuant to Table 1 or 2 of 49 CFR 172.504.

Political subdivision. A municipality, public agency or other instrumentality of one or more States, or a public corporation, board, or commission established under the laws of one or more States.

Radioactive material. Any material having a specific activity greater than 0.002 microcuries per gram (uCi/g), as defined in 49 CFR 173.403.

Routing agency. The State highway agency or other State agency designated by the Governor of that State, or an agency designated by an Indian tribe, to supervise, coordinate, and approve the NRHM routing designations for that State or Indian tribe.

Routing designations. Any regulation, limitation, restriction, curfew, time of travel restriction, lane restriction, routing ban, port-of-entry designation, or route weight restriction, applicable to the highway transportation of NRHM over a specific highway route or portion of a route.

Secretary. The Secretary of Transportation.

State. A State of the United States, the District of Columbia, the Commonwealth of Puerto Rico, the Commonwealth of the Northern Mariana Islands, the Virgin Islands, American Samoa or Guam.

§397.67 Motor carrier responsibility for routing.

(a) A motor carrier transporting NRHM shall comply with NRHM routing designations of a State or Indian tribe pursuant to this subpart.

(b) A motor carrier carrying hazardous materials required to be placarded or marked in accordance with 49 CFR 177.823 and not subject to a NRHM routing designations pursuant to this subpart, shall operate the vehicle over routes which do not go through or near heavily populated areas, places where crowds are assembled, tunnels, narrow streets, or alleys, except where the motor carrier determines that:

(1) There is no practicable alternative;

(2) A reasonable deviation is necessary to reach terminals, points of loading and unloading, facilities for food, fuel, repairs, rest, or a safe haven; or

(3) A reasonable deviation is required by emergency conditions, such as a detour that has been established by a highway authority, or a situation exists where a law enforcement official requires the driver to take an alternative route.

(c) Operating convenience is not a basis for determining whether it is practicable to operate a motor vehicle in accordance with paragraph (b) of this section.

(d) Before a motor carrier requires or permits a motor vehicle containing explosives in Class 1, Divisions 1.1, 1.2, 1.3, as defined in 49 CFR 173.50 and 173.53 respectively, to be operated, the carrier or its agent shall prepare a written route plan that complies with this section and shall furnish a copy to the driver. However, the driver may prepare the written plan as agent for the motor carrier when the trip begins at a location other than the carrier's terminal.

§397.69 Highway routing designations; preemption.

(a) Any State or Indian tribe that establishes or modifies a highway routing designation over which NRHM may or may not be transported on or after November 14, 1994, and maintains or enforces such designation, shall comply with the highway routing standards set forth in §397.71 of this subpart. For purposes of this subpart, any highway routing designation affecting the highway transportation of NRHM, made by a political subdivision of a State is considered as one made by that State, and all requirements of this subpart apply.

(b) Except as provided in §§397.75 and 397.219, a NRHM route designation made in violation of paragraph (a) of this section is preempted pursuant to section 105(b)(4) of the Hazardous Materials Transportation Act (49 U.S.C. app. 1804(b)(4)). This provision shall become effective after November 14, 1996.

(c) A highway routing designation established by a State, political subdivision, or Indian tribe before November 14, 1994 is subject to preemption in accordance with the preemption standards in paragraphs (a)(1) and (a)(2) of §397.203 of this subpart.

(d) A State, political subdivision, or Indian tribe may petition for a waiver of preemption in accordance with §397.213 of this part.

§397.71 Federal standards.

(a) A State or Indian tribe shall comply with the Federal standards under paragraph (b) of this section when establishing, maintaining or enforcing specific NRHM routing designations over which NRHM may or may not be transported.

(b) The Federal standards are as follows:

(1) Enhancement of public safety. The State or Indian tribe shall make a finding, supported by the record to be developed in accordance with paragraphs (b)(2)(ii) and (b)(3)(iv) of this section, that any NRHM routing designation enhances public safety in the areas subject to its jurisdiction and in other areas which are directly affected by such highway routing designation. In making such a finding, the State or Indian tribe shall consider:

(i) The factors listed in paragraph (b)(9) of this section; and

(ii) The DOT "Guidelines for Applying Criteria to Designate Routes for Transporting Hazardous Materials," DOT/RSPA/OHMT-89-02, July 1989[1] or its most current version; or an equivalent routing analysis which adequately considers overall risk to the public.

(2) Public participation. Prior to the establishment of any NRHM routing designation, the State or Indian tribe shall undertake the following actions to ensure participation by the public in the routing process:

(i) The State or Indian tribe shall provide the public with notice of any proposed NRHM routing designation and a 30-day period in which to comment. At any time during this period or following review of the comments received, the State or Indian tribe shall decide whether to hold a public hearing on the proposed NRHM route designation. The public shall be given 30 days prior notice of the public hearing which shall be conducted as described in paragraph (b)(2)(ii) of this section. Notice for both the comment period and the public hearing, if one is held, shall be given by publication in at least two newspapers of general circulation in the affected area or areas and shall contain a complete description of the proposed routing designation, together with the date, time, and location of any public hearings. Notice for both the comment period and any public hearing may also be published in the official register of the State.

(ii) If it is determined that a public hearing is necessary, the State or Indian tribe shall hold at least one public hearing on the record during which the public will be afforded the opportunity to present their views and any information or data related to the proposed NRHM routing designation. The State shall make available to the public, upon payment of prescribed costs, copies of the transcript of the hearing, which shall include all exhibits and documents presented during the hearing or submitted for the record.

---

1. This document may be obtained from Safety Technology and Information Management Division, HHS-10, Federal Highway Administration, U.S. Department of Transportation, 400 7th Street, SW., Washington, D.C. 20590-0001.

(3) Consultation with others. Prior to the establishment of any NRHM routing designation, the State or Indian tribe shall provide notice to, and consult with, officials of affected political subdivisions, States and Indian tribes, and any other affected parties. Such actions shall include the following:

(i) At least 60 days prior to establishing a routing designation, the State or Indian tribe shall provide notice, in writing, of the proposed routing designation to officials responsible for highway routing in all other affected States or Indian tribes. A copy of this notice may also be sent to all affected political subdivisions. This notice shall request approval, in writing, by those States or Indian tribes, of the proposed routing designations. If no response is received within 60 days from the day of receipt of the notification of the proposed routing designation, the routing designation shall be considered approved by the affected State or Indian tribe.

(ii) The manner in which consultation under this paragraph is conducted is left to the discretion of the State or Indian tribe.

(iii) The State or Indian tribe shall attempt to resolve any concern or disagreement expressed by any consulted official related to the proposed routing designation.

(iv) The State or Indian tribe shall keep a record of the names and addresses of the officials notified pursuant to this section and of any consultation or meeting conducted with these officials or their representatives. Such record shall describe any concern or disagreement expressed by the officials and any action undertaken to resolve such disagreement or address any concern.

(4) Through routing. In establishing any NRHM routing designation, the State or Indian tribe shall ensure through highway routing for the transportation of NRHM between adjacent areas. The term "through highway routing" as used in this paragraph means that the routing designation must ensure continuity of movement so as to not impede or unnecessarily delay the transportation of NRHM. The State or Indian tribe shall utilize the procedures established in paragraphs (b)(2) and (b)(3) of this section in meeting these requirements. In addition, the State or Indian tribe shall make a finding, supported by a risk analysis conducted in accordance with paragraph (b)(1) of this section, that the routing designation enhances public safety. If

the risk analysis shows—

(i) That the current routing presents at least 50 percent more risk to the public than the deviation under the proposed routing designation, then the proposed routing designation may go into effect.

(ii) That the current routing presents a greater risk but less than 50 percent more risk to the public than the deviation under the proposed routing restriction, then the proposed routing restriction made by a State or Indian tribe shall only go into effect if it does not force a deviation of more than 25 miles or result in an increase of more than 25 percent of that part of a trip affected by the deviation, whichever is shorter, from the most direct route through a jurisdiction as compared to the intended deviation.

(iii) That the current route has the same or less risk to the public than the deviation resulting from the proposed routing designation, then the routing designation shall not be allowed.

(5) Agreement of other States; burden on commerce. Any NRHM routing designation which affects another State or Indian tribe shall be established, maintained, or enforced only if:

(i) It does not unreasonably burden commerce, and

(ii) It is agreed to by the affected State or Indian tribe within 60 days of receipt of the notice sent pursuant to paragraph (b)(3)(i) of this section, or it is approved by the Administrator pursuant to §397.75.

(6) Timeliness. The establishment of a NRHM routing designation by any State or Indian tribe shall be completed within 18 months of the notice given in either paragraph (b)(2) or (b)(3) of this section, whichever occurs first.

(7) Reasonable routes to terminals and other facilities. In establishing or providing for reasonable access to and from designated routes, the State or Indian tribe shall use the shortest practicable route considering the factors listed in paragraph (b)(9) of this section. In establishing any NRHM routing designation, the State or Indian tribe shall provide reasonable access for motor vehicles transporting NRHM to reach:

(i) Terminals,

(ii) Points of loading, unloading, pickup and delivery, and

(iii) Facilities for food, fuel, repairs, rest, and safe havens.

(8) Responsibility for local compliance. The States shall be responsible for ensuring that all of their political subdivisions comply with the provisions of this subpart. The States shall be responsible for resolving all disputes between such political subdivisions within their jurisdictions. If a State or any political subdivision thereof, or an Indian tribe chooses to establish, maintain, or enforce any NRHM routing designation, the Governor, or Indian tribe, shall designate a routing agency for the State or Indian tribe, respectively. The routing agency shall ensure that all NRHM routing designations within its jurisdiction comply with the Federal standards in this section. The State or Indian tribe shall comply with the public information and reporting requirements contained in §397.73.

(9) Factors to consider. In establishing any NRHM routing designation, the State or Indian tribe shall consider the following factors:

(i) Population density. The population potentially exposed to a NRHM release shall be estimated from the density of the residents, employees, motorists, and other persons in the area, using United States census tract maps or other reasonable means for determining the population within a potential impact zone along a designated highway route. The impact zone is the potential range of effects in the event of a release. Special populations such as schools, hospitals, prisons, and senior citizen homes shall, among other things, be considered when determining the potential risk to the populations along a highway routing. Consideration shall be given to the amount of time during which an area will experience a heavy population density.

(ii) Type of highway. The characteristics of each alternative NRHM highway routing designation shall be compared. Vehicle weight and size limits, underpass and bridge clearances, roadway geometrics, number of lanes, degree of access control, and median and shoulder structures are examples of characteristics which a State or Indian tribe shall consider.

(iii) Types and quantities of NRHM. An examination shall be made of the type and quantity of NRHM normally transported along highway routes which are included in a proposed NRHM routing designation, and consideration shall be given to the relative impact zone and risks of each type and quantity.

(iv) Emergency response capabilities. In consultation with

the proper fire, law enforcement, and highway safety agencies, consideration shall be given to the emergency response capabilities which may be needed as a result of a NRHM routing designation. The analysis of the emergency response capabilities shall be based upon the proximity of the emergency response facilities and their capabilities to contain and suppress NRHM releases within the impact zones.

(v) Results of consultation with affected persons. Consideration shall be given to the comments and concerns of all affected persons and entities provided during public hearings and consultations conducted in accordance with this section.

(vi) Exposure and other risk factors. States and Indian tribes shall define the exposure and risk factors associated with any NRHM routing designations. The distance to sensitive areas shall be considered. Sensitive areas include, but are not limited to, homes and commercial buildings; special populations in hospitals, schools, handicapped facilities, prisons and stadiums; water sources such as streams and lakes; and natural areas such as parks, wetlands, and wildlife reserves.

(vii) Terrain considerations. Topography along and adjacent to the proposed NRHM routing designation that may affect the potential severity of an accident, the dispersion of the NRHM upon release and the control and clean up of NRHM if released shall be considered.

(viii) Continuity of routes. Adjacent jurisdictions shall be consulted to ensure routing continuity for NRHM across common borders. Deviations from the most direct route shall be minimized.

(ix) Alternative routes. Consideration shall be given to the alternative routes to, or resulting from, any NRHM route designation. Alternative routes shall be examined, reviewed, or evaluated to the extent necessary to demonstrate that the most probable alternative routing resulting from a routing designation is safer than the current routing.

(x) Effects on commerce. Any NRHM routing designation made in accordance with this subpart shall not create an unreasonable burden upon interstate or intrastate commerce.

(xi) Delays in transportation. No NRHM routing designations may create unnecessary delays in the transportation of NRHM.

(xii) Climatic conditions. Weather conditions unique to a highway route such as snow, wind, ice, fog, or other climatic conditions that could affect the safety of a route, the dispersion of the NRHM upon release, or increase the difficulty of controlling it and cleaning it up shall be given appropriate consideration.

(xiii) Congestion and accident history. Traffic conditions unique to a highway routing such as: traffic congestion; accident experience with motor vehicles, traffic considerations that could affect the potential for an accident, exposure of the public to any release, ability to perform emergency response operations, or the temporary closing of a highway for cleaning up any release shall be given appropriate consideration.

§397.73 Public information and reporting requirements.

(a) Public information. Information on NRHM routing designations must be made available by the States and Indian tribes to the public in the form of maps, lists, road signs or some combination thereof. If road signs are used, those signs and their placements must comply with the provisions of the Manual on Uniform Traffic Control Devices,[2] published by the FHWA, particularly the Hazardous Cargo signs identified as R14-2 and R14-3 shown in Section 2B-43 of that Manual.

(b) Reporting and publishing requirements. Each State or Indian tribe, through its routing agency, shall provide information identifying all NRHM routing designations which exist within their jurisdictions on November 14, 1994 to the FHWA, HHS-30, 400 7th St., SW., Washington, D.C. 20590-0001 by March 13,1995. The State or Indian tribe shall include descriptions of these routing designations, along with the dates they were established. This information may also be published in each State's official register of State regulations. Information on any subsequent changes or new NRHM routing designations shall be furnished within 60 days after establishment to the FHWA. This information will be available from the FHWA, con-

---

2.This publication may be purchased from the Superintendent of Documents, U.S. Government Printing Office (GPO), Washington, D.C. 20402 and has Stock No. 050-001-81001-8. It is available for inspection and copying as prescribed in 49 CFR part 7, appendix D. See 23 CFR 655, subpart F.

solidated by the FHWA, and published annually in whole or as updates in the *Federal Register.* Each State may also publish this information in its official register of State regulations.

(Approved by the Office of Management and Budget under control number 2125-0554)

§397.75 Dispute resolution.

(a) Petition. One or more States or Indian tribes may petition the Administrator to resolve a dispute relating to an agreement on a proposed NRHM routing designation. In resolving a dispute under these provisions, the Administrator will provide the greatest level of safety possible without unreasonably burdening commerce, and ensure compliance with the Federal standards established at §397.71 of this subpart.

(b) Filing. Each petition for dispute resolution filed under this section must:

(1) Be submitted to the Administrator, Federal Highway Administration, U.S. Department of Transportation, 400 7th Street, SW., Washington, DC 20590-0001. Attention: HCC-10 Docket Room, Hazardous Materials Routing Dispute Resolution Docket.

(2) Identify the State or Indian tribe filing the petition and any other State, political subdivision, or Indian tribe whose NRHM routing designation is the subject of the dispute.

(3) Contain a certification that the petitioner has complied with the notification requirements of paragraph (c) of this section, and include a list of the names and addresses of each State, political subdivision, or Indian tribe official who was notified of the filing of the petition.

(4) Clearly set forth the dispute for which resolution is sought, including a complete description of any disputed NRHM routing designation and an explanation of how the disputed routing designation affects the petitioner or how it impedes through highway routing. If the routing designation being disputed results in alternative routing, then a comparative risk analysis for the designated route and the resulting alternative routing shall be provided.

(5) Describe any actions taken by the State or Indian tribe to resolve the dispute.

(6) Explain the reasons why the petitioner believes that the Administrator should intervene in resolving the dispute.

(7) Describe any proposed actions that the Administrator should take to resolve the dispute and how these actions would provide the greatest level of highway safety without unreasonably burdening commerce and would ensure compliance with the Federal standards established in this subpart.

(c) Notice.

(1) Any State or Indian tribe that files a petition for dispute resolution under this subpart shall mail a copy of the petition to any affected State, political subdivision, or Indian tribe, accompanied by a statement that the State, political subdivision, or Indian tribe may submit comments regarding the petition to the Administrator within 45 days.

(2) By serving notice on any other State, political subdivision, or Indian tribe determined by the Administrator to be possibly affected by the issues in dispute or the resolution sought, or by publication in the *Federal Register*, the Administrator may afford those persons an opportunity to file written comments on the petition.

(3) Any affected State, political subdivision, or Indian tribe submitting written comments to the Administrator with respect to a petition filed under this section shall send a copy of the comments to the petitioner and certify to the Administrator as to having complied with this requirement. The Administrator may notify other persons participating in the proceeding of the comments and provide an opportunity for those other persons to respond.

(d) Court actions. After a petition for dispute resolution is filed in accordance with this section, no court action may be brought with respect to the subject matter of such dispute until a final decision has been issued by the Administrator or until the last day of the one- year period beginning on the day the Administrator receives the petition, whichever occurs first.

(e) Hearings; alternative dispute resolution. Upon receipt of a petition filed pursuant to paragraph (a) of this section, the Administrator may schedule a hearing to attempt to resolve the dispute and, if a hearing is scheduled, will notify all parties to the dispute of the date, time, and place of the hearing. During the hearing the parties may offer any information pertinent to the resolution of the dispute. If an agreement is reached, it may be stipulated by the parties, in writing, and, if the Administrator agrees, made part of the decision in paragraph (f) of this section. If no agreement is reached, the Administrator may take the matter under consideration and announce his or her decision in accordance with paragraph (f) of this section. Nothing in this section shall be construed as prohibiting the parties from settling the dispute or seeking other methods of alternative dispute resolution prior to the final decision by the Administrator.

(f) Decision. The Administrator will issue a decision based on the petition, the written comments submitted by the parties, the record of the hearing, and any other information in the record. The decision will include a written statement setting forth the relevant facts and the legal basis for the decision.

(g) Record. The Administrator will serve a copy of the decision upon the petitioner and any other party who participated in the proceedings. A copy of each decision will be placed on file in the public docket. The Administrator may publish the decision or notice of the decision in the *Federal Register.*

§397.77 Judicial review of dispute decision.

Any State or Indian tribe adversely affected by the Administrator's decision under §397.75 of this subpart may seek review by the appropriate district court of the United States under such proceeding only by filing a petition with such court within 90 days after such decision becomes final.

Subpart D — Routing of Class 7 (Radioactive) Materials

§397.101 Requirements for motor carriers and drivers.

(a) Except as provided in paragraph (b) of this section or in circumstances when there is only one practicable highway route available, considering operating necessity and safety, a carrier or any person operating a motor vehicle that contains a Class 7 (radioactive) material, as defined in 49 CFR 172.403, for which placarding is required under 49 CFR part 172 shall:

(1) Ensure that the motor vehicle is operated on routes that minimize radiological risk;

(2) Consider available information on accident rates, transit time, population density and activities, and the time of day and the day of week during which transportation will occur to deter-

mine the level of radiological risk; and

(3) Tell the driver which route to take and that the motor vehicle contains Class 7 (radioactive) materials.

(b) Except as otherwise permitted in this paragraph and in paragraph (f) of this section, a carrier or any person operating a motor vehicle containing a highway route controlled quantity of Class 7 (radioactive) materials, as defined in 49 CFR 173.403(l), shall operate the motor vehicle only over preferred routes.

(1) For purposes of this subpart, a preferred route is an Interstate System highway for which an alternative route is not designated by a State routing agency; a State-designated route selected by a State routing agency pursuant to §397.103; or both of the above.

(2) The motor carrier or the person operating a motor vehicle containing a highway route controlled quantity of Class 7 (radioactive) materials, as defined in 49 CFR 173.403(l) and (y), shall select routes to reduce time in transit over the preferred route segment of the trip. An Interstate System bypass or Interstate System beltway around a city, when available, shall be used in place of a preferred route through a city, unless a State routing agency has designated an alternative route.

(c) A motor vehicle may be operated over a route, other than a preferred route, only under the following conditions:

(1) The deviation from the preferred route is necessary to pick up or deliver a highway route controlled quantity of Class 7 (radioactive) materials, to make necessary rest, fuel or motor vehicle repair stops, or because emergency conditions make continued use of the preferred route unsafe or impossible;

(2) For pickup and delivery not over preferred routes, the route selected must be the shortest-distance route from the pickup location to the nearest preferred route entry location, and the shortest-distance route to the delivery location from the nearest preferred route exit location. Deviation from the shortest-distance pickup or delivery route is authorized if such deviation:

(i) Is based upon the criteria in paragraph (a) of this section to minimize the radiological risk; and

(ii) Does not exceed the shortest-distance pickup or delivery route by more than 25 miles and does not exceed 5 times the length of the shortest-distance pickup or delivery route.

(iii) Deviations from preferred routes, or pickup or delivery routes other than preferred routes, which are necessary for rest, fuel, or motor vehicle repair stops or because of emergency conditions, shall be made in accordance with the criteria in paragraph (a) of this section to minimize radiological risk, unless due to emergency conditions, time does not permit use of those criteria.

(d) A carrier (or a designated agent) who operates a motor vehicle which contains a package of highway route controlled quantity of Class 7 (radioactive) materials, as defined in 49 CFR 173.403(l), shall prepare a written route plan and supply a copy before departure to the motor vehicle driver and a copy to the shipper (before departure for exclusive use shipments, as defined in 49 CFR 173.403(i), or within fifteen working days following departure for all other shipments). Any variation between the route plan and routes actually used, and the reason for it, shall be reported in an amendment to the route plan delivered to the shipper as soon as practicable but within 30 days following the deviation. The route plan shall contain:

(1) A statement of the origin and destination points, a route selected in compliance with this section, all planned stops, and estimated departure and arrival times; and

(2) Telephone numbers which will access emergency assistance in each State to be entered.

(e) No person may transport a package of highway route controlled quantity of Class 7 (radioactive) materials on a public highway unless:

(1) The driver has received within the two preceding years, written training on:

(i) Requirements in 49 CFR parts 172, 173, and 177 pertaining to the Class 7 (radioactive) materials transported;

(ii) The properties and hazards of the Class 7 (radioactive) materials being transported; and

(iii) Procedures to be followed in case of an accident or other emergency.

(2) The driver has in his or her immediate possession a certificate of training as evidence of training required by this section, and a copy is placed in his or her qualification file (see §391.51 of this subchapter), showing:

(i) The driver's name and operator's license number;

(ii) The dates training was provided;

(iii) The name and address of the person providing the training;

(iv) That the driver has been trained in the hazards and characteristics of highway route controlled quantity of Class 7 (radioactive) materials; and

(v) A statement by the person providing the training that information on the certificate is accurate.

(3) The driver has in his or her immediate possession the route plan required by paragraph (d) of this section and operates the motor vehicle in accordance with the route plan.

(f) A person may transport irradiated reactor fuel only in compliance with a plan if required under 49 CFR 173.22(c) that will ensure the physical security of the material. Variation for security purposes from the requirements of this section is permitted so far as necessary to meet the requirements imposed under such a plan, or otherwise imposed by the U.S. Nuclear Regulatory Commission in 10 CFR part 73.

(g) Expect for packages shipped in compliance with the physical security requirements of the U.S. Nuclear Regulatory Commission in 10 CFR part 73, each carrier who accepts for transportation a highway route controlled quantity of Class7 (radioactive) material (see 49 CFR 173.401 (l)), shall, within 90 days following the acceptance of the package, file the following information concerning the transportation of each such package with the Associate Administrator for Safety and System Applications, Federal Highway Administration, Attn: Traffic Control Division, HHS-32, room 3419, 400 Seventh Street, SW., Washington, DC 20590-0001:

(1) The route plan required under paragraph (d) of this section including all required amendments reflecting the routes actually used;

(2) A statement identifying the names and addresses of the shipper, carrier and consignee; and

(3) A copy of the shipping paper or the description of the Class 7 (radioactive) material in the shipment required by 49 CFR 172.202 and 172.203.

§397.103 Requirements for State routing designations.

(a) The State routing agency, as defined in §397.201(c), shall select routes to minimize radiological risk using "Guidelines for Selecting Preferred Highway Routes for Highway Route Controlled Quantity Shipments of Radioactive Materials," or an equivalent routing analysis which adequately considers overall risk to the public. Designations must be preceded by substantive consultation with affected local jurisdictions and with any other affected States to ensure consideration of all impacts and continuity of designated routes.

(b) State routing agencies may designate preferred routes as an alternative to, or in addition to, one or more Interstate System highways, including interstate system bypasses, or Interstate System beltways.

(c) A State-designated route is effective when—

(1) The State gives written notice by certified mail, return receipt requested, to the Associated Administrator for Safety and System Applications, Federal Highway Administration, Attn: Traffic Control Division, HHS-32, Room 3419, Registry of State-designated routes, at the address above; and

(2) Receipt thereof is acknowledged in writing by the Associate Administrator.

(d) Upon request, the Office of Highway Safety, Traffic Control Division, HHS-32, room 3419, at the address above, will provide a list of State-designated preferred routes and a copy of the "Guidelines for Selecting Preferred Highway Routes for Highway Route Controlled Quantity Shipments of Radioactive Materials."

Emergency Phone Numbers

DOT National Emergency Response Center:	(800) 424-8802
Center for Disease Control:	(800) 232-0124
Chemtrec®:	(800) 424-9300
Chem-Tel, Inc.:	(800) 255-3924
Infotrac:	(800) 535-5053
3E Company:	(800) 451-8346
U.S. Military Shipments	
Explosives/ammunition incidents:	(703) 697-0218
All other dangerous goods incidents:	(800) 851-8061
Nationwide Poison Control Center:	(800) 222-1222

NOTES

NOTES

NOTES

LABELS

CLASS 1

CLASS 2

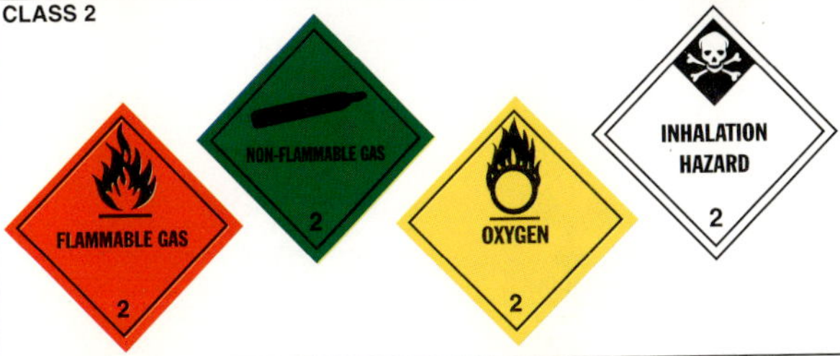

CLASS 3

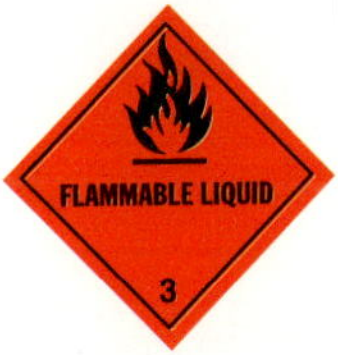

CLASS 4

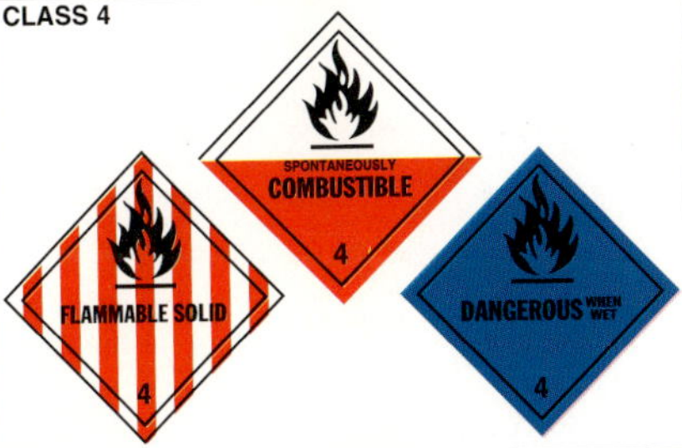

CLASS 5

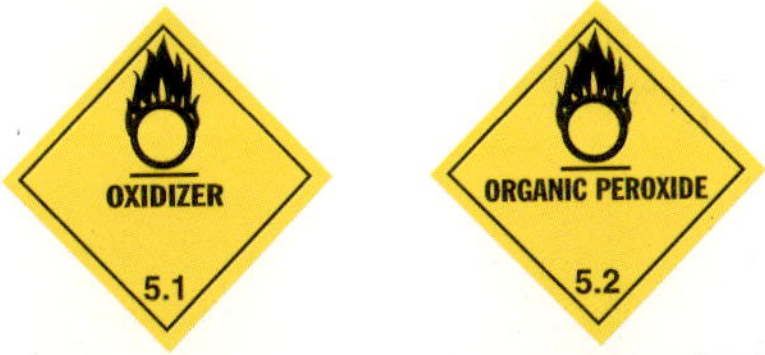

LABELS

CLASS 6

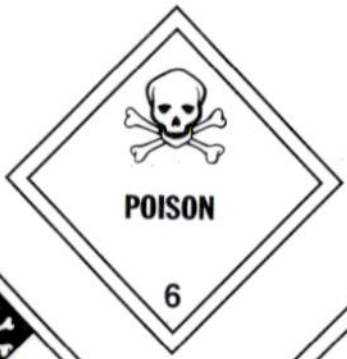

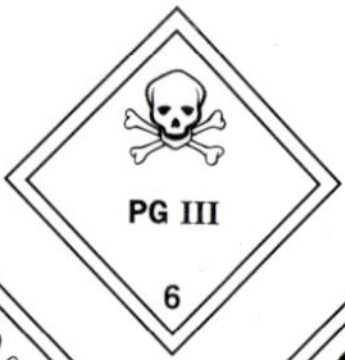

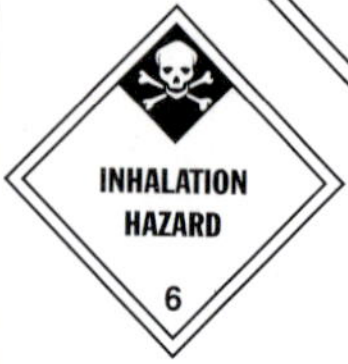

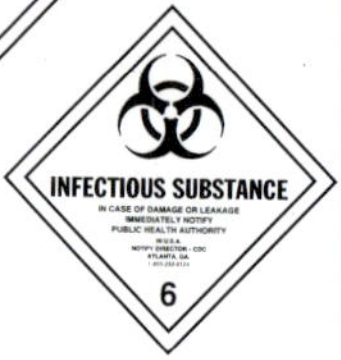

CLASS 7

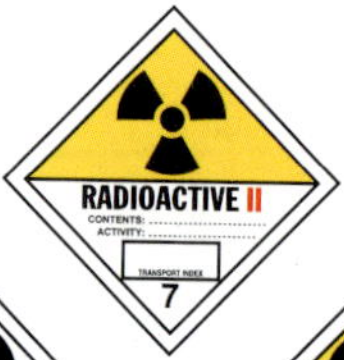

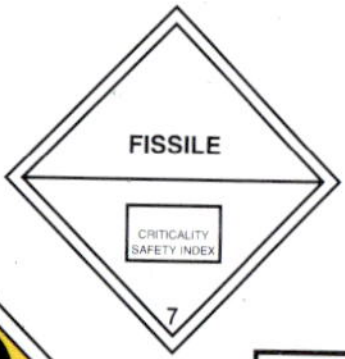

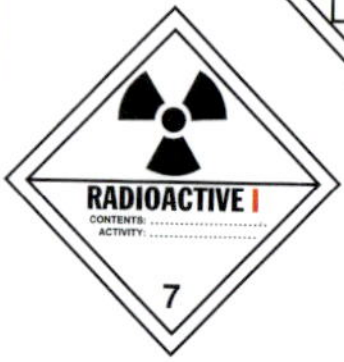

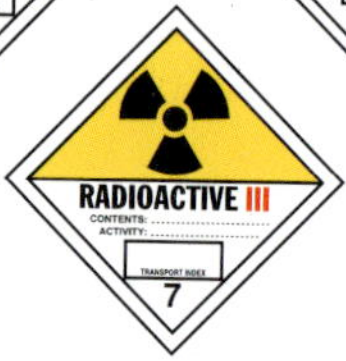

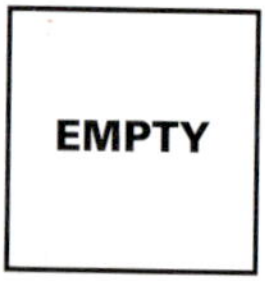

CLASS 8

CLASS 9

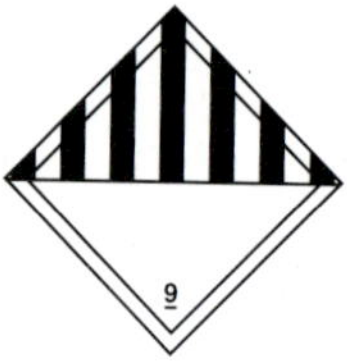

AIRCRAFT

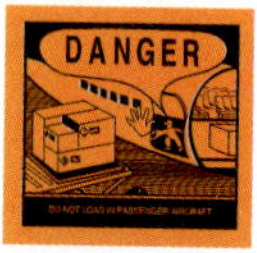

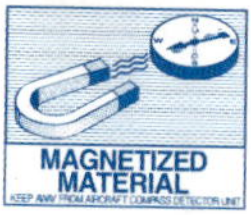

PLACARDS

CLASS 1

EXPLOSIVES 1.1, 1.2, & 1.3

* The Division number 1.1, 1.2 or 1.3 and compatibility group (when required) are in black ink. Placard any quantity of Division number 1.1, 1.2, or 1.3 material.

CLASS 1

EXPLOSIVES 1.4

* The compatibility group (when required) is in black ink. Placard 454 kg (1001 lbs.) or more of 1.4 Explosives.

CLASS 1

EXPLOSIVES 1.5

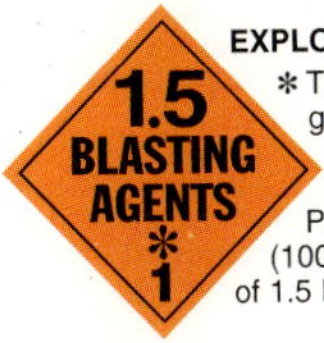

* The compatibility group (when required) is in black ink. Placard 454 kg (1001 lbs.) or more of 1.5 Blasting Agents.

CLASS 1

EXPLOSIVES 1.6

* The compatibility group (when required) is in black ink. Placard 454 kg (1001 lbs.) or more of 1.6 Explosives.

CLASS 2 **Division 2.1**

FLAMMABLE GAS

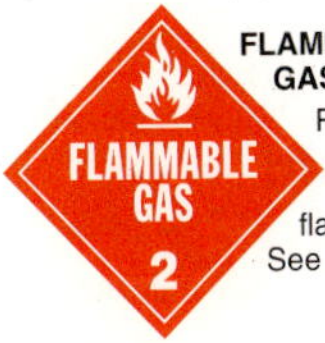

Placard 454 kg (1001 lbs.) or more of flammable gas. See DANGEROUS.

CLASS 2 **Division 2.2**

NON-FLAMMABLE GAS

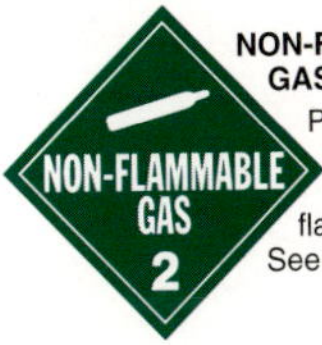

Placard 454 kg (1001 lbs.) or more of non-flammable gas. See DANGEROUS.

CLASS 2

OXYGEN

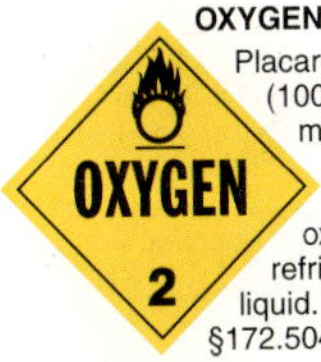

Placard 454 kg (1001 lbs.) or more of either oxygen compressed or oxygen, refrigerated liquid. See §172.504(f)(7).

CLASS 2 **Division 2.3**

POISON GAS

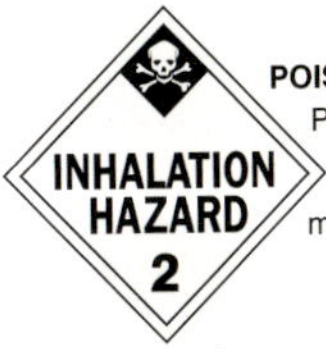

Placard any quantity of Division 2.3 material.

PLACARDS

CLASS 3

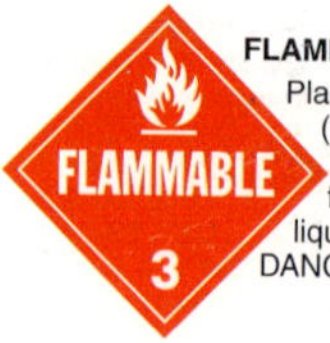

FLAMMABLE
Placard 454 kg (1001 lbs.) or more of flammable liquid. See DANGEROUS.

CLASS 3

GASOLINE
May be used in place of FLAMMABLE on a placard displayed on a cargo tank or a portable tank being used to transport gasoline by highway. See §172.542(c).

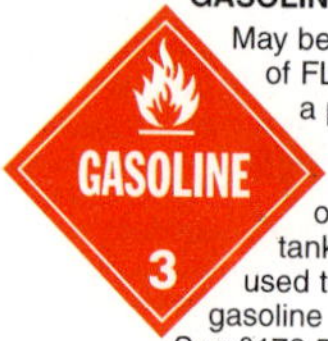

CLASS 3

COMBUSTIBLE
Placard a combustible liquid when transported in bulk. A FLAMMABLE placard may be used in place of a COMBUSTIBLE placard on a cargo tank or portable tank or a compartmented tank car which contains both flammable and combustible liquids. See §172.504(f)(2). No placard is required for a combustible liquid transported in a non-bulk packaging (450 L (119 gal.) or less).

CLASS 3

FUEL OIL
May be used in place of COMBUSTIBLE on a placard displayed on a cargo tank or portable tank being used to transport, by highway, fuel oil not classed as a flammable liquid. See §172.544(c).

CLASS 4 **Division 4.1**

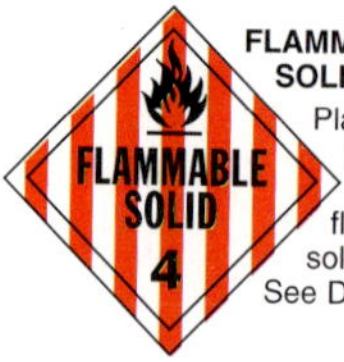

FLAMMABLE SOLID
Placard 454 kg (1001 lbs.) or more of flammable solid. See DANGEROUS.

CLASS 4 **Division 4.2**

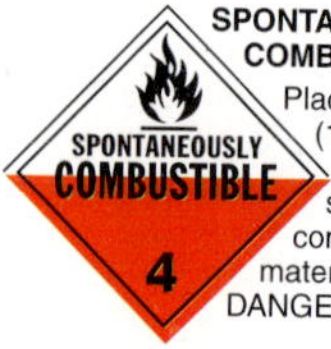

SPONTANEOUSLY COMBUSTIBLE
Placard 454 kg (1001 lbs.) or more of spontaneously combustible material. See DANGEROUS.

CLASS 4 **Division 4.3**

DANGEROUS WHEN WET
Placard any quantity of Division 4.3 material.

PLACARDS

CLASS 5 — **Division 5.1**

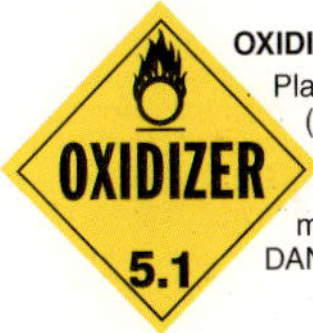

OXIDIZER
Placard 454 kg (1001 lbs.) or more of oxidizing material. See DANGEROUS.

CLASS 5 — **Division 5.2**

ORGANIC PEROXIDE

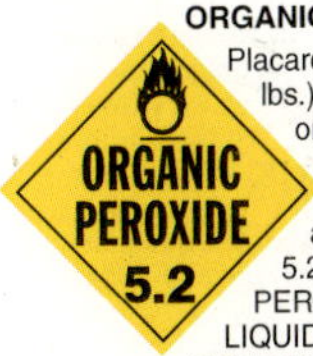

Placard 454 kg (1001 lbs.) or more of organic peroxide. See DANGEROUS. Placard any quantity of 5.2, ORGANIC PEROXIDE, TYPE B, LIQUID OR SOLID, TEMPERATURE CONTROLLED.

CLASS 6 — **Division 6.1**
Inhalation Hazard

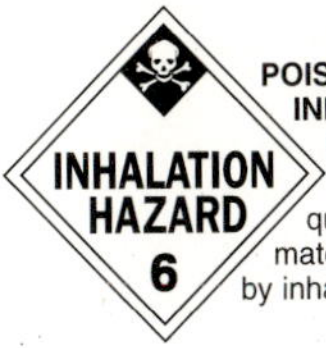

POISON INHALATION HAZARD
Placard any quantity of material poisonous by inhalation.

CLASS 6 — **Division 6.1**
Other Than Inhalation Hazard

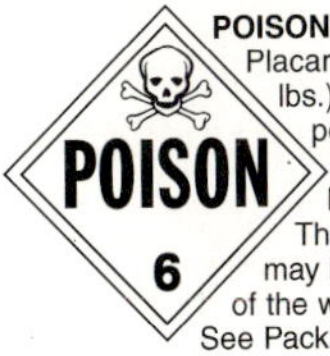

POISON
Placard 454 kg (1001 lbs.) or more of poison (not PIH). See DANGEROUS. The word "TOXIC" may be used in place of the word "POISON." See Packing Group III.

CLASS 6 — **Division 6.1**
Packing Group III

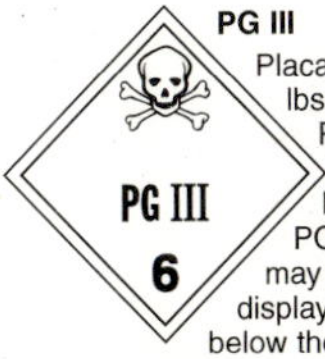

PG III
Placard 454 kg (1001 lbs.) or more of Packing Group III. See DANGEROUS. A POISON placard may be modified to display the text "PG III" below the mid line of the placard.

CLASS 7

RADIOACTIVE

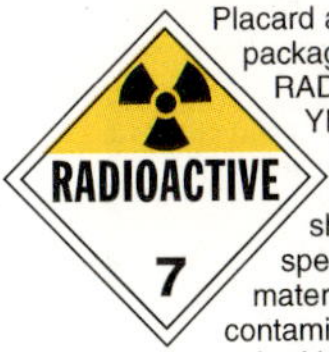

Placard any quantity of packages bearing the RADIOACTIVE YELLOW III label. Placard exclusive use shipments of low specific activity material and surface contaminated objects as required by §173.427.

CLASS 8

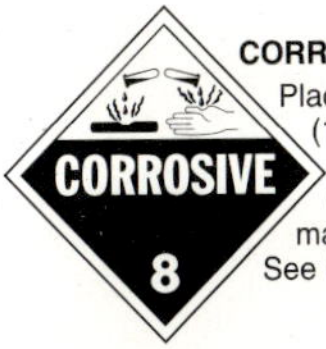

CORROSIVE
Placard 454 kg (1001 lbs.) or more of corrosive material. See DANGEROUS.

CLASS 9

MISCELLANEOUS

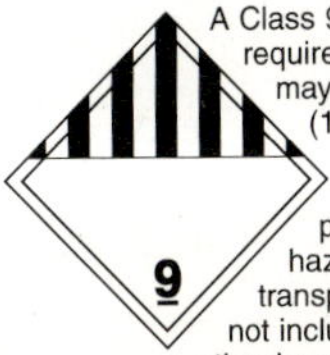

A Class 9 placard is not required. However, you may placard 454 kg (1001 lbs.) or more of a material which presents a hazard during transport, but which is not included in any other hazard class. See DANGEROUS.

PLACARDS

DANGEROUS

Placard 454 kg (1001 lbs.) gross weight of two or more categories of hazardous materials listed in Table 2.

A freight container, unit load device, transport vehicle, or rail car which contains non-bulk packages with two or more categories of hazardous materials that require different placards, as specified in Table 2, may be placarded with a DANGEROUS placard instead of the separate placarding specified for each of the materials in Table 2. However, when 1,000 kg (2,205 pounds) aggregate gross weight or more of one category of material is loaded therein at one loading facility on a freight container, unit load device, transport vehicle, or rail car, the placard specified in Table 2 for that category must be applied.

DISPLAY OF IDENTIFICATION NUMBER

The display of an identification number on a placard is allowed, except for Class 1, Class 7, DANGEROUS, or subsidiary hazard placards.

For a COMBUSTIBLE placard used to display an identification number, the entire background below the identification number must be white for transportation by rail and may be white for transportation by highway.

The white square background is required for the following placards when on rail cars: EXPLOSIVES 1.1 or 1.2; POISON GAS (Division 2.3, Hazard Zone A); POISON INHALATION HAZARD (Division 6.1, PG I, Hazard Zone A) and

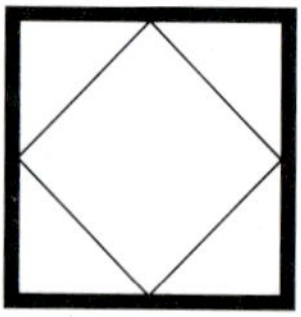

for DOT 113 tank cars FLAMMABLE GAS. The white square background is required for placards on motor vehicles transporting highway route controlled quantities of Class 7 (radioactive) materials.

SUBSIDIARY RISK

NUMBERED

UNNUMBERED

Allowed for rail or highway transport until October 1, 2005. See §172.519(b)(4).

Placard not required for:

1. Class 7 (radioactive) White I and Yellow II labels.
2. Division 6.2 materials (infectious substances).
3. ORM–D materials.
4. Any hazardous material identified on shipping papers as a "limited quantity."
5. Combustible liquid in a non-bulk packaging (450 L (119 gal.) or less).
6. Class 9 materials (domestic shipments).